NEW
TECHNIQUES
IN ONCOLOGIC
IMAGING

NEW TECHNIQUES IN ONCOLOGIC IMAGING

edited by

Anwar R. Padhani, F.R.C.P., F.R.C.R.
Mount Vernon Cancer Centre
London, U.K.

Peter L. Choyke, M.D.
Molecular Imaging Program
National Cancer Institute
Bethesda, Maryland, U.S.A.

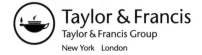
Taylor & Francis
Taylor & Francis Group
New York   London

Published in 2006 by
CRC Press
Taylor & Francis Group
6000 Broken Sound Parkway NW, Suite 300
Boca Raton, FL 33487-2742

International Standard Book Number-10: 0-8493-9274-8 (Hardcover)
International Standard Book Number-13: 978-0-8493-9274-0 (Hardcover)

Library of Congress Cataloging-in-Publication Data

Catalog record is available from the Library of Congress

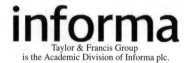

informa
Taylor & Francis Group
is the Academic Division of Informa plc.

Visit the Taylor & Francis Web site at
http://www.taylorandfrancis.com

and the CRC Press Web site at
http://www.crcpress.com

To

Our mentors—Janet Husband and Andrew Dwyer
Our wives—Femeeda and Lynda
Our children—Shahid, Sabiha, Aliya and Adam, Sarah

For their patience and continued support

Foreword

As the wealth of laboratory and clinical research in cancer takes us beyond today's practice into the new paradigm for 21st century medicine in which malignant disease will be detected much earlier, where tumors will be genotypically profiled and factors influential in phenotype will become known, and where treatments will be targeted according to abnormalities in specific molecular pathways and directed to eradication of small volume disease using highly sophisticated surgical and radiotherapy techniques, so medical imaging will take center stage. Thus we are at the dawn of a new era in medicine and the vision of imaging in this new era has been captured by Drs. Padhani and Choyke in their book *New Techniques in Oncologic Imaging*.

The goal of cancer imaging is to provide a detailed portrait of a tumor by combining exquisite morphological information with pathophysiological and metabolic measurements. The elegant anatomical detail provided by three-dimensional, multi-slice computed tomography (CT) is likely to continue as the mainstay for providing morphological information on the presence and extent of tumor, tumor volume, and anatomic relationships. Morphological information provided by magnetic resonance imaging (MRI) surpasses CT in well-defined anatomical sites and in the evaluation of specific tumors, so the role of MRI in this context continues to evolve. However, the fundamental requirement remains—the need to provide detailed morphological information about relevant biological processes including angiogenesis, hypoxia, apoptosis, cellular membrane integrity, necrosis, and other malignancy specific processes. Based on these parameters, clinicians will be able to make more precise management decisions noninvasively, thereby fine-tuning cancer therapy whether it be with targeted drugs, surgery, or radiotherapy. Such developments in imaging will also allow new therapies to be developed such as robotic surgical procedures and focused physical therapies.

This text is aimed at those who are or wish to be engaged in advanced imaging including scientists, physicists, chemists, biologists; radiologists, and clinicians—all of whom have an increasing need for the latest information on advances in cancer imaging techniques that will underpin much of the future developments in clinical practice.

Drs. Padhani and Choyke have recognized and responded to this exciting challenge in *New Techniques in Oncologic Imaging*. A major advantage of this text is that the editors have brought together state-of-the-art evidence in all the different imaging modalities being applied to cancer research and, in so doing, have provided a comprehensive review of the whole field of morphological and functional measurement of tumors. This text will not only allow those focused on one aspect of research to acquaint themselves with progress in other modalities, but will set the scene for functional imaging to be viewed as a whole rather than as a topic of measurement confined to one modality. At this time of staggering advances in imaging, this approach provides an outstanding contribution to medical literature. Surely this will guide and inform future clinical practice, which will be based on integrated morphology, pathophysiological, and metabolic information rather than being confined to measurement provided by a single technique.

Drs. Padhani and Choyke are both outstanding experts in cancer imaging who have contributed individually to the growing body of literature in the field of functional imaging. They have brought their expertise and experience together in *New Techniques in Oncologic Imaging,* and have recruited a superb team of experts from many different fields of cancer imaging from the United States and Europe. The text covers ultrasound, CT, magnetic resonance, nuclear medicine, and positron emission tomography, and looks to the future with reviews on electron spin resonance, optical imaging, and bioluminescence.

The important issue of image processing, central to the development and effective use of modern imaging, is also appropriately considered. The editors are to be congratulated for their vision and commitment in bringing this exciting project to fruition.

Janet E. Husband, OBE. FMedSci, FRCP, FRCR
Professor of Diagnostic Radiology
Royal Marsden NHS Foundation Trust
President, Royal College of Radiologists
London, U.K.

Foreword

The nexus between oncology and imaging grows continually stronger. Today, imaging is a key enabling biomarker for modern oncologic practice. The traditional requirement of oncologists was to stage disease; i.e., to define the extent of involvement by cancer. With structurally oriented imaging, it is now possible to obtain images from head to toe within minutes by computed tomography (CT) and magnetic resonance imaging (MRI). We today have imaging technologies that enable assessment at multiple levels of resolution from the whole body to a targeted molecular pathway. Moreover, these powerful imaging methods can now be harnessed to guide the delivery of therapeutic interventions such as minimal invasive surgery, high precision radiotherapy, or percutaneous ablations. Modern multi-slice spiral CT and fast gradient MRI are now routinely available in most cancer centers and both physicians and patients have high expectations that these methodologies will continue to rapidly improve and to deliver tangible clinical benefits.

Despite their continued and rapid improvement in resolution, structural imaging modalities like X-ray, CT, and static MRI rely on morphology that is fundamentally non-specific. The past decade has now seen the addition of functional or physiologic information on top of excellent anatomic depiction. The best example of this is fluorodeoxyglucose (FDG) imaging, which has revolutionized the practice of oncology. While its clinical development and acceptance has taken more than ten years, it is now possible and accepted to classify lesions according to their level of glucose metabolism. In some cases, this directly relates to treatment response and prognosis. Additionally, dynamic contrast enhanced MRI (DCE-MRI) and MR spectroscopy (MRS) have provided novel insights into the behavior of disease at diagnosis and during treatment. Functional imaging represents a major step forward in the evolution of oncologic imaging and it will rapidly continue to evolve with targeted molecular and nano-compound enabled imaging.

Novel imaging methodologies, currently being developed seek to identify neoplasms at the limits of their detectability. Methods such as optical imaging and radionuclide and PET imaging are capable of detecting biochemical compounds at the nano to pico-molar concentration level. This sensitivity is matched only by the specificity with which such targeted imaging probes are able to seek out and label cancers. The promise of the non-invasive "virtual biopsy," in which all of the metabolic, proteomic, and genomic information needed to make management decisions can be derived from imaging, is not as far fetched today as it was ten years ago. Indeed, reporter gene strategies have proved the principle that highly specific imaging probes can selectively enhance targeted tissue.

Ultimately, it is hoped that these new imaging methods will aid in the detection of pre-malignant conditions, early detection of cancer, early monitoring of therapeutic interventions, and in discovering recurrence before it causes irreparable damage. As a complement to drug therapy, imaging biomarkers truly have the potential that they may soon help select patients for particular therapies, identify proper dosing, and aid in drug discovery processes.

The future of imaging in oncology is exciting and filled with technologic and biologic wonders. *New Techniques in Oncologic Imaging* captures this spirit of innovation and wonder. Written and edited by experts from around the world representing major cancer centers, it fills a void by providing an up-to-date resource for oncologists and imagers. One hopes that it will stimulate the reader to higher levels of understanding of the capabilities of advanced imaging, and will motivate further exploration of the promising possibilities and capabilities in oncology. Imaging has come a long way from the original discovery of X-rays by Wilhelm Röntgen at the end of the 19th century. *New Techniques in Oncologic Imaging* represents an excellent resource to update one's knowledge of the uninterrupted progress in oncologic imaging over the last 100 years.

Michael V. Knopp, M.D., Ph.D.
Professor and Chairman
Department of Radiology
Ohio State University
Columbus, Ohio, U.S.A.

Preface

Twenty years ago diagnostic radiology departments were far simpler places. The cancer patient could expect to undergo a series of radiographic studies or fluoroscopy, perhaps an ultrasound or simple axial computed tomography all of which were recorded on film. Now, cancer patients undergo any number of highly specialized computed tomography or MRI scans, positron emission tomography, radionuclide, or sonographic studies in order to characterize their disease and for staging and treatment planning purposes. Traditionally, each examination was evaluated and the next recommended on the basis of the results obtained. Today, speed seems to be of the essence and multiple examinations are often quickly performed in succession "according to protocols." A computed tomographic scan that may have taken 30 minutes in the past now takes only seconds to complete and can be reformatted into non-orthogonal planes without loss of resolution or even used to create three-dimensional models. Moreover, today's patient may be offered a bewildering array of minimally invasive diagnostic and therapeutic interventional procedures. All of the images obtained will be recorded and displayed electronically. The increased sophistication of oncologic imaging demands increased understanding on the part of health care providers and consumers about the strengths and limitations of the choices available. This book helps readers gain that understanding. We have gathered experts from Europe and the United States to discuss their areas of expertise in a readable format and to quickly convey the theory and technology underlying their particular speciality.

Just as yesterday's technology was considered optimal in its time (but soon became outdated), so today's technology is just a step away from obsolescence. Newer technologies will surely replace older ones at an increasing pace. Already, there are indications of major shifts in the direction of oncologic imaging. Previously imaging focused on improving spatial resolution and data acquisition speed to achieve excellence in anatomic resolution that we take for granted today, there is an increasing recognition that imaging must provide more than just sharp pictures. Increasing importance is now placed on "functional imaging information"; that is, imaging that depicts critical physiologic processes within tumors, such as angiogenesis or metabolism, which can then be spatially matched with anatomic images. Thus, we see the development of clinically relevant "functional" imaging such as position emission tomography (PET), dynamic contrast enhanced MRI, and MR spectroscopy fused to "conventional imaging" like computed tomography and MRI. Looking further ahead, the future clearly points to molecularly targeted imaging agents that bind specifically to particular tumors or reporter gene systems, where transfected cells "report" the status of therapeutic genes by inserting imaging "beacons" or enzymes that entrap exogenously delivered imaging "beacons" intracellularly. The prospect of such systems in the clinical environment is enticing and is encouraging the development of research programs around the world.

Much of the current enthusiasm is prompted by the expected interplay between imaging and therapy in the future. Molecular imaging, the name that has been used to describe imaging that reflects biologic or molecular processes in vivo, will be an important adjunct to targeted molecular therapies. As we move toward personalized medicine where cancer patients are treated not by the anatomical site of the tumor but by its phenotype or molecular signature, so it is hoped that molecular imaging will guide patient selection and will tailor therapy to the individual patient's needs. Once such therapies are begun, these same imaging techniques will be used to determine whether drug delivery to the target system or cell has occurred, whether specific molecular pathways are suitably modulated, and whether underlying pathophysiological processes are being altered—all before anatomic improvements are visible. If treatments are successful, then patients will still need to be monitored for recurrent disease that may be detected before morphological alternations have taken place. Thus, molecular imaging will be highly integrated with molecular therapies. At this point in its development, an understanding of the basic precepts of molecular imaging will help prepare the reader for the coming revolution in molecular medicine.

This book is composed of chapters written by experts in their respective fields from Europe and the United States. Each chapter provides an overview of the current status of the modality or technology but cannot be comprehensive in scope. A wealth of information is available on each topic and guidance is supplied in the references. It is hoped that this effort will whet the appetites of interested readers for more knowledge.

We are indebted to the many contributors to this book and the helpfulness of our Editor, Geoffrey Greenwood and his editorial and production teams, in seeing this project to its completion.

Peter L. Choyke
Anwar R. Padhani

Contents

Contributors

Jeffry R. Alger Department of Radiological Sciences, Ahmanson-Lovelace Brain Mapping Center, Brain Research Institute, Jonsson Comprehensive Cancer Center, David Geffen School of Medicine at UCLA, University of California, Los Angeles, California, U.S.A.

Jelle Barentsz Department of Radiology, Radboud University Medical Center Nijimegen, Nijimegen, The Netherlands

Martin Blomley Imaging Sciences Department, Imperial College, Hammersmith Hospital, London, U.K.

John Butman Diagnostic Radiology Department, Warren G. Magnusson Clinical Center, National Institutes of Health, Bethesda, Maryland, U.S.A.

Kevin Camphausen Radiation Oncology Branch, CCR, NCI, NIH, DHHS, Bethesda, Maryland, U.S.A.

Peter L. Choyke Molecular Imaging Program, National Cancer Institute, Bethesda, Maryland, U.S.A.

Deborah Citrin Radiation Oncology Branch, CCR, NCI, NIH, DHHS, Bethesda, Maryland, U.S.A.

Norman C. Coleman Radiation Oncology Sciences Program, NCI, NIH, DHHS, Bethesda, Maryland, U.S.A.

David J. Collins Cancer Research UK Clinical Magnetic Resonance Research Group, Institute of Cancer Research and The Royal Marsden NHS Trust, Sutton, Surrey, U.K.

Gary J. R. Cook Department of Nuclear Medicine, Royal Marsden Hospital, Sutton, Surrey, U.K.

John A. Cook Radiation Biology Branch, Center for Cancer Research, National Cancer Institute, Bethesda, Maryland, U.S.A.

David Cosgrove Imaging Sciences Department, Imperial College, Hammersmith Hospital, London, U.K.

Nallathamby Devasahayam   Radiation Biology Branch, Center for Cancer Research, National Cancer Institute, Bethesda, Maryland, U.S.A.

James Deye   Radiation Oncology Sciences Program, NCI, NIH, DHHS, Bethesda, Maryland, U.S.A.

Antonia Dimitrakopoulou-Strauss   Medical PET Group—Biological Imaging, Clinical Cooperation Unit Nuclear Medicine, German Cancer Research Center, Heidelberg, Germany

Simon Doran   University of Surrey, Guildford, Surrey, U.K.

Andrew J. Dwyer   Diagnostic Radiology Department, National Institutes of Health, Bethesda, Maryland, U.S.A.

Andrzej Dzik-Jurasz   CR UK Clinical Magnetic Resonance Research Group, Institute of Cancer Research and Royal Marsden NHS Trust, Sutton, U.K.

Rob Eckersley   Imaging Sciences Department, Imperial College, Hammersmith Hospital, London, U.K.

Sean J. English   Radiation Biology Branch, Center for Cancer Research, National Cancer Institute, Bethesda, Maryland, U.S.A.

Sanjiv S. Gambhir   The Crump Institute for Molecular Imaging, Departments of Molecular and Medical Pharmacology and Biomathematics, and UCLA-Johnsson Comprehensive Cancer Center, David Geffen School of Medicine, University of California at Los Angeles, Los Angeles, California, U.S.A.; and Department of Radiology and the Bio-X Program, Stanford University School of Medicine, Stanford, California, U.S.A.

Alexander M. Gorbach   Department of Diagnostic Radiology, National Institutes of Health, Bethesda, Maryland, U.S.A.

Mukesh Harisinghani   Division of Abdominal Imaging and Interventional Radiology, Department of Radiology, Massachusetts General Hospital, Boston, Massachusetts, U.S.A.

Chris Harvey   Imaging Sciences Department, Imperial College, Hammersmith Hospital, London, U.K.

E. Edmund Kim   Division of Diagnostic Imaging, The University of Texas M.D. Anderson Cancer Center, Houston, Texas, U.S.A.

Myles Koby   Diagnostic Radiology Department, Warren G. Magnusson Clinical Center, National Institutes of Health, Bethesda, Maryland, U.S.A.

Murali C. Krishna   Radiation Biology Branch, Center for Cancer Research, National Cancer Institute, Bethesda, Maryland, U.S.A.

Tarik F. Massoud   The Crump Institute for Molecular Imaging, David Geffen School of Medicine, University of California at Los Angeles, Los Angeles, California, U.S.A.; Departments of Radiology and Oncology, University of Cambridge School of Clinical Medicine, Cambridge, U.K.

Cynthia Ménard   Radiation Oncology Branch, CCR, NCI, NIH, DHHS, Bethesda, Maryland, U.S.A.

Ken Miles   Brighton and Sussex Medical School, Falmer, Brighton, U.K.

James B. Mitchell   Radiation Biology Branch, Center for Cancer Research, National Cancer Institute, Bethesda, Maryland, U.S.A.

Rendon C. Nelson   Duke University Medical Center, Durham, North Carolina, U.S.A.

Vasilis Ntziachristos   Massachusetts General Hospital, Harvard Medical School, Boston, Massachusetts, U.S.A.

Anwar R. Padhani   Mount Vernon Cancer Centre, London, U.K.

Lev T. Perelman   Beth Israel Deaconess Medical Center, Harvard Medical School, Boston, Massachusetts, U.S.A.

Koen Reijnders   Radiation Biology Branch, Center for Cancer Research, National Cancer Institute, Bethesda, Maryland, U.S.A.

Simon P. Robinson   Division of Basic Medical Sciences, St. George's, University of London, London, U.K.

Anuradha Saokar   Division of Abdominal Imaging and Interventional Radiology, Department of Radiology, Massachusetts General Hospital, Boston, Massachusetts, U.S.A.

Ludwig G. Strauss   Medical PET Group—Biological Imaging, Clinical Cooperation Unit Nuclear Medicine, German Cancer Research Center, Heidelberg, Germany

Sankaran Subramanian   Radiation Biology Branch, Center for Cancer Research, National Cancer Institute, Bethesda, Maryland, U.S.A.

Robert C. Susil   Department of Biomedical Engineering, Johns Hopkins University Schoool of Medicine, Baltimore, Maryland, U.S.A.

David Thomassen   Diagnostic Radiology Department, National Institutes of Health, Bethesda, Maryland, U.S.A.

Wai Lup Wong   Paul Strickland Scanner Centre, Mount Vernon Hospital, Northwood, Middlesex, U.K.

Kenichi Yamada   Radiation Biology Branch, Center for Cancer Research, National Cancer Institute, Bethesda, Maryland, U.S.A.

David J. Yang   Division of Diagnostic Imaging, The University of Texas M.D. Anderson Cancer Center, Houston, Texas, U.S.A.

Jianhua Yao   Department of Diagnostic Radiology, Warren G. Magnusson Clinical Center, National Institutes of Health, Bethesda, Maryland, U.S.A.

1

Advances in Computed Tomography

Rendon C. Nelson
Duke University Medical Center, Durham, North Carolina, U.S.A.

A Note from the Editors

*C*omputed tomography (CT) is the mainstay of cancer imaging outside of the central nervous system. Advances in multidetector CT (MDCT) technology have had a profound impact on its diagnostic capabilities. Such techniques as multiphase, single breath-hold imaging, CT angiography (CTA), volume rendering and virtual colonography owe their success to the development of multidetector arrays with continuously moving gantries. However, to achieve these advantages without incurring the penalty of increased radiation exposure, care must be exercised in selecting the optimum combination of slice thickness, X-ray beam collimation, and table speed.

When discussing computed tomography (CT), it is interesting and useful to review the evolution of this technology since its inception. In the early 1970s, axial scanners were first introduced. These scanners had large cables attaching the X-ray tube to the power supply (1–3). This limitation resulted in intermittent X-ray exposures (eventually as short as two seconds) and incremental table motion. With these scanners, it was difficult to obtain more than about 10 slices per minute and slices were typically on the order of 10 mm in thickness. As a result, imaging of the chest and abdomen, for example, was primarily performed during the longer and more sustaining venous and/or equilibrium phases. Furthermore, since the chest and upper abdomen was scanned during multiple breath-holds, respiratory misregistration was a significant problem.

In the early 1990s, helical scanners were introduced, having a slip-ring connection between the X-ray tube and the power supply (4–10). This allowed for both continuous tube rotation and continuous table motion. As a result, a volumetric dataset was acquired consisting of up to 75 slices per minute with a slice thickness that was typically about 5 mm. Owing to the speed of these scanners, dynamic multiphasic imaging was introduced which was particularly advantageous in organs such as the liver and pancreas, where imaging during both the arterial and venous phases improved both the detection and the characterization of various tumors (Fig. 1) (11–19). Because an entire organ, such as the liver and pancreas, could be scanned during a single breath-hold, there was also a marked reduction in respiratory misregistration artifacts. Furthermore, noninvasive CT–angiography (CTA) became a reality, although in the initial stages anatomic coverage was somewhat limited because of the relatively slow table speeds (20–24). In the early- to mid-1990s, dual slice helical CT scanners were introduced which allowed for either twice the anatomic coverage or half the acquisition time. There was otherwise little change in CT parameters and, as a result, the quality of the datasets was relatively similar to single slice helical scanners. In the late 1990s, four-slice helical scanners were introduced, resulting in a precipitous increase in table speeds (25). With these scanners, for example, one could image the entire abdomen and pelvis (approximately

(A)   **(B)**

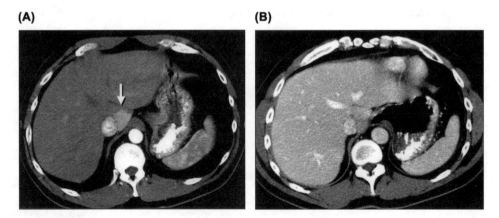

Figure 1   Biphasic liver imaging: (**A**) Axial image through the upper abdomen during the late hepatic arterial phase reveals a hyper-enhancing mass in the caudate lobe (segment I) (*arrow*). The mass is relatively homogenous and there is no evidence of either a central scar or a capsule. (**B**) During the portal venous phase, the mass demonstrates subtle hypo-attenuation and is much less conspicuous. This is a metastasis from an endocrine primary tumor.

400 mm of longitudinal coverage) during a single breath-hold with slices as thin as 2.50 mm (26,27). When less anatomic coverage was needed, slices as thin as 1.25 mm could be acquired. This resulted in a dramatic improvement in both the temporal resolution for multiphasic examinations and in the spatial resolution for CTA examinations. As certain regions of the body such as the entire abdomen and pelvis could be imaged during a single breath-hold, there were essentially no misregistration artifacts. The trade-off, however, was an increase in the radiation dose compared to single detector CT scanners.

In the early 2000s, 8- and 16-slice multidetector helical scanners were introduced (28). Compared to four-slice scanners, these scanners had the following imaging options: (i) scan much faster while obtaining a helical dataset of similar image quality, (ii) scan slightly faster while obtaining a dataset of slightly better image quality, and (iii) scan during a similar time while obtaining a much better helical dataset. Overall, the result was much higher quality three-dimensional (3D) and multiplanar reformations, which could be obtained in virtually every patient. Furthermore, on the sixteen-slice scanners the voxels can be nearly isotropic, meaning that the dimensions in the x-, y-, and z-axes are similar. Radiation doses could actually be reduced slightly on the 8 and 16 slice compared to four-slice multidetector scanners, although they continue to be higher than single detector scanners.

PRINCIPLES OF MULTIDETECTOR CT

Differences Between Single Detector and Multidetector CT

On a single detector CT (SDCT) scanner, the detector consists of a single slab of ceramic material and the slice thickness is simply determined by the collimator (Fig. 2). In comparison, on a multidetector CT (MDCT) scanner the detector has a matrix array, which consists of a ceramic detector divided into small individual pieces separated by thin metallic septae (29,30). With these scanners, the slice thickness is determined not only by the collimator but also by the detector configuration (Fig. 3). In addition, multidetector CT scanners have X-ray tubes with a much higher heat-loading capacity and have shorter gantry rotation times (e.g.,

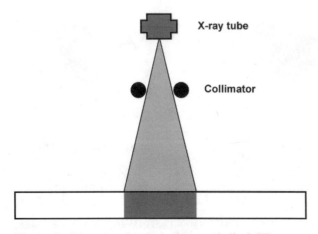

Figure 2 Diagram of a single detector helical CT scanner: It is noted that the detector consists of a single slab of ceramic material (e.g., total of 20 mm in the z-axis) and that the slice thickness is determined by the collimation width.

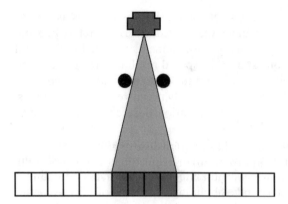

Figure 3 Diagram of a MDCT (multidetector computed tomography) scanner. It is noted that the detector consists of a row of small individual squares of ceramic material (e.g., four slice scanner consisting of 16 detectors each measuring 1.25 mm in the z-axis for a combined footprint of 20 mm) and that the slice thickness is determined both by the collimation width and the detector configuration.

0.75–1.0 seconds for SDCT vs. 0.4–0.8 seconds for MDCT). These short gantry rotation times are in part facilitated by shorter tube-to-isocenter distances, which effectively reduce rotational inertia (31). An additional advantage of a shorter tube-to-isocenter distance is the fact that there is less X-ray flux thereby requiring lower mAs. For example, reducing the distance from 630 to 541 mm increases the X-ray flux by 36% $[(630/541)^2 = 1.36]$, thereby allowing for a 74% $(1/1.36 = 0.74)$ reduction in the mA (32).

One of the interesting features of MDCT scanners is the phenomenon of focal spot wobble (32). This focal spot motion causes the X-ray beam to move back-and-forth on the detector so that the collimators must be opened to irradiate the specified detectors consistently within the matrix (Fig. 4). As a result, focal spot wobble can cause a substantial increase in radiation dose. Currently, all of the manufactures provide hardware and software solutions to this problem.

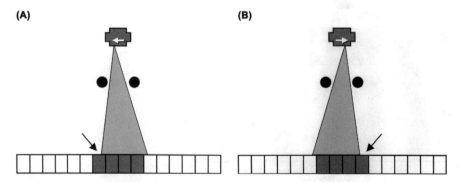

Figure 4 Focal spot wobble. Because of rotational factors the focal spot moves back-and-forth on the anode (*white arrow*). This causes the X-ray beam to move back-and-forth on the detector, as well. To prevent partial radiation of key detectors (*black arrow*) the collimators are opened, thus further increasing the radiation dose.

In general, radiation doses are significantly higher on MDCT scanners compared to SDCT scanners (32). First, the X-ray beam is collimated to a much wider width. For example, on a SDCT scanner the beam collimation to achieve a 5-mm thick slice X-ray width is 5 mm. On a MDCT scanner, the beam collimation for a 5-mm thick slice width can vary from 10 to 20 mm. To minimize this effect, the combination of a narrower collimation and a higher pitch is preferred over the combination of a wider collimation and a slower pitch. For example, comparing the 4×5.00 mm detector configuration at a pitch of 0.75 to that of a 4×2.50 mm detector configuration at a pitch of 1.5, one diminishes the radiation dose by about 25% without changing the table speed (15 mm per gantry rotation) or acquisition time (33). Second, is the effect of the penumbra. The X-ray beam has two components, (i) the umbra that is the central and most usable portion of the X-ray beam and (ii) the penumbra, which is the peripheral and unusable portion of the beam (Fig. 5). On the four-slice MDCT scanner, the penumbra represents a significant percentage of the beam; therefore, the collimation width must be increased to irradiate specified detectors with the umbra. Fortunately, on 8- and 16-slice scanners, the penumbra, represents a much smaller percentage of the total beam and therefore, has a lesser effect.

The thin septations in a matrix detector are in the order of 90 to 100 μm in thickness and represent dead space since X-ray photons striking these metallic septae do not contribute to the image. This results in a higher radiation dose. Furthermore, scanners with 8- and 16-slice capability have more septations resulting in more dead space and a further increase in radiation dose. Fortunately, these scanners can partially counteract this effect by using higher pitches and as a result, faster table speeds.

Detector Configurations

An example of the various detector configurations on a four-slice MDCT scanner manufactured by General Electric (Milwaukee, Wisconsin, U.S.A.) is as follows (26): The matrix array on this particular scanner consists of sixteen 1.25-mm thick

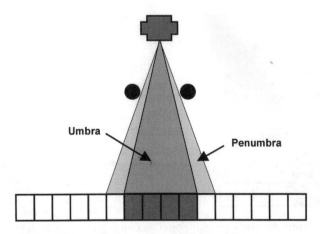

Figure 5 The X-ray beam consists of the umbra, the constant and usable portion of the beam, and the penumbra, the tapering and unusable portion of the beam. As the width of the penumbra is relatively the same, it has less of an impact with wide compared to narrow collimation as well as with 8 or 16 slice compared to 4-slice MDCT scanners.

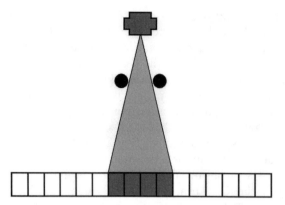

Figure 6 Depiction of the 4×1.25 mm detector configuration. It is noted that the outer 12 detectors do not contribute to image reconstruction. With this configuration, 1.25, 2.50, 3.75, and 5.00-mm thick slices can be reconstructed. This configuration is associated with the slowest table speeds, the fewest artifacts, and the highest quality dataset. Owing to limited anatomic coverage, it is mainly used for single organ CT angiography.

detectors oriented in the z-axis and having a maximum footprint of 20 mm. With the 4×1.25 mm detector configuration, the four central detectors are irradiated and slice thicknesses of 1.25, 2.50, 3.75, or 5.00 mm can be reconstructed (Fig. 6). The maximum table speed using a pitch of 1.5 with this configuration is 7.5 mm per gantry rotation (up to 15 mm per second using a 0.5-second gantry rotation time). As a result, even though this yields the best spatial resolution in the z-axis, slower table speeds limit anatomic coverage. In the abdomen, for example, this is an acceptable trade-off for certain organ-specific applications such as in the liver, kidneys, or pancreas.

With the 4×2.50 mm detector configuration, the central eight detectors are irradiated and slice thicknesses of 2.50, 3.75, and 5.00 mm can be reconstructed (Fig. 7). It is noted that a slice thickness of 1.25 mm is not available with this configuration. The maximum table speed using a pitch of 1.5 is 15 mm per gantry rotation (30 mm per

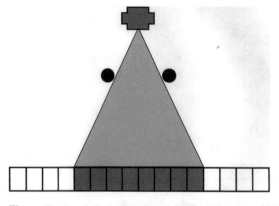

Figure 7 Depiction of the 4×2.50 mm detector configuration. It is noted that the outer eight detectors do not contribute to image reconstruction. With this configuration, 2.50-, 3.75-, and 5.00-mm thick slices can be reconstructed. A slice thickness of 1.25 mm is not available. Due to an excellent combination of slice thickness and table speed, this configuration is widely used for CT angiography.

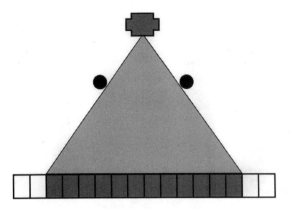

Figure 8 Depiction of the 4×3.75 mm detector configuration. It is noted that the outer four detectors do not contribute to image reconstruction. With this configuration, 3.75 and 5.00-mm thick slices can be reconstructed. Slice thicknesses of 1.25 and 2.50 mm are not available. This configuration is widely used in pediatric patients. It is not a good choice for CT angiography.

second using a gantry rotation time of 0.5 seconds). As a result, this configuration and pitch is an excellent compromise between slice thickness in the z-axis and anatomic coverage, and for example, is widely used for routine imaging of the abdomen and pelvis (single breath-hold in 12 to 20 seconds) as well as CTA. With CTA, the images are reconstructed with a thickness of 2.50 mm at a 1.00 mm interval (60% overlap) (34,35).

    With the 4×3.75 mm detector configuration, the central 12 detectors are irradiated, yielding slice thicknesses of 3.75, 5.00, and 7.50 mm (Fig. 8). It is to be noted that at the higher pitch of 1.5 the minimum slice thickness is 5.00 mm because of the slice broadening in the z-axis and that slice thicknesses of 1.25 and 2.50 mm are not available, regardless of the pitch. This configuration is primarily used for pediatric imaging since a slice thickness of 3.75 mm is popular in these smaller individuals. Furthermore, it is used with a higher pitch (e.g., 1.5) when faster table speeds are required during the fleeting hepatic arterial phase of liver imaging (22.5 mm per rotation or up to 45 mm per second using a 0.5 second gantry rotation time). Although there tends to be more streak artifacts at the faster table speeds, they are acceptable at 22.5 mm per rotation.

    With the 4×5.00 mm detector configuration, all 16 detectors are irradiated yielding slice thicknesses of 5.00 and 7.50 mm (Fig. 9). It is to be noted that a slice thickness of 1.25, 2.50, or 3.75 mm is not available at this configuration. This particular configuration is used infrequently since at the lower pitch radiation doses are inordinately high (compared to the 4×2.50 detector configuration at a pitch of 1.5) and at the higher pitch, images are significantly degraded by streak artifacts (because of aliasing).

Definitions of Pitch

There are two definitions of pitch, (i) the slice pitch and (ii) the beam pitch. The slice pitch was the original but less meaningful definition, which is defined as:

    Table travel (per gantry rotation)/Thickness of one of multiple slices.

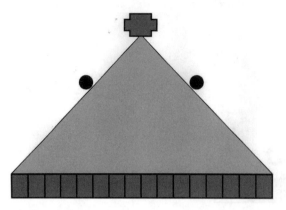

Figure 9 Depiction of the 4 × 5.00 mm detector configuration. It is noted that all 16 detectors contribute to image reconstruction. With this configuration, only 5.00-mm thick slices can be reconstructed. Slice thicknesses of 1.25, 2.50, and 3.75 mm are not available. This configuration is associated with the fastest table speed but the most artifacts. It will not yield an adequate dataset for either 3D or multiplanar reformations.

For example, if the detector configuration is 4 × 2.50 mm and the table travel is 15 mm per gantry rotation, the pitch is $15/2.50 = 6$.

The beam pitch is a more meaningful definition, which is defined as:

Table travel (per gantry rotation)/Collimation width

(additive thickness of all slices).

For example, using a 4 × 2.50 mm detector configuration and a table travel of 15 mm per gantry rotation (same as above), the pitch is $15/10 = 1.5$. The reason "beam pitch" is the preferred term since a pitch of less than one is associated with an overlap or redundancy in radiating some of the detectors following two gantry rotations. This results in an inordinate increase in the radiation dose. For example, with a pitch of 0.75 there is redundancy or oversampling of 25% of the slices (one slice on a 4-slice scanner, 2 slices on an 8-slice scanner, and 4 slices on a 16-slice scanner) (Fig. 10). With a pitch of 1.5, there is no overlap between the first and second gantry rotations and in fact, there is a 50% gap (Fig. 11). However, this does not imply that there is a gap in data acquisition but it does mean that the radiation dose is lower. The trade-off is that with higher pitches the number of photons per voxel is diminished resulting in more noise. An exception for using a pitch less than one is in applications such as the staging of pancreatic adenocarcinoma, when high spatial resolution is needed and radiation dose is less of an issue.

Formula for Determining the Detector Configuration

Knowledge of what detector configuration is being used for a specific application is helpful, not only for understanding the table and the acquisition speed but also for determining what slice thicknesses are available for retrospective reconstruction. To calculate the detector configuration, one must determine two parameters, (i) the pitch and (ii) the table speed. Then, by simply dividing the table speed by the pitch (preferably the beam pitch), the collimation width can be determined. For example,

Beam Pitch = 0.75

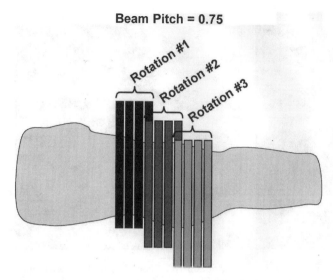

Figure 10 Beam pitch: example of a beam pitch of 0.75. It is noted that there is a 25% overlap (1 slice in a 4-slice scanner, 2 slices in an 8-slice scanner, and 4 slices in a 16-slice scanner) following two gantry rotations. This overlap improves the quality of the dataset but increased the radiation dose.

using a pitch of 1.5 and a table speed of 15 mm per gantry rotation, the collimation width is $15/1.5 = 10$ mm. The detector configuration using this example would be 4×2.50, 8×1.25, and 16×0.625 mm on 4-slice, 8-slice, and 16-slice scanners, respectively. It is possible to reconstruct slices thicker but not thinner than acquired (minimum thickness of 2.50, 1.25, and 0.625 mm, respectively, in the above example).

Beam Pitch = 1.50

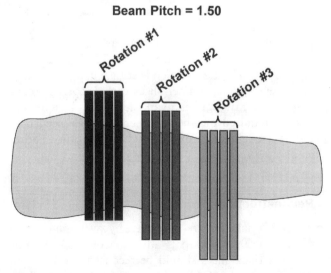

Figure 11 Beam pitch: example of a beam pitch of 1.50. It is noted that there is a 50% separation rather than an overlap following two gantry rotations. This lack of overlap diminishes the quality of the dataset but decreased the radiation dose.

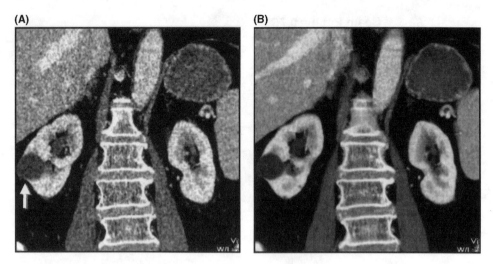

Figure 12   Coronal reformations of the upper abdomen. (**A**) There is a well-circumscribed low attenuation mass in the lower pole of the right kidney suggesting a simple cyst (*arrow*). It is noted that the image is quite noisy since it has been reconstructed with a thickness of 1 mm in the z-axis (antero–posterior direction). (**B**) When the same coronal image is reconstructed with a thickness of 5 mm in the z-axis, there is a significant decrease in noise. The trade-off, however, is an increase in partial volume average, which can make lesion characterization difficult. This is especially problematic for small lesions.

Principles of Reconstructing Images Thicker than Acquired

The goal with MDCT is to obtain the best possible volumetric dataset by choosing a detector configuration, which couples the thinnest possible slices with a pitch that yields a table speed and an acquisition time that is compatible with the patient's breath-holding capacity. One of the strategies to reduce image noise on the axial images is to reconstruct the slices thicker than acquired. For example, 2.50 or 5.00 mm thick images are reconstructed from images that are acquired from 4×1.25, 8×1.25, or 16×0.625 mm detector configurations (Fig. 12). This also has the added benefit of reducing the number of images, which is critical in practices that print and read from film. With these datasets, thinner slices can always be reconstructed retrospectively (as long as the raw data is available) when high quality 3D or multiplanar reformations are required or when thinner slices are needed to reduce the effects of partial volume averaging (for example, characterizing an adrenal nodule or a cystic renal mass).

Principles of Overlapping Reconstructions

For CTA, it has been shown that 3D datasets are improved by overlapping slice reconstructions. In general, a 50% to 60% overlap is advantageous (34,35). For example, on a SDCT scanner, 3-mm thick slices should be reconstructed at 1 mm intervals resulting in a 67% overlap. On a MDCT scanner, 2.50-mm thick slices should be reconstructed at 1.00 mm intervals yielding a 60% overlap (Figs. 13 and 14). It has to be kept in mind that with overlapping reconstructions there is

3 mm thick at 3 mm intervals
(no overlap)

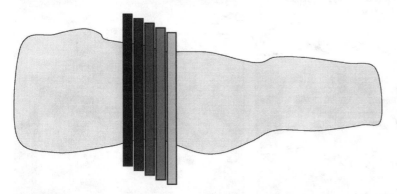

Figure 13 Nonoverlapping reconstruction: example of a nonoverlapping reconstruction, where 3 mm thick slices are reconstructed at 3 mm intervals. This would be acceptable for axial image review but not for either 3D or multiplanar reformations.

no change in the slice thickness, although the number of slices is dramatically increased because of the overlap.

Evolution in Voxel Sizes Toward Isotropia

In making the transition from four to eight slices per gantry rotation, there is no change in the nominal voxel size. For example, using a field-of-view of 360 mm and a detector configuration of 4 or 8×1.25 mm, the voxel size is $360/512 = 0.7$ mm in

3 mm thick at 1 mm intervals
(67% overlap)

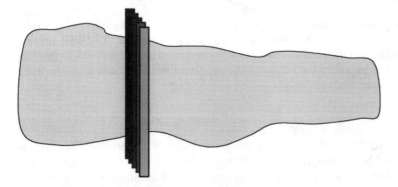

Figure 14 Overlapping reconstruction: example of overlapping reconstruction, where 3 mm thick slices are reconstructed at 1 mm intervals. It is noted that while there is a change in the reconstruction interval (e.g., 1 mm), there is no change in the slice thickness (e.g., 3 mm). An overlap of 60% or more is optimal for 3D or multiplanar reformations.

(A)   (B)

(C)   (D)

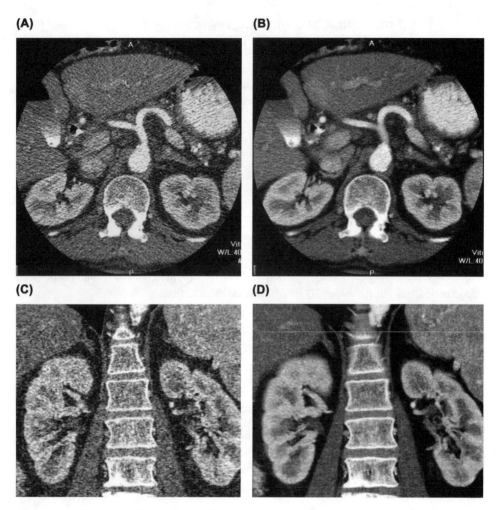

Figure 15 Examples of images acquired with a 16×0.625 mm detector configuration and reconstructed at various slice thicknesses. (**A**) An axial images reconstructed at 0.625 mm thick has increased noise due to fewer photons per voxel. There is, however, much less partial volume averaging in the z-axis (cranio-caudal direction). (**B**) The same axial image reconstructed at 5.00 mm thick has much less noise but more partial volume averaging. To make off-axis reformations, the axial images are first reconstructed 0.625 mm thick at 0.50 mm interval. This dataset was then rendered in either a straight or curved format. (**C**) In this coronal image, the slice thickness in the z-axis (antero–posterior direction) is 0.625 mm. (**D**) In this coronal image, the slice thickness in the z-axis is 5.00 mm, dramatically reducing the noise while increasing partial volume averaging.

the x-axis, 0.7 mm in the y-axis, and 1.25 mm in the z-axis (plus nominal slice broadening as determined by the pitch). When making the transition from 8 to 16 slices per gantry rotation, the nominal voxel size can be smaller. For example, using a 360 mm field-of-view and a detector configuration of 16×0.625 mm, the voxel size is 360/ $512 = 0.7$ mm in the x-axis, 0.7 mm in the y-axis and 0.625 mm in the z-axis (plus nominal slice broadening as determined by the pitch). For the first time in the history of CT, the voxels can be isotropic, meaning that the dimensions of the voxel are

(A)   (B)

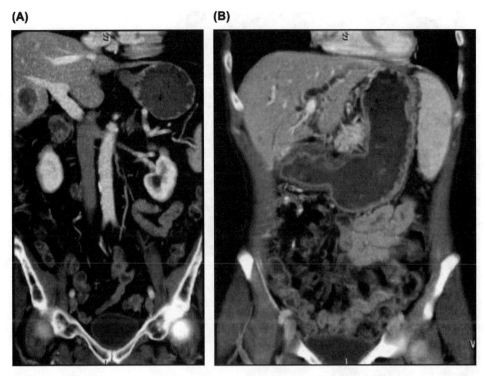

Figure 16 Coronal reformations of the entire abdomen and pelvis acquired with an
8 × 1.25 mm detector configuration and pitch of 1.68. The axial images are reconstructed with
a thickness of 1.25 mm at 0.50-mm intervals. A coronal image is then reformatted with a thickness of 5.00 mm in the z-axis (antero–posterior direction) to decrease noise. (**A**) There is a large
metastasis in the right hepatic lobe. (**B**) No masses are noted on an image obtained more anteriorly, but there is excellent depiction of the stomach due to distention of the lumen with water
and enhancement of the wall with intravenous contrast material.

equal in the x-, y-, and z-axes. Although spatial resolution in all three axes is
improved, the trade-off is fewer photons per voxel and higher image noise. Since
kV and mA are set to near maximum on an eight-slice MDCT scanner to achieve
adequate image quality with low noise, there are few options to increase the technique further on a 16-slice scanner. As a result, until, X-ray tubes with higher heat
loading capacity are available, images acquired at 16 × 0.625 mm will be inherently
noisy, which may limit some applications, such as CT angiography (Fig. 15).

Fundamental Advantages of MDCT

The first advantage of MDCT is the ability to scan a lot faster while acquiring a
dataset with similar slice thickness and image quality to that of SDCT. Faster table
speeds are particularly advantageous in patients with reduced breath-holding
capacity since table speeds on the order of 50 to 70 mm per second are achievable.
Fast table speeds are often chosen in the setting of trauma, in patients with dyspnea,
in young children or in those patients in whom there are communication difficulties
such as a language barrier or deafness.

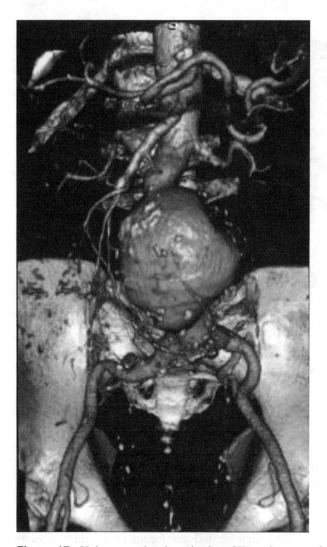

Figure 17 Volume rendered projection CT angiogram of the abdominal aorta and iliac arteries revealing a large infrarenal aortic aneurysm. It is noted that the entire dataset was acquired during a single breath-hold on the order of 15 seconds.

The second advantage of MDCT is the ability to scan faster while acquiring a dataset with a similar slice thickness but better image quality, compared to SDCT. For example, this is the strategy used for routine imaging of the abdomen and pelvis in patients with average breath holding capacity. With these parameters, the entire abdomen and pelvis (350–400 mm of longitudinal coverage) can be scanned in a single breath-hold of 12 to 20 seconds in duration (Fig. 16). It is recommended that faster gantry rotation speeds (e.g., 0.5 seconds per rotation) should be selected whenever possible. Although images acquired using shorter gantry rotation times are reconstructed using fewer trajectories in the algorithm (i.e., undersampling), image quality is not significantly degraded (31). An exception might be encountered when scanning through the shoulders and bony pelvis or in large patients where aliasing in the form of streak artifacts may be encountered.

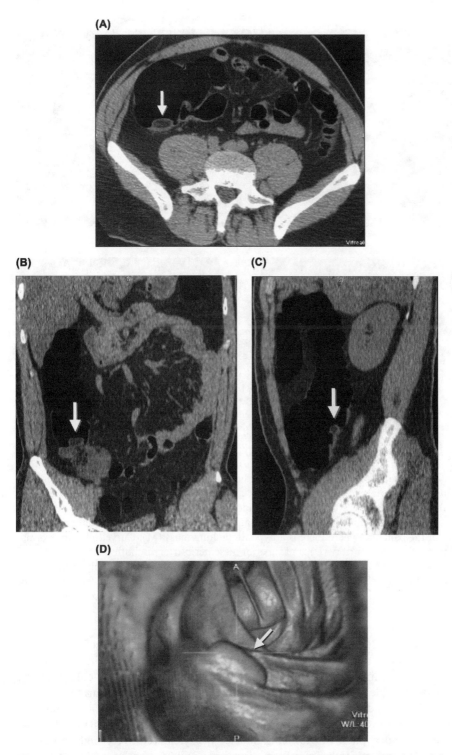

Figure 18 (**A**) Axial CT colonographic image acquired following insufflation of the entire colon with air. A moderate-sized polyp is noted in the cecum (*arrow*). It is noted that the internal attenuation of the polyp is similar to adjacent retroperitoneal fat, consistent with a lipoma. The lipoma is also well visualized on the coronal (**B**) and the sagittal (**C**) reformation and on a virtual endoscopic view (**D**).

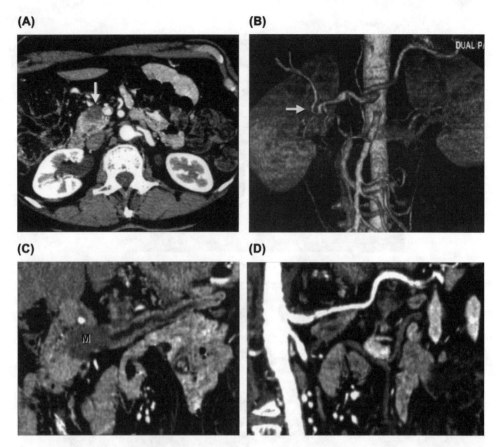

Figure 19 (**A**) An axial image through the upper abdomen reveals an approximately 2 cm hypoattenuating mass in the pancreatic head (*arrow*). The mass abuts the superior mesenteric vein but does not appear to invade the wall or lumen. (**B**) Antero–posterior volume rendered projection image reveals conventional anatomy as well as an unusual "hairpin" course of the proximal proper hepatic artery, without evidence of narrowing or irregularity (*arrow*). (**C**) Curved planar reformation through the main pancreatic duct reveals dilatation down to the head of the pancreas where there is a hypoattenuating mass (**M**). Curved planar reformations through the splenic artery (**D**), and superior mesenteric artery in both the coronal (**E**) and sagittal (**F**) planes reveal no evidence of tumor encasement or adjacent lymphadenopathy. (**G**) Curved planar reformation through the hepatic artery reveals circumferential tumor encasement at the level of the "hairpin" tortuosity (*arrow*). (*Continued on next page*).

The second advantage of MDCT noted above is particularly useful for multi-planar reformations and CTA (36). When large areas of anatomy need to be scanned such as the abdominal aorta and iliac arteries (Fig. 17) or in CT-colonography (Fig. 18), faster table speeds are selected to complete the acquisition during a reasonable breath-hold and/or during peak arterial enhancement (37,38). On a four-slice scanner, the parameters for such a protocol would include a 4×2.50 mm detector configuration and a pitch of 1.5. This dataset will yield relatively high-resolution images for 3D and multiplanar reformations, particularly for larger blood vessels that are perpendicular to the axial plane.

The third advantage of MDCT includes the ability to scan during a similar time with either thinner slices and/or much better quality images, compared to

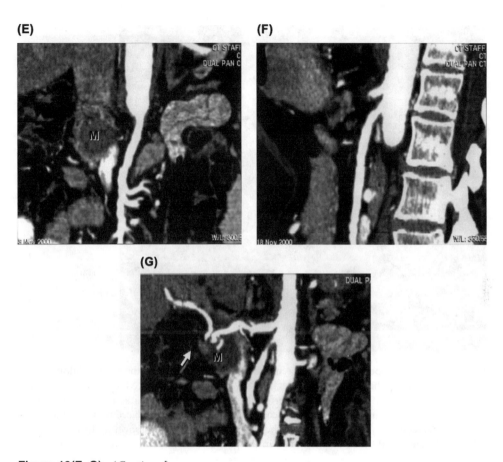

Figure 19(E–G) (*Continued*).

SDCT. These datasets can be acquired during a comfortable breath-hold (10–20 seconds) with reasonable anatomic coverage (200–300 mm). For example, in the abdomen, this advantage is particularly applicable when evaluating single organs such as the liver, pancreas, or kidneys. As less anatomic coverage is needed to scan these organs, slower table speeds and thinner slices can be used to provide very high quality datasets for 3D and multiplanar reformations (28). Specific applications include the staging of pancreatic adenocarcinoma (Fig. 19), evaluation of the liver prior to hepatic tumor resection (Fig. 20) or transplantation, and the evaluation of the kidney prior to partial or donor nephrectomy.

THE FUTURE OF CT

In the future, CT scanners that have much faster image reconstruction, higher heat-loading capacity X-ray tubes, even faster table speeds, and automatic volume rendering of the datasets may be expected. The latter feature will give the radiologist the ability to change the slice thickness, location, and orientation during interpretation, interactively. There will be ongoing efforts to reduce the radiation dose without

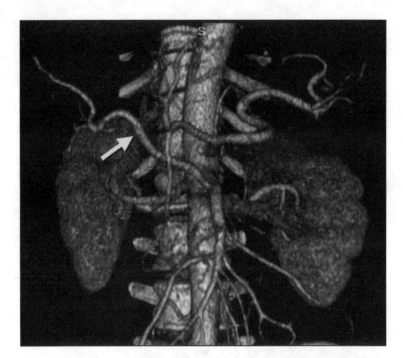

Figure 20 Antero–posterior volume rendered projection image of the upper abdomen in a patient anticipating hepatic tumor resection reveals a large replaced right hepatic artery (*arrow*). The entire left hepatic lobe is perfused from the proper hepatic artery. If placement of a chemotherapy infusion pump was indicated in this patient, the replaced right hepatic artery would be ligated to allow collaterals from the left hepatic artery to crossover to the right hepatic lobe. A catheter would then be positioned in the gastroduodenal artery for drug infusion.

sacrificing image quality and to improve reconstruction algorithms. Improvement in the *x*- and *y*-axis dimension of the voxel may even be witnessed, which have not changed since the inception of this useful technology.

REFERENCES

1. Hounsfield GN. Computerized transverse axial scanning (tomography). Brit J Radiol 1973; 46:1016–1022.
2. Brooks RA, DiChiro G. Theory of image reconstruction in computed tomography. Radiology 1975; 117:561–572.
3. McCullough EC, Payne JT, Baker HL, et al. Performance evaluation and quality assurance of computed tomography scanners with illustrations from the EMI, ACTA and Delta scanners. Radiology 1976; 120:173–188.
4. Heiken JP, Brink JA, Vannier MW. Spiral (helical) CT. Radiology 1993; 189:647–656.
5. Brink JA. Technical aspects of helical (spiral) CT. Radiol Clin North Am 1995; 33:825–841.
6. Kalender WA, Seissler W, Klotz E, Vock P. Spiral volumetric CT with single-breath-hold technique, continuous transport, and continuous scanner rotation. Radiology 1990; 176:181–183.
7. Polacin A, Kalender WA, Marchal C. Evaluation of section sensitivity profiles and image noise in spiral CT. Radiology 1992; 185:29–35.

8. Costello P, Anderson W, Blume D. Pulmonary nodule: evaluation with spiral volumetric CT. Radiology 1991; 179:875–876.
9. Costello P, Ecker CP, Tello R, Hartnell GG. Assessment of the thoracic aorta by spiral CT. Am J Roentgenol 1992; 158:1127–1130.
10. Heiken JP, Brink JA, Sagel SS. Helical CT: abdominal applications. Radiographics 1994; 14:919–924.
11. Bluemke DA, Fishman EK. Spiral CT of the liver. Am J Roentgenol 1992; 160:787–792.
12. Bonaldi VM, Bret PM, Reinhold C, Mostafa A. Helical CT of the liver: value of an early hepatic arterial phase. Radiology 1995; 197:357–363.
13. Hollett MD, Jeffrey RB Jr, Nino-Murcia M, Jorgensen MJ, Harris DP. Dual-phase helical CT of the liver: value of arterial phase scans in the detection of small malignant hepatic neoplasms. Am J Roentgenol 1995; 164:879–884.
14. Oliver JH III, Baron RL, Federle MP, et al. Detecting hepatocellular carcinoma: value of unenhanced or arterial phase CT imaging or both used in conjunction with conventional portal venous phase contrast-enhanced CT imaging. Am J Roentgenol 1996; 167:71–77.
15. Baron RL, Oliver JH III, Dodd GD III, Nalesnik M, Holbert BL, Carr B. Hepatocellular carcinoma: evaluation with biphasic, contrast-enhanced, helical CT. Radiology 1996; 199:505–511.
16. van Leeuwen MS, Noordzij J, Feldberg MA, Hennipman AH, Doornewaard H. Focal liver lesions: characterization with triphasic spiral CT. Radiology 1996; 201:327–336.
17. Hollett MD, Jorgensen MJ, Jeffrey RB. Quantitative evaluation of pancreatic enhancement during dual-phase helical CT. Radiology 1995; 195:359–361.
18. Dupuy DE, Costello P, Ecker CP. Spiral CT of the pancreas. Radiology 1992; 183: 815–818.
19. Lu DSK, Vendantham S, Krasny RM, Kadell B, Berger WL, Reber HA. Two-phase helical CT for pancreatic tumor: pancreatic versus hepatic phase enhancement of tumor, pancreas and vascular structures. Radiology 1996; 199:697–701.
20. Napel S, Marks MP, Rubin GD, et al. CT angiography with spiral CT and maximum intensity projection. Radiology 1992; 185:607–610.
21. Diedrichs CG, Keating DP, Glatting G, Oestmann JW. Blurring of vessels in spiral CT angiography: effects of collimation width, pitch, viewing plane and windowing in maximum intensity projection. J Comput Assist Tomogr 1996; 20:965–974.
22. Galanski M, Prokop M, Chavan A, Schaefer CM, Jandeleit K, Nischelsky JE. Renal arterial stenosis: spiral CT angiography. Radiology 1993; 189:185–192.
23. Rubin GD, Dake MD, Napel S, et al. Spiral CT of renal artery stenosis: comparison of three-dimensional rendering techniques. Radiology 1994; 190:181–189.
24. Raptopoulos V, Rosen MP, Kent KC, Kuestner LM, Sheiman RG, Pearlman JD. Sequential helical CT angiography of aortoiliac disease. Am J Roentgenol 1996; 166:1347–1354.
25. McCollough CH, Zink FE. Performance evaluation of a multislice CT system. Med Phys 1999; 26:2223–2230.
26. Killius JS, Nelson RC. Logistic advantages of four-section helical CT in the abdomen and pelvis. Abdom Imaging 2000; 25:643–650.
27. Cuomo FA, Brink JA. Radiation dose with multidetector row CT: comparison of high and low pitch scanning strategies for abdominal imaging [Abstract]. Radiology 2000; 81:505.
28. Gupta AK, Nelson RC, Johnson GA, Paulson EK, Delong DM, Yoshizumi TT. Optimization of eight-element multidetector row helical CT technology for evaluating the abdomen. Radiology 2003; 227:739–745.
29. Hu H, He HD, Foley WD, Fox SH. Four multidetector-row helical CT: image quality and volume coverage speed. Radiology 2000; 215:55–62.
30. Hu H. Multislice CT: scan and reconstruction. Med Phys 1999; 26:5–18.

31. Bergin D, Heneghan JP, Ho LM, Nelson RC. Multidetector helical CT of the chest, abdomen and pelvis: does increasing the gantry rotation speed from 0.8 to 0.5 seconds affect image quality? [Abstract]. Am J Roentgenol 2002; 178:43.

32. Yoshizumi TT, Nelson RC. Radiation issues with multidetector row helical CT. Crit Rev Comput Tomogr 2003; 44:95–117.

33. General Electric Light Speed Protocol Simulator; Proprietary data.

34. Urban BA, Fishman EK, Kuhlman JE, Kawashima A, Hennessey JG, Siegelman SS. Detection of focal hepatic lesions with spiral CT: comparison of 4- and 8-mm interscan spacing. Am J Roentgenol 1993; 160:783–785.

35. Brink JA, Wang G, McFarland EG. Optimal section spacing in single-detector helical CT. Radiology 2000; 214:575–578.

36. Schoepf UJ, Becker CR, Bruening RD, et al. Multislice CT angiography. Brit Inst Radiol 2001; 13:357–365.

37. Rubin GD, Shiau MC, Leung AN, Kee ST, Logan LJ, Sofilos MC. Aorta and iliac arteries: single versus multiple detector-row helical CT angiography. Radiology 2000; 215:670–676.

38. McFarland EG, Brink JA, Pilgram TK, et al. Spiral CT colonography: reader agreement and diagnostic performance with two- and three-dimensional image-display techniques. Radiology 2001; 218:375–383.

2

Advances in MRI of the Brain

John Butman and Myles Koby
*Diagnostic Radiology Department, Warren G. Magnusson Clinical Center,
National Institutes of Health, Bethesda, Maryland, U.S.A.*

Peter L. Choyke
*Molecular Imaging Program, National Cancer Institute, Bethesda,
Maryland, U.S.A.*

A Note from the Editors

P
*ractically every innovation in magnetic resonance
imaging (MRI) has been applied first to the brain.
The brain's well-defined anatomy, MR characteristics, and relative absence of motion make it ideal for MRI.
Advances in hardware, such as higher field strengths, high
performance gradients, and advanced coil designs have led to
brain scans with more contrast obtained at higher speeds.
Pulse sequence advances such as echo planar imaging, fluid
attenuated inversion recovery, diffusion weighted, perfusion
imaging, and spectroscopic images have expanded the
diagnostic range of MRI. Image processing and image
management have also had a profound impact on MRI of the
brain. This chapter reviews these developments and provides
illustrative examples.*

INTRODUCTION

Magnetic resonance imaging (MRI) is the premier modality for evaluating brain tumors. The relatively small size of the brain along with the relative absence of motion makes high-resolution imaging routinely possible. Moreover, the well-known MRI behavior of white and gray matter and cerebrospinal fluid (CSF) makes them ideal for optimizing contrast parameters. The paucity of air and fat reduces the artifacts often seen with body MRI. For these reasons, MRI of the brain has been the focus of most new developments in technology. Such developments are often introduced in MRI of the brain before they are attempted in other parts of the body. These natural advantages of MRI of the brain create an excellent platform for the study of brain tumors.

The advances in MRI technology of the brain can be divided into hardware, software, and image processing improvements. These advances combine to create rapid, high-resolution scans that provide unique biologic information. This chapter will review these recent advances.

HARDWARE ADVANCES

Advances in magnet technology, gradient speed and strength, coil design and parallel processing, and table control have been instrumental in improving the capabilities of brain MRI. Here we consider each separately.

Magnet Design

Perhaps the most significant recent advance in MRI of the brain has been the development of high-field strength magnets. "High-field" now generally refers to field strengths of 3T or higher, since most superconducting magnets have 1.5T. Commercial high-field MR units now range from 3 to 8T, and experimental units of 12T have been designed.

The principal advantage of high-field strength is the higher signal-to-noise ratio (SNR) resulting from the higher proportion of spins that align with the magnetic field as opposed to spins that align against the magnetic field (1). This gain in signal can be used in a variety of applications, including higher resolution scans, faster scans, more highly resolved NMR spectroscopy, and blood oxygen level determination (BOLD) studies (2).

Excellent spatial resolution is important for detecting small lesions in the brain (e.g., metastases) and fine structures such as the cranial nerves or inner ear structures that may be affected by brain tumors (3). However, increasing spatial resolution is more demanding of signal strength; a 50% increase in resolution requires a four-fold increase in signal to maintain a constant SNR. Similarly, faster imaging speeds, are required for dynamic contrast-enhanced (DCE) studies, which are more demanding of signal strength; a 50% reduction in scan time requires a doubling of signal to maintain SNR. Enhancement may be greater at higher field strengths for the same dose of contrast (4). MR spectroscopy, discussed in detail later in this chapter and in a separate chapter, is also improved by higher field strength because individual metabolite peaks can be resolved at higher field, whereas at lower field these metabolites may be combined into a single peak (5). BOLD imaging, which is used to identify functionally critical regions of the brain that must be spared during surgical therapies, is also improved by the higher SNR of high-field strengths. BOLD depends on subtle shifts in the relative ratio of oxyhemoglobin to deoxyhemoglobin within tissue and the signal change is often quite small (1–3%) (2,3). Thus, changes in local blood flow occurring in response to performing a specific task are more easily and reliably detected at higher field. Time-of-flight magnetic resonance angiography (MRA), which depicts the vessels of the circle of Willis, is also improved at higher fields since the in-flow enhancement effects are greater.

There are a number of potential disadvantages to higher MR fields. In addition to the added costs of the magnet and the difficulties in siting the unit due to larger fringe fields and heavier magnets, there are increased safety concerns at high-field strength. Heating deposition, which is measured in units of specific absorbed radiation (SAR), is a greater concern at higher fields. SAR depends on radiofrequency absorption and tissue attenuation which is greater at the higher resonance frequencies required by higher field strengths. Thus, pulse sequences that might be perfectly safe at 1.5 T may produce unacceptable heating due to SAR at higher field strengths. As a result, pulse sequences normally performed at 1.5 T must be altered to prevent overheating the patient. For instance, the substitution of lower SAR gradient echo images at 3 T for higher SAR T1-weighted spin echo images at 1.5 T has made interpretation of the bone marrow within the skull for possible metastatic disease more difficult. Additionally, some patients experience dizziness or nausea due to stronger and faster magnetic gradient switching. This is due to small induced currents within the semicircular canals of the inner ear leading to inappropriate stimulation of the mechanism of balance. A final disadvantage of high fields is that there are more susceptibility artifacts due to air–tissue interfaces.

Open Systems

While in some settings there is a growing trend toward the use of higher field strengths in enclosed circular magnets, in other settings, open MRI systems, which utilize lower field strengths (0.15–1.0 T) have become more widespread. These magnets are considered "open" because the magnets consist of two opposing magnetic plates with a space in between. Consequently, they do not require the patient to be enclosed by the bore of a magnet. Lack of image quality, previously a significant limitation of open systems, has been overcome to some degree by improved coil designs and better magnet designs.

Open MRIs have a number of advantages over conventional enclosed units. Claustrophobic patients and children can be scanned in an open MRI without sedation. Some open MRI systems are configured so that the patient may stand during the scan thus loading the spine in a physiologic manner. This is primarily useful for vertebral disk disease and may find application in back pain related to potential metastatic disease and vertebral body instability.

Open systems are generally preferred by patients. However, they also allow interventional procedures to be performed under MR guidance. For instance, stereotactic biopsies can be performed under real-time guidance, and this could permit more accurate needle guidance, minimizing risk to the patient while maximizing the diagnostic yield. Intraoperative open MRI systems can also be used to guide neurosurgery and other interventions (6–8).

Open MRIs have recently improved in quality. However, due to their lower field strength they suffer from intrinsically lower SNR which results in longer scan times to preserve image quality. Furthermore, the lower field makes it difficult to perform studies such as spectroscopy and diffusion-weighted MRI, thus limiting the capabilities of the magnet.

High Performance Gradients

Many of the features most desired by clinicians such as resolution, slice thickness, and speed are determined not only by magnetic *field strength* but also by the strength and speed of the magnetic *gradients*. Magnetic gradients are small fields that are superimposed on the main magnetic field in order to change the resonance frequency of water, which in turn, allows the signal from the MRI to be localized and thereby generate images. Magnetic gradients are usually applied for very short periods during the scanning process. Stronger magnetic gradients permit thinner slices and higher matrices to be acquired thus improving the image resolution. The speed with which these strong gradients are applied, known as the slew rate, can improve the speed of scanning and also allow for extended spin and gradient echoes to be acquired, resulting in highly efficient scans in which images with varying T1 and T2 weighting can be obtained during a single acquisition.

The sudden bursts of energy created by rapidly changing the local magnetic field of tissue induce small currents in the body. When strong gradients change quickly ("high performance gradients"), they may exceed the threshold of stimulation of peripheral nerves resulting in tingling or a "pins and needles" sensation in the arms and legs. Such peripheral nerve stimulation, while unpleasant is not dangerous. Much care is taken in the design of gradients to avoid peripheral nerve stimulation.

Parallel Coil Imaging

A recent hardware/software innovation in acquisition MRI has been parallel coil imaging. Coils can be thought of as receiver antennas. In parallel imaging, instead of relying on one coil or even one set of many coils to collect a single data set, each coil in an array simultaneously collects a different part of the total image data ("k-space"); these parts are combined to form an image. As a result of this "parallel" processing, dramatic improvements in imaging speed can be achieved (9–11). For instance, if two coils are actively parallel, the scan time can be cut by a factor of two, and if four coils are active in the array, the scan time can, in theory, be cut by a factor of four and so forth. Parallel processing is possible only because of high-bandwidth receivers that allow the simultaneous acquisition of data from multiple coils and a custom-designed software that permits different coils to sample different parts of k-space.

In this manner, head-spine arrays can be designed so that acquisitions can be greatly accelerated and are much more convenient for technologists since multiple coil changes are not necessary (11). Thus, a survey of the brain and spinal cord for metastatic disease can be performed in a single imaging session. Parallel imaging also permits higher temporal resolution in applications such as MRA, dynamic contrast enhancement, diffusion-weighted imaging (DWI), and spectroscopy. High bandwidth receivers also permit shorter pulse sequences.

The primary disadvantage of parallel imaging is loss of signal and in applications where signal is already low (e.g., phosphorous spectroscopy), parallel imaging may not be feasible. Fortunately, this is of less concern in the brain where SNR is usually more than adequate.

Moving Table

The ability to control the speed and direction of table motion over wide areas of the body has enabled total body screening studies to be contemplated. Although not yet in wide use, total body imaging has been proposed for monitoring populations at high risk of developing primary or secondary tumors. Thus, head-to-toe scanning is technically feasible in less than one hour. Such scans are still considered experimental because risks and benefits to individuals as well as costs to society are yet to be rigorously analyzed.

Largely due to considerations of time, it can be difficult to optimize the imaging parameters for each body part. Thus, the field of view used for chest imaging may also be used in the brain imaging, which lowers the effective resolution of brain imaging. Such scans are generally performed with fast sequences and compromises are made in resolution and contrast in order to achieve efficient coverage. The efficacy of total body screening has not yet been proven in large studies.

SOFTWARE ADVANCES

Equally important as advances in hardware are advances in software or pulse sequence design. MR images are the final product of a carefully orchestrated sequence of radiofrequency pulses and magnetic gradients known as pulse sequences. Pulse sequences are designed to extract specific types of data about the brain. As a consequence they are often not optimized for other types of data. Thus, a complete MRI is composed of several complementary sequences from which a diagnosis can usually be made. Generic pulse sequences include those that are T1-weighted or T2-weighted. This designation simply means that although both T1 and T2 effects contribute to the image contrast, the image is dominated by either the T1 or T2 relaxation properties of the tissue.

3D SPOILED GRADIENT ECHO

Stronger gradients have made possible ultrashort 3D imaging sequences that are T1-weighted. Scans that are less than 1 mm thick can be obtained through the entire brain. Because they depict the anatomy with exquisite detail they can be fused with images of lower resolution but have functional attributes such as positron emission tomography (PET) scans, which have lower spatial resolution but may be more sensitive for detecting pathology.

High-resolution MR scans are termed "isotropic," since they demonstrate the same resolution along any plane of section. Thus, a single isotropic 3D acquisition obtained in the coronal plane can be reformatted without loss of anatomic detail along any arbitrary line of section. These scans are used for surgical planning, intraoperative guidance, and radiotherapy planning. 3D images of brain tumors, after intravenous contrast, are obtained to accurately determine tumor volume during treatment.

Rapid Acquisition Relaxation-Enhanced and Fast Spin Echo

A conventional T2-weighted spin echo sequence typically yields one echo for every 90° pulse which is then detected by a receiver coil. The rapid acquisition relaxation-enhanced (RARE) or fast spin echo (FSE) sequence shortens the time needed to acquire T2-weighted scans by obtaining multiple echoes for every 90° pulse. Whereas traditional T2-weighted scans require 6 to 10 minutes for scanning whole brain; T2-weighted RARE or FSE images are often acquired in two to five minutes. Although it was initially felt that such scans were not as sensitive to early pathology as peritumoral edema, in fact this has proven to be a minor disadvantage compared with the gain in speed and RARE and FES are now routine. The increased speed of acquisition can also be employed to generate higher resolution images and thus improve detection of small brain lesions. These sequences have the desirable property of reducing artifacts caused by susceptibility and thus are less influenced by surgical clips or air adjacent to the brain.

Echo Planar Imaging

Echo planar imaging (EPI) is used to generate fast whole brain images within one to two seconds. EPI produces multiple echoes, similar to FSE but with many more echoes while the readout gradient is varying. This is known as an echo train, and it dramatically reduces scan time. To achieve such rapid scans, however, image resolution is generally compromised, and image quality is not as good as traditional sequences due to susceptibility artifacts. EPI is primarily used during 3D acquisitions for BOLD or diffusion imaging.

Gradient and Spin Echo

Gradient and spin echo (GRASE) imaging is a recent innovation primarily used at high-field strengths to overcome some of the heating concerns that occur with T2-weighted scans at higher field strengths (12–14). By combining gradient echo and spin echo images in a single sequence, SAR can be reduced and T2-like contrast can be achieved within reasonable time constraints. Thus, sequences normally performed at 1.5 T can be modified to GRASE-type sequences at 3.0 T.

T2* Perfusion Imaging

Susceptibility imaging for measurement of brain perfusion is performed by intravenously injecting a gadolinium chelate at a high rate (e.g., 5 cc/sec) and observing a decrease in signal related to the T2* effects of the rapidly administered gadolinium chelate within the brain parenchyma (15). This is accomplished by rapidly acquiring T2* EPI images and then analyzing these images on a pixel-by-pixel basis. The rapid drop in signal intensity followed by a rapid restoration of signal within the brain is related to the first pass of the gadolinium chelate bolus. The signal intensity-time curve is used to derive regional cerebral blood volume (rCBV), mean transit time (MTT), and regional cerebral blood flow (rCBF) (Figs. 1–3) (15–17). These are usually used in the context of strokes; however, their use in measuring brain tumor response to therapy is being explored (18). The breakdown of the blood brain barrier reduces the T2* effects by allowing dilution of the contrast bolus, thus leading to errors in rCBV and rCBF measurements, however, this property has been exploited to calculate vascular permeability within tumors.

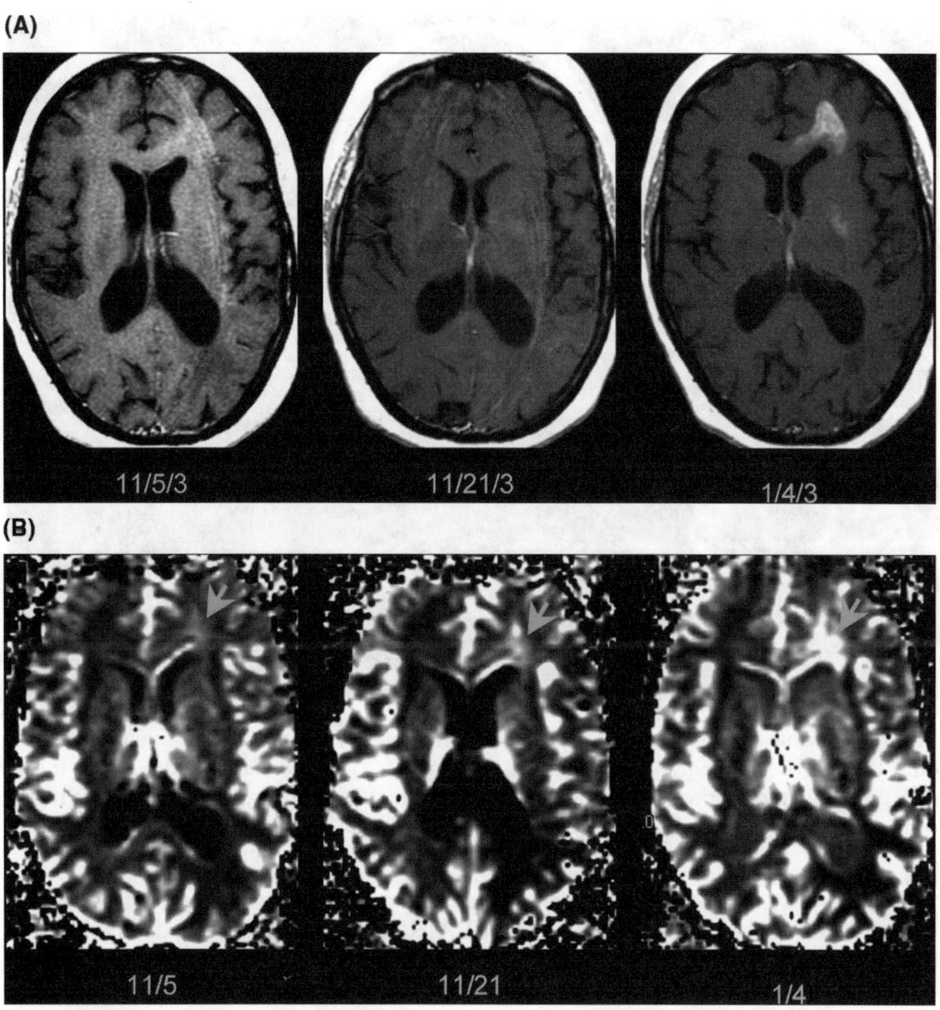

(A)

(B)

Figure 1   Transition of glioblastoma from low grade to high grade was first detected on T2*
perfusion blood volume map. (A) Contrast-enhanced T1-weighted MRIs at three different
dates demonstrates leakage of contrast media only on the third scan indicative of a high-grade
tumor. (B) Blood volume maps, however, obtained with T2* perfusion demonstrate that
abnormal blood volume could be detected earlier (*arrow*) than with the T1-weighted images.

Fluid-Attenuated Inversion Recovery

Fluid-attenuated inversion recovery (FLAIR) is an MR sequence that suppresses
CSF by applying an initial inverting 180° pulse, which negatively magnetizes the
CSF and then waiting approximately for the T1 of CSF so that its magnetization
(and hence signal) crosses a zero point just as the imaging data begins to be acquired
(19). Thus, water signal is suppressed. It can be used in conjunction with long time-
to-echo (T2-weighted) or short time-to-echo (T1-weighted) fast spin echo sequences.
FLAIR suppresses signal from CSF and any other fluid with a comparable T1, thus
it is nonspecific.

   FLAIR T2-weighted images improve the conspicuity of lesions, especially those
located near CSF spaces, such as near the cerebral ventricles. Moreover, because fluid

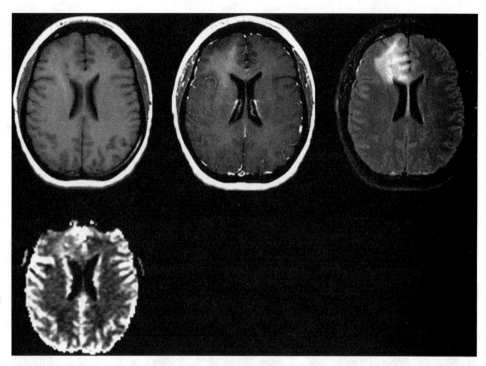

Figure 2 Value of blood volume maps in assessing brain tumors. Glioblastoma multiforme on T1-weighted (*upper left*), T1-weighted postcontrast (*upper middle*), and FLAIR (*upper right*) demonstrate, respectively, no abnormality, subtle enhancement, and edema in the region of the tumor indicative of a low grade tumor. The T2* perfusion blood volume map (*lower left*), however, demonstrates increased blood volume suggesting a higher-grade tumor.

is present along the cerebral convexities, FLAIR greatly improves the detectability of lesions located near the dura. Thus, FLAIR T2-weighting has become a new standard in imaging the brain (20,21).

Contrast enhancement is a critical component of brain MRI, because it identifies sites of breakdown in the blood brain barrier which is often associated with

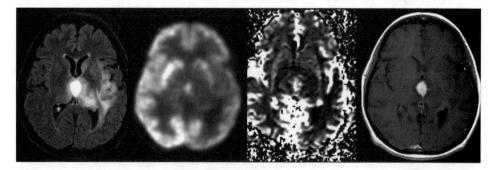

Figure 3 Comparison of MRI, PET, and blood volume maps. *Left to right*: FLAIR image, FDG PET, blood volume, and postcontrast T1-weighted image. Respectively these images depict: a lesion in the mass intermedia demonstrating high signal on FLAIR, relatively low metabolic activity on PET but increased blood volume despite absence of enhancement in the thalamus and insula suggesting a large, high-grade glioma.

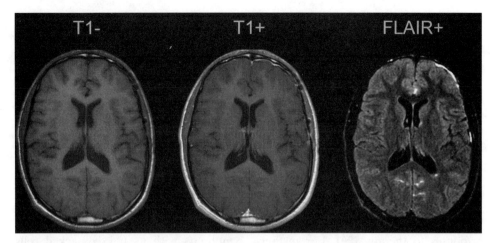

Figure 4 Advantage of FLAIR for detecting leptomeningeal metastases. Left to right: T1-weighted MRI before contrast, the T1-weighted MRI after intravenous contrast, and the FLAIR after contrast. Note that the enhancement of the subarachnoid space indicative of leptomeningeal involvement of the occipital lobe is seen only on the FLAIR.

tumor. Conventional T1-weighted imaging depicts enhancing lesions as foci of increased signal. For the brain parenchyma, T1-weighting alone is usually sufficient, however, it can be difficult to detect leptomeningeal invasion on conventional T1-weighted scans (Fig. 4). By using FLAIR sequences after contrast administration, it is easier to detect enhancement in the meninges or parenchyma since the CSF is suppressed in this sequence (Fig. 5) (19).

Diffusion Weighted Imaging

DWI is a technique that applies a series of increasingly strong magnetic gradients during acquisition. Water molecules that are restricted in their motion will not wander over these gradients during the acquisition and so will tend to retain signal; whereas tissues with highly diffusing water molecules will quickly lose signal with the

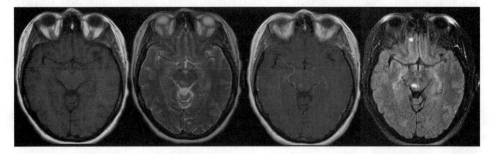

Figure 5 Advantage of FLAIR for detecting parenchymal lesions. Occasionally, FLAIR can depict parenchymal lesions better than other methods, although this is unusual. Left to right: T1-weighted MRI without contrast, T2-weighted MRI, T1-weighted MRI after intravenous contrast, and FLAIR after contrast. Note that two subtle lesions, one in the midbrain and one in the frontal lobe, are best seen on the FLAIR sequence.

application of progressively stronger gradients as the signal is dissipated by the gradients (22). The loss of signal as a function of diffusion gradient strength can be quantified by the apparent diffusion coefficient (ADC) which becomes a convenient measure of diffusion.

DWI has primarily been employed in evaluating early brain infarcts where the lower temperature within ischemic strokes decreases water diffusion, and therefore results in higher signal even before changes in tissue T1 and T2 can be detected (23–25). Therefore, DWI is used as a method of confirming the presence of a suspected brain infarct in its early hours. Its role in cancer imaging is more controversial. It is thought that intact tumors with their dense cellularity and intact cellular membranes have restricted diffusion due to these structural barriers. However, after treatment, as cell membranes become more disrupted and permeable, water is less restricted and is able to diffuse further, a process detectable as signal loss on DWI. This property of DWI makes it attractive as a method of demonstrating early responses to therapy (26). For instance, lymphoma with its tightly packed cells usually has restricted diffusion and is relatively bright on DWI compared to the detection of other tumors. Following treatment, however, the signal within lymphoma will drop on DWI indicating cellular membrane breakdown. Additionally, when attempting to differentiate between an abscess and a glioblastoma, DWI is often used because the water molecules within infected pocket of an abscess exhibit restricted diffusion (cellularity, mucus, proteinaceous debris, cytokines), and thus abscesses tend to be much higher in signal than do glioblastomas (27,28). However, ADC maps generated using the images obtained with different gradient field strengths can clarify the nature of the lesion (Fig. 6).

Dynamic Contrast Enhanced-MRI

DCE-MRI generally refers to a rapidly acquired T1-weighted volume acquisition before, during, and after the administration of a gadolinium chelate. This is distinct from the $T2^*$-weighted dynamic sequences described previously. These sequences require a rapid injection of contrast and ultrafast imaging, and are complete within a minute of injection after the first pass. T1-weighted, dynamic contrast-enhanced images are 3D volume acquisitions obtained every 2 to 10 seconds for a period of minutes and the kinetics reflect perfusion and permeability as well as vascular volume. The kinetics of the time–signal curve can be fit to a pharmacokinetic model from which parameters can be derived which relate to vessel permeability and relative vascular volume (Fig. 7). The theory of these models is covered in another chapter in this book. Since most MRI studies performed in oncology utilize gadolinium chelates, this functional test adds little total time to the imaging (29).

Applications of DCE-MRI include attempting to distinguish radiation necrosis from recurrent disease. Tumors tend to have rapid enhancement and relatively rapid washout while necrosis enhances less intensely and more slowly, and therefore washes out more slowly. DCE-MRI has also been used to monitor therapies, particularly those directed against angiogenesis, because changes on DCE-MRI directly relate to changes in vascular permeability (30).

MR Spectroscopic Imaging

Brain tissue is complex and is composed of many metabolites, some of which have unique magnetic resonance frequencies. However, most conventional MRI scans

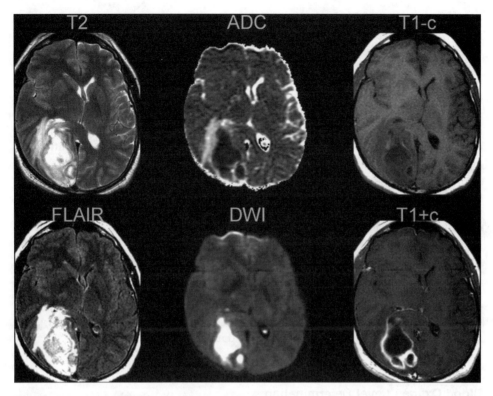

Figure 6 Value of DWI and ADC maps. Left to right and top to bottom: T2, ADC, T1 without contrast, FLAIR, DWI, and T1 after intravenous contrast. Note that there is a ring-enhancing lesion in the right occipital lobe. The central portion is high in signal on DWI likely due to "T2 shine through," since the T2-weighted scan show similar high signal. This alone could not differentiate a tumor from an abscess. The ADC map, however, demonstrates low signal indicating low diffusion in the center; higher in the periphery, indicative of pus-containing abscess.

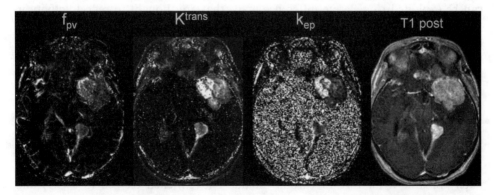

Figure 7 Value of DCE-MRI for brain tumors. Left to right: f_{pv} map, K^{trans} map, and k_{ep} map as well as the standard T1-weighted contrast enhanced image. The f_{pv} and K^{trans} maps indicate that this is a highly vascular tumor with high vascular permeability. The histologic diagnosis was meningioma. (*See color insert.*)

depend only on water and fat peaks to generate sufficient signal to generate an image. By selectively measuring the peaks of other metabolites relative to water, a spectrum can be generated that contains important clinical information. Two metabolites of particular importance in the brain are N-acetyl acetate (NAA) and choline (Ch) (31). NAA is a structural component of intact neural tissue. Choline is a membrane component of cells. In tumors, NAA would be expected to decrease in concentration whereas choline would be expected to increase in concentration. Thus, the ratio of NAA/Ch decreases in tumors compared to normal brain tissue, and this ratio appears to have prognostic information. Tumors with low NAA/Ch ratio have poorer prognoses.

MR spectroscopic imaging (MRSI) can be used to detect tumors which are otherwise not visible. Many brain tumors particularly in the brainstem will not disturb the blood brain barrier and will not be detectable by T1-weighted, T2-weighted, or enhanced T1-weighted images (32). MRSI can be used to target biopsies and detect the true borders of tumors beyond the enhancing rim. It is also useful in distinguishing radiation necrosis and tumor recurrence (33,34). It has been used to direct radiation therapy of brain tumors.

Recently, 3D multivoxel acquisitions have become possible so that spectra localized to specific brain regions can be obtained in a relatively time efficient manner. Color-encoded images reflecting precalculated metabolite ratios such as NAA/Ch simplify the interpretation of these complex data sets.

Blood Oxygen Level Determination

Functional MRI (fMRI) refers to MRI of the brain performed while the subject is performing a specific task. For instance, a patient may be asked to repeatedly touch their thumb and forefinger together while being scanned, and this action causes a small change in blood flow to a specific motor center in the brain. The change in blood flow induced by this action causes a change in the ratio of deoxyhemoglobin to oxyhemoglobin. Deoxyhemoglobin is paramagnetic and relaxes relatively faster on $T2^*$-weighted images than does oxyhemoglobin. This small change in signal can be detected and is known as "blood oxygen level determination" scans as it depends on the deoxy/oxy hemoglobin ratio. The differential in $T2^*$ relaxation can be exploited to generate difference maps that are thought to reflect activity in the brain. It is important to note that this technique does not necessarily measure tissue oxygenation, i.e., the partial pressure of oxygen within tissue. Rather, it reflects the available oxygen carrying capacity within the hemoglobin of red blood cells within tissue; therefore, it does not necessarily reflect tissue hypoxia.

BOLD imaging has been used to map motor, language, and sensory regions of the brain prior to neurosurgery in an effort to spare vital functions. It can be performed prior to surgery for removal of a tumor to modify the surgical approach, if the tumor is close to an important functional center.

Instead of functionally challenging the brain, an extrinsic contrast agent can be given to augment hemoglobin saturation with oxygen. Making the patient to alternately breathe a mixture of carbon dioxide and enriched oxygen (5% CO_2 and 95% O_2), a mixture called carbogen, and room air can depict regions of hypoxia within tumors. Presumably, oxygen-deprived regions of a tumor will demonstrate larger changes in signal than do regions that are already satisfactorily served by an oxygenated blood supply. Thus, this technique may reflect tissue hypoxia.

Magnetization Transfer

MRI depends on a resonance phenomenon in which tissue at a specific magnetic field will resonate at a specific radiofrequency. However, some tissue resonates at slightly different frequency due to local influences on the magnetic field. This is known as "magnetization transfer (MT)." Off resonance, pulses will stimulate water protons in restricted spaces such as within cells, and these "bound" protons will then exchange with "free" water protons. If there is an exchange, it will serve to lower the signal from the target. This technique is especially useful in suppressing background tissue, and thus increases the conspicuity of white matter lesions. By suppressing background, there is also increased sensitivity to small enhancing lesions, however, because vessels are also high in signal on MT studies, it may be difficult to interpret such studies (35).

IMAGE MANAGEMENT

The increasingly sophisticated imaging capabilities of MRI necessitate the development of equally advanced image processing tools. Many of the techniques described above generate huge amounts of data. To be useful, these images must be synthesized into formats that are accessible to clinicians.

Image management in MRI can be viewed as a series of events. After image acquisition, the images are sent to electronic workstations. Here they are stored in digital imaging and communications in medicine (DICOM) format, and then are processed using one or more different software tools. Since this is an increasingly time-consuming process, often a radiology department will form an image processing team comprising one or more individuals. Once the images are processed, they are sent back to the picture archiving and communications system (PACS) for storage and distribution. Current studies may generate between 1000 and 5000 images, and thus tax the storage capabilities of many conventional PACS systems. Fortunately, new hardware is beginning to address this critical issue.

CHALLENGES IN NEURORADIOLOGY

While routine imaging of the brain for metastatic disease or for primary brain tumors is highly developed and considered generally to be quite successful, there remain a number of challenges. One of the most vexing issues is that concerning the nonenhancing brain lesion. As mentioned, these may require the acquisition of an MR spectroscopy in order to detect the lesion. However, such lesions raise perplexing problems. For instance, to what extent can one rely on imaging findings to dictate therapy, if the actual lesion can be detected only by a ratio of metabolites?

Among lesions that are easily seen on MRI, there remain a number of significant challenges. For instance, having detected a small lesion how long should it be watched and when should surgery be performed? This topic is the subject of intense research and it is hoped answers will emerge in the near future.

Therapy is influenced by tumor grade. Perfusion MR, DCE-MRI, and MR spectroscopy can be used to estimate grade based on a constellation of findings. MR results can be added to PET results to further refine the estimate of tumor grade. The coordination of this data and the synthesis of it into a coherent and reproducible algorithm are the subject of current research. Ultimately, bioinformatics, the management of quantitative biologic information combined with available clinical data may prove useful in helping to determine the nature of a lesion.

Even with the numerous techniques available, radiation necrosis is still difficult to differentiate from progressive disease. Perfusion scans, MR spectroscopy, and DCE-MRI have been used in this setting, although none of these techniques is fully satisfactory. Again, multiparametric imaging may provide better answers in the future.

CONCLUSIONS

MRI of the brain is a vital part of modern oncology. In addition to very accurate T1-weighted, T2-weighted, and gadolinium-enhanced T1-weighted MRI, a number of other techniques including FLAIR, BOLD, DCE MRI, T2* perfusion imaging, MRSI, and DWI add diagnostic value. The increasing complexity of interpreting and teaching neuroradiology has led to increased specialization and the development of customized software tools. Hardware and image processing advances have combined to improve the diagnostic capabilities of brain MRI. Future developments include the discovery of molecular imaging probes with specificity for brain tumors, the ability to image tumors with intact blood brain barriers, and the development of early biomarkers of therapeutic success or failure that will aid in the treatment monitoring of patients undergoing therapy.

REFERENCES

1. Frayne R, Goodyear BG, Dickhoff P, Lauzon ML, Sevick RJ. Magnetic resonance imaging at 3.0 Tesla: challenges and advantages in clinical neurological imaging. Invest Radiol 2003; 38:385–402.
2. Di Salle F, Esposito F, Elefante A, et al. High field functional MRI. Eur J Radiol 2003; 48:138–145.
3. Yacoub E, Duong TQ, Van de Moortele PF, et al. Spin-echo fMRI in humans using high spatial resolutions and high magnetic fields. Magn Reson Med 2003; 49:655–664.
4. Nobauer-Huhmann IM, Ba-Ssalamah A, Mlynarik V, et al. Magnetic resonance imaging contrast enhancement of brain tumors at 3 tesla versus 1.5 tesla. Invest Radiol 2002; 37:114–119.
5. Di Costanzo A, Trojsi F, Tosetti M, et al. High-field proton MRS of human brain. Eur J Radiol 2003; 48:146–153.
6. McGirt MJ, Villavicencio AT, Bulsara KR, Friedman AH. MRI-guided stereotactic biopsy in the diagnosis of glioma: comparison of biopsy and surgical resection specimen. Surg Neurol 2003; 59:277–281.
7. Nabavi A, Gering DT, Kacher DF, et al. Surgical navigation in the open MRI. Acta Neurochir Suppl 2003; 85:121–125.
8. Nimsky C, Ganslandt O, Gralla J, Buchfelder M, Fahlbusch R. Intraoperative low-field magnetic resonance imaging in pediatric neurosurgery. Pediatr Neurosurg 2003; 38: 83–89.
9. de Zwart JA, Ledden PJ, van Gelderen P, Bodurka J, Chu R, Duyn JH. Signal-to-noise ratio and parallel imaging performance of a 16-channel receive-only brain coil array at 3.0 Tesla. Magn Reson Med 2004; 51:22–26.
10. Pruessmann KP, Weiger M, Scheidegger MB, Boesiger P. SENSE: sensitivity encoding for fast MRI. Magn Reson Med 1999; 42:952–962.
11. European Federation of Neurological Societies Task Force. The future of magnetic resonance-based techniques in neurology. Eur J Neurol 2001; 8:17–25.

12. Patel MR, Klufas RA. Gradient- and spin-echo MR imaging of the brain. Am J Neuro-radiol 1999; 20:1381–1383.

13. Umek W, Ba-Ssalamah A, Prokesch R, Mallek R, Heimberger K, Hittmair K. Imaging of the brain using the fast-spin-echo and gradient-spin-echo techniques. Eur Radiol 1998; 8:409–415.

14. Hittmair K, Umek W, Schindler EG, Ba-Ssalamah A, Pretterklieber ML, Herold CJ. Fast flair imaging of the brain using the fast spin-echo and gradient spin-echo technique. Magn Reson Imaging 1997; 15:405–414.

15. Moseley ME, Wendland MF, Kucharczyk J. Magnetic resonance imaging of diffusion and perfusion. Top Magn Reson Imaging 1991; 3:50–67.

16. Kucharczyk J, Vexler ZS, Roberts TP, et al. Echo-planar perfusion-sensitive MR imaging of acute cerebral ischemia. Radiology 1993; 188:711–717.

17. de Crespigny AJ, Tsuura M, Moseley ME, Kucharczyk J. Perfusion and diffusion MR imaging of thromboembolic stroke. J Magn Reson Imaging 1993; 3:746–754.

18. Lee SJ, Kim JH, Kim YM, et al. Perfusion MR imaging in gliomas: comparison with his-tologic tumor grade. Korean J Radiol 2001; 2:1–7.

19. Herlihy AH, Hajnal JV, Curati WL, et al. Reduction of CSF and blood flow artifacts on FLAIR images of the brain with k-space reordered by inversion time at each slice posi-tion (KRISP). Am J Neuroradiol 2001; 22:896–904.

20. Castillo M, Mukherji SK. Clinical applications of FLAIR, HASTE, and magnetization transfer in neuroimaging. Semin Ultrasound CT MR 2000; 21:417–427.

21. Rumboldt Z, Marotti M. Magnetization transfer, HASTE, and FLAIR imaging. Magn Reson Imaging Clin N Am 2003; 11:471–492.

22. Bammer R. Basic principles of diffusion-weighted imaging. Eur J Radiol 2003; 45:169–184.

23. Li TQ, Chen ZG, Hindmarsh T. Diffusion-weighted MR imaging of acute cerebral ische-mia. Acta Radiol 1998; 39:460–473.

24. Schaefer PW, Grant PE, Gonzalez RG. Diffusion-weighted MR imaging of the brain. Radiology 2000; 217:331–345.

25. Roberts TP, Rowley HA. Diffusion weighted magnetic resonance imaging in stroke. Eur J Radiol 2003; 45:185–194.

26. van Rijswijk CS, Kunz P, Hogendoorn PC, Taminiau AH, Doornbos J, Bloem JL. Diffusion-weighted MRI in the characterization of soft-tissue tumors. J Magn Reson Imaging 2002; 15:302–307.

27. Nadal Desbarats L, Herlidou S, de Marco G et al. Differential MRI diagnosis between brain abscesses and necrotic or cystic brain tumors using the apparent diffusion coeffi-cient and normalized diffusion-weighted images. Magn Reson Imaging 2003; 21:645–650.

28. Dorenbeck U, Butz B, Schlaier J, Bretschneider T, Schuierer G, Feuerbach S. Diffusion-weighted echo-planar MRI of the brain with calculated ADCs: a useful tool in the differ-ential diagnosis of tumor necrosis from abscess? J Neuroimaging 2003; 13:330–338.

29. Taylor JS, Reddick WE. Evolution from empirical dynamic contrast-enhanced magnetic resonance imaging to pharmacokinetic MRI. Adv Drug Deliv Rev 2000; 41:91–110.

30. Yang S, Law M, Zagzag D, et al. Dynamic contrast-enhanced perfusion MR imaging measurements of endothelial permeability: differentiation between atypical and typical meningiomas. Am J Neuroradiol 2003; 24:1554–1559.

31. Smith JK, Castillo M, Kwock L. MR spectroscopy of brain tumors. Magn Reson Ima-ging Clin N Am 2003; 11:415–429, v–vi.

32. Smith JK, Londono A, Castillo M, Kwock L. Proton magnetic resonance spectroscopy of brain-stem lesions. Neuroradiology 2002; 44:825–829.

33. Nelson SJ. Multivoxel magnetic resonance spectroscopy of brain tumors. Mol Cancer Ther 2003; 2:497–507.

34. Rand SD, Prost R, Li SJ. Proton MR spectroscopy of the brain. Neuroimaging Clin N Am 1999; 9:379–395.

35. Mathews VP, Caldemeyer KS, Ulmer JL, Nguyen H, Yuh WT. Effects of contrast dose, delayed imaging, and magnetization transfer saturation on gadolinium-enhanced MR imaging of brain lesions. J Magn Reson Imaging 1997; 7:14–22.

3
Advances in Ultrasound

David Cosgrove, Chris Harvey, Martin Blomley, and Rob Eckersley
Imaging Sciences Department, Imperial College, Hammersmith Hospital, London, U.K.

A Note from the Editors

*U*ltrasound remains the key imaging modality for the routine assessment of patients with cancers. The last few years have seen notable developments on the ease of use of these machines, but have also heralded the introduction of new techniques that will expand the roles played by ultrasound. These arise from developments in contrast media that are based on gas filled microbubbles (now available in Europe and Japan), the development of elasticity imaging, and the use of ultrasound for therapy. The latter includes the use of ultrasound as a means of inducting heat-mediated tissue coagulation and as a way to target the tumor circulation.

INTRODUCTION

Ultrasound (US) has undergone impressive technical developments since the earliest static scanners with the progressive introduction of gray scale (1970), real time (1975), multi-element arrays (1975), pulsed Doppler (1970), color Doppler (1985), and the conversion to digital systems (1985); all of which have extended its reliability and ease of use so that now almost 25% of all clinical imaging studies worldwide are US examinations (1). The last five years have seen an emphasis on ease of use, with control panel ergonomics greatly improved and the development of systems to improve imaging such as automatic time gain compensation (TGC) and Doppler settings, which not only speed examinations but also improve reproducibility. Radical innovations of particular importance in oncology are the development of safe and effective contrast agents for US in the form of microbubbles, the development of elasticity imaging (elastography), and the use of US in therapy, both as a means of heat-coagulating tissue (high intensity focused ultrasound, HIFU) and as a way to improve drug delivery, either on its own or in combination with microbubbles.

IMAGING AND DOPPLER

Both gray scale and Doppler imaging have been greatly improved by the combination of new transducer technologies and digital signal processing.

Transducers

Transducers remain crucial to obtaining high quality images and Doppler, and have been the focus of extensive development. The piezoelectric material used is paramount in the performance of the transducer. Lead zirconate titanate (PZT) has been used for decades but it has a much higher acoustic impedance than that of tissue. This impedance mismatch results in strong reflections at the skin–probe interface; these decrease sensitivity and increase the ring down time of the transducer, which lengthens the transmitted pulses thus reducing spatial resolution. Multiple reflections between the surfaces of the transducer can also be transmitted into the tissue to produce reverberation artifacts. One solution is to combine PZT with a material of low acoustic impedance, such as epoxy resin, to form a composite transducer. Channels are cut into the PZT and filled with resin, thus reducing the acoustic impedance mismatch with tissue and simultaneously preventing waves traveling along the PZT, which otherwise confuse the clean shape of the transmitted beam. New piezoelectric materials, such as ferroelectric relaxors, are currently under evaluation (2). They are much more efficient in their conversion of electrical to sound energy, with acoustic impedance better matched to tissue than PZT.

US transducers have a limited range of frequencies over which they are effective, their "bandwidth." A large bandwidth improves the axial spatial resolution, and offers the possibility of using two or more frequencies in a single probe with cost and ergonomic savings. It is also essential for harmonic imaging. Bandwidth has been increased by applying multiple matching layers to the front of the transducer; these optimize electromechanical coupling so that the transduction of electrical energy to sound energy (and vice versa) is more efficient. Analogous matching layers on camera lenses lend them iridescent blue or yellow tints.

Transducer technology has also addressed the problem of lack of control of the beam's shape in the Z axis (orthogonal plane). Conventionally, the slice thickness is reduced by fixed focusing using a lens or by curving the transducer. However, if the transducer material is sliced across as well as along the block and appropriate electrodes applied, the inner elements across the array can be fired with a slight delay relative to the outer ones and the beam is electronically focused in the Z plane exactly as is normally performed in the X plane. This adds flexibility to the orthogonal focus so that the beam thickness can be controlled for different depths. These so-called "matrix arrays" are now becoming widely available despite the manufacturing challenge they pose and the added cabling and electronic complexity.

An elegant way of achieving a similar effect without these overheads is the plano-concave transducer known as the Hanafy lens, after its inventor. The front of the transducer is made concave so that its edges are thicker than the central strip. Thus, the edges respond to lower frequencies and the center to higher; since lower frequencies penetrate to greater depths, the focus in the Z plane is progressively and automatically optimized.

Signal Processing

Harnessing the power of fast digital computers to US has resulted in a number of important improvements in imaging and in convenience and reproducibility (3).

Harmonics

The discovery that sound propagates through the tissue in a nonlinear fashion to produce overtones of the transmitted signal (harmonics) has improved contrast resolution and reduced artifacts that result from beam imperfections (4). The principle is simple: tissue is slightly compressed during the positive pressure phase of the ultrasonic wave (and vice versa); sound travels faster in a denser medium and so the compression part of the cycle travels faster so that the wave looses its original symmetry. Such an asymmetric wave contains harmonics, which can be selected from the returning echoes either by applying a frequency filter or by comparing the echoes from a pair of pulses transmitted with opposite phase; the linear signals cancel, leaving the harmonics for image formation. Because these tissue harmonics are more strongly elicited by higher power US, artifacts caused by the side lobes and reverberations are relatively reduced, resulting in a cleaner, less noisy image (Fig. 1). In effect, the imaging beam is generated from within the tissue itself.

Compounding

Compounding is a technique in which two or more images acquired simultaneously from the same tissue are superimposed; this reduces the speckle content, which has a random distribution and gives a smoother, more anatomically correct image (Fig. 2) (5). An obvious way is to collect two images from different angles, a method that was widely used with the original articulated arm static scanners. Using the electronic beam steering of an array transducer, overlapping scans (varying from three to nine frames) from different angles can be acquired in real time with only a modest loss of frame rate. Alternatively, the same effect can be achieved by collecting data at different frequencies and the two methods can be combined. The scans are then averaged to produce real-time compound images.

(A)

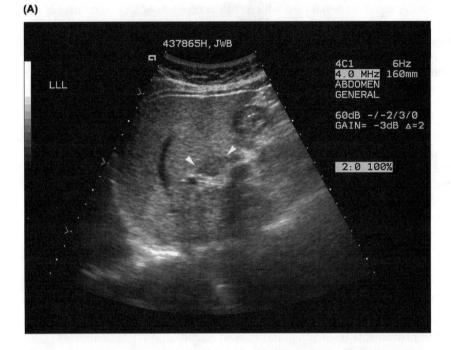

(B)

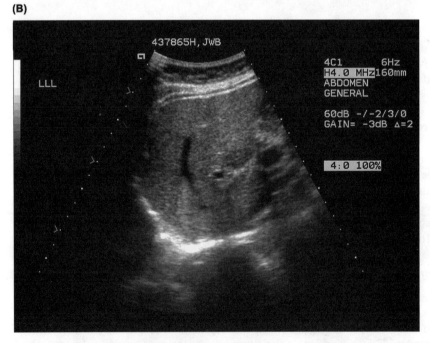

Figure 1 Tissue harmonics. The echo-poor region in segment 4 (*arrowheads* in **A**) has the appearances of focal fatty sparing but its outlines are more clearly seen when imaged with tissue harmonics (**B**) using the same settings. Tissue harmonics improves contrast by reducing side lobe and reverberation artifacts. The patient was being staged for breast cancer; the typical benign appearances made further investigation unnecessary.

(A)

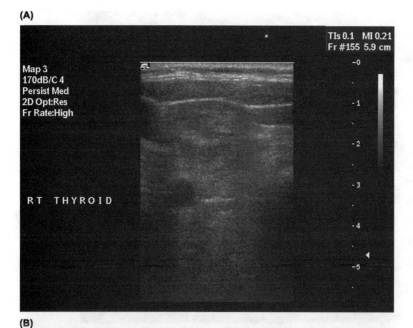

(B)

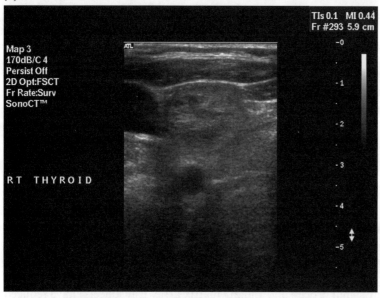

Figure 2 Compound scan. Compared with the conventional image of this thyroid cancer (**A**), the compounded image (**B**) shows more detail because the information from beams at three different angles has been combined, and also there is more contrast because the speckle noise has been reduced.

Display

Extended Field of View (EFOV)

When US was introduced into clinical practice in the 1970s, the transducer was mounted on an articulated arm and swept to produce extended field of view images but this was sacrificed when real-time US was developed. Advances in computing

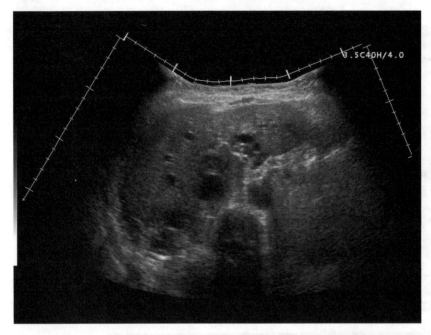

Figure 3 Extended field-of-view. In this patient with extensive polycystic liver disease, the liver was too large to fit on a single scan. However, using the extended field of view technique (Sciescape, Siemens, Germany) the entire liver could be measured.

that track the speckle pattern of the images as the transducer is swept across extended anatomical regions now allow high-resolution EFOV images to be created in gray-scale or color Doppler (Fig. 3). Large lesions can be included in a single image and also provides a better display of their anatomical relationships. It is an excellent teaching aid; it allows measurements of large structures to be performed and serves as a useful record for follow-up.

3D Imaging

Until comparatively recently US has lagged behind both CT and MR in three-dimensional (3D) imaging. The 3D US is based on reconstruction algorithms and is therefore dependent on high quality 2D data, which has been limited by speckle, side lobes, clutter, and other artifacts. Recent improvements in imaging (harmonic imaging, nonlinear signal processing, and 2D matrix array transducers) have reduced these problems and paved the way for useful 3D imaging, while fast computing has allowed the production of real-time 3D scans (so-called 4D US imaging) (Voluson® 730, GE-Kretz). A position sensor attached to the transducer or an arrangement whereby the transducer is swept across the volume by a motor provides the necessary positional data. Volumes can be displayed as either series of multiplanar reformats or rendered 3D images, which improve appreciation of the relative position of structures, including flowing blood. Currently, the main clinical application is in obstetrics but the approach shows promise in breast and prostate cancer, and reveals the complexity of tumor vascularity in an elegant way (Fig. 4) (6). In interventional procedures, 4D US is promising for needle biopsy guidance while 3D US is used to guide radioactive seed implants in the prostate and for breast

(A)

(B)

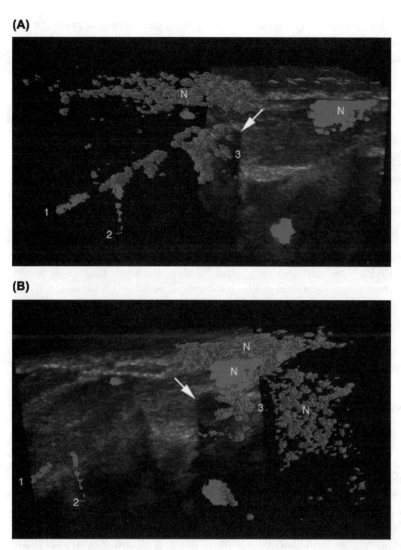

Figure 4 Three-dimensional scan with Doppler. In this three-dimensional reconstruction of a breast mass (*arrows*), the image has been duplicated and opposite halves of the gray scale portion removed from the opposing sides to reveal the arrangement of the blood vessels using power Doppler (shown in red). Corresponding portions of the vasculature are numbered. This form of display allows the vessels to be seen in their relationship to the mass. *Source*: Photos courtesy of Drs. W.E. Svensson, S. Kyriazi, and K. Humphries. (*See color insert.*)

biopsy and a stereotactic system has been developed for needle delivery using electromagnetic position sensors (7).

Coded Excitation

One of the limits to the sensitivity of US imaging is the amount of acoustic energy that can be deposited in the tissues. Rather than increasing the transmit power, one way to get around this limitation is to use longer pulses. Generally, longer pulses mean poorer spatial resolution along the beam but this can be overcome if the acoustic pulses are digitally encoded: the received signals are then processed to recover the spatial information. Examples of coding strategies include varying the frequency (e.g., as a chirp of rising frequency) or amplitude (complex shapes that are similar to those used in mobile phone technology to allow a band to carry multiple signals and retain their integrity). Using this approach the sensitivity of the US scanner to weaker echoes can be improved. Therefore, higher frequencies can be used and still separate it from noise to give better spatial resolution down to greater depths.

Automatic Optimization Systems

Automatic Gain Compensation Modes set the correct gain in 2D at any point across the image with a single switch. This is achieved by the processor analyzing the distribution of gray levels in each part of the image and adjusting the level of each pixel to optimize local contrast. This not only improves image quality rapidly but also offers better consistency between operators, thus reducing operator dependence. Automatic optimization systems are also available for color and spectral Doppler where they unwrap aliasing by shifting the baseline and optimizing the pulse repetition frequency (PRF). They can also automatically place the angle correction cursor by "looking at" the walls of the vessel in which the sample volume has been placed and noting their position. Dhotopic Ultrasound Imaging (Elegra; Siemens, Germany) is a real-time post processing technology, which takes advantage of the eye's perception of light to optimize gray-scale tissue differentiation. X-res (Philips-ATL, U.S.A.) is a postprocessing system that seeks to display the image brightness in an optimal fashion; it derives from MRI display processing and reduces speckles.

Contrast Agents

US, unlike all other imaging modalities, has lacked effective contrast agents until comparatively recently. This was rectified with the introduction of microbubbles in the 1990s; they have revolutionized clinical and research applications in this field and provided the stimulus for the development of harmonic modes to improve conventional imaging as well as microbubble-specific modes that have proved useful for staging and for characterizing tumors among other applications (8,9). They also provide opportunities for unique functional studies (10,11). Their small size and short life in the blood as well as their inert composition has meant that they are very safe with no significant adverse effects; in particular, they are not nephrotoxic and do not cause cardiovascular changes. A large number of agents have been developed and several have been introduced into clinical practice (Table 1).

Principles

The microbubbles used as contrast agents for US are made to be smaller than 7 μm in diameter so that they can cross capillary beds. When administered intravenously, these agents flood the blood pool and (usually) remain within the vascular compartment. They must survive passage through the cardiopulmonary circulation to produce useful systemic enhancement. An ingenious range of methods has been deployed to achieve the required stability and to provide a clinically useful duration of enhancement. Both the gas contain usually air or a perfluoro gas and the stabilizing shell (denatured albumin, phospholipids, surfactants, or cyanoacrylate) are critical in this respect. The first agent for cardiac use, Albunex, had an albumen shell and contained air. The first generally used agent, Levovist, consists of galactose microcrystals whose surfaces provide nidation sites on which air bubbles form when they are

Table 1 Classification of Ultrasound Microbubbles

Microbubble	Gas	Stabilization	Company
Air-based agents			
Agitated saline	Air	None	N/A
Albunex[a]	Air	Sonicated albumin	Tyco
Echovist[b]	Air	None	Schering
Levovist[b] *SHU 508A*	Air	Palmitic acid	Schering
Quantison[a]	Air	Dried albumin	Andaris Ltd.
Perfluoro agents			
BR14	Perfluorobutane	Phospholipids	Bracco
Echogen[a] *QW3600*	Dodecafluoropentane	Emulsion, surfactants	Sonus
Definity *perflutren*	Perfluoropropane	Phospholipids	Bristol-Myers Squibb
Imagent *AFO150*	Perfluorohexane	Surfactants	Schering
Optison	Perfluoropropane	Albumen	Amersham Health
Perfluorocarbon Exposed Sonicated Dextrose Albumin *PESDA*	Perfluorobutane	Sonicated albumin	University of Nebraska
Quanfuxian *QFX*	Perfluoro	Sonicated albumin	Nanfang Hospital, Guangzhou, China
SonoVue *BR1*	Sulfur hexafluoride	Phospholipids	Bracco
Liver trophic agents			
Levovist *SHU 508A*	Air	Palmitic acid	Schering
Sonavist[a] *SHU 563A*	Air	Cyanoacrylate	Schering
Sonazoid[a] *NC100100*	Perfluorocarbon	Not published	Amersham (Nycomed)

[a]No longer under development or marketed.
[b]Licensed for clinical use.

suspended in water; the resulting microbubbles are stabilized by a trace of a surfactant, palmitic acid. An improved version of Albunex, Optison, is filled with perfluoropropane while a family of perfluoro gas containing agents such as SonoVue and Definity use phospholipids as the membrane are becoming important in clinical practice.

Interactions of Microbubbles with US Waves

The interactions of microbubbles with an US beam are complex (12–14). Their gas content makes them much more compressible than soft tissue and so, when exposed to the compression–rarefaction wave of an ultrasonic pulse, they undergo alternate contractions and expansions. Like all oscillating systems, they vibrate most readily at a particular frequency, their resonance frequency. For microbubbles $<10\,\mu m$ in diameter this turns out to correspond to the frequencies actually used in diagnostic US (2–10 MHz). It is this fortunate coincidence that underpins the extraordinary effectiveness of microbubbles as US contrast agents. When the ultrasound beam used is weak (power <0.1 MPa corresponding to a mechanical index (MI) of around 0.01), these oscillations are symmetrical (i.e., their behavior is "linear") and the frequency of the returned signal is unaltered. However, as the acoustic power is increased (MI, 0.1–1.0), the expansion and contraction phases become unequal because the microbubbles resist compression more strongly than expansion. This "nonlinear" behavior means that the signals they return contain multiples of the insonating frequency. These higher frequency components are known as harmonics as the phenomenon is identical to the overtones produced by a musical instrument. (It is to be noted that microbubble harmonics are produced when the ultrasound is reflected by the microbubbles, not during ultrasound propagation, as is the case with tissue harmonics.) At still higher powers (though within accepted limits for diagnostic imaging), highly nonlinear behavior occurs and the microbubbles are disrupted and disappear from the sound field.

Harmonics may be used to image US contrast agents by tuning the receiver to listen to a band of frequencies centered on a harmonic signal (usually the second harmonic at double the fundamental frequency) so that the harmonics can be separated from the fundamental signals from tissue. However, as noted above, tissues also produce harmonics, especially when higher acoustic powers are used and distinguishing between them is challenging. In practice, in many of the simple contrast modes available, the two are inextricably mixed together.

The goal of separating them completely can be achieved in two ways. In the first approach to be discovered, a high MI beam is used and the microbubbles are deliberately disrupted (15). When using a color Doppler mode, the sudden disappearance of a signal from its previous location (loss of correlation between sequential echoes) is seen as a major Doppler shift and registered as color signals, rather like aliasing. This method works well for the more fragile air-based agents such as Levovist and modified color Doppler software has been developed to optimize the display. This approach, often known a Stimulated Acoustic Emission (SAE), is particularly successful in the late phase of contrast agents that show liver/spleen tropism, which develops a few minutes after injection. Because it highlights the normal liver and spleen, lesions that do not contain functioning tissue, such as malignancies, appear as obvious voids in the color map. This method has the advantage of high sensitivity (it can probably detect a single microbubble being disrupted) and of showing the microbubble signature exclusively in the color layer of the registered image with the conventional gray scale image as an under layer for reference purposes. However, it does destroy the contrast agent rapidly, and this precludes the use of real time, so a sweep-and-review approach has to be adopted.

The alternative approach, and increasingly the mode of choice for contrast studies, relies on the fact that with newer microbubbles (particularly those with phospholipid shells), harmonics can be elicited at much lower acoustic powers than are necessary to generate tissue harmonics (16). Thus, if a very low acoustic power can be used without the image being lost in noise, the microbubble signals (harmonics) can be separated from the tissue signal (fundamental). An important step in the progress to this ideal was the development of phase inversion techniques, which evolved from the need to detect microbubble harmonics but to avoid frequency filtering because the narrow bandwidth that this method requires degrades spatial resolution. In the phase inversion mode (PIM), a pair of pulses is sent sequentially along each scan line, the second being inverted in phase from the first. The returning echoes from the pair are summed so that the linear echoes cancel because they are out of phase, leaving only non linear components, which are used for image formation. Because the transmitted pulses are the same as those used for conventional imaging (except for the phase inversion), spatial resolution is not impaired—in fact, this method is sometimes termed "wideband harmonics." PIM gives excellent quality images in both vascular and late phases and, like the high

MI approach, detects the presence of microbubble without relying on their motion. Thus, both these modes can detect contrast in the microcirculation (though, of course, vessels smaller than the resolution limit of ultrasound—some 200 μm at best—cannot be resolved as discrete structures).

As initially implemented, PIM deployed a relatively high MI and therefore tissue harmonics contaminated the microbubble signal. Special approaches are required to operate PIM at the very low powers needed to avoid tissue harmonics without too much noise in the images. One solution is to send a stream of alternating phase pulses and use color Doppler circuitry to pick out the harmonics; essentially this method (known as Power Pulse Inversion, PPI) exploits the high sensitivity of Doppler to overcome the signal-to-noise limitation. Because the Doppler circuitry is used for the microbubble signature, PPI achieves the twin goals of complete separation of the contrast from the tissue information and of displaying each in a separate image layer (PPI in color, B-mode in gray), which can be viewed separately or as a mix. Another approach to solve the problem also uses a series of pulses, though usually only around three per line. Here, as well as inverting the phase, the amplitude of the pulses is also changed. This method preserves more of the nonlinear content of the received signals and, importantly nonlinear signals at the fundamental frequency, which are discarded in PIM, can be detected. Since these fall within the most sensitive band of the transducers, this can improve the sensitivity of this mode. Implemented as Contrast Pulse Sequences (CPS, Siemens), the harmonics are displayed in a color tint over the B-mode picture and, as with PPI, either one or both can be viewed as required.

In another approach, the direction of flow of the microbubbles (and therefore of blood) in larger vessels is detected with low MI velocity Doppler, while slow moving and stationary microbubbles are shown in green using power Doppler. This combined mode, known as vascular recognition imaging (VRI, Toshiba), also allows the microbubble signature to be displayed separately from or combined with the B-mode and has the advantage of providing additional information on the flow direction in larger vessels.

If the sequence of images obtained using a low MI mode is cumulated over a period of a minute or so after the injection, the tracks of individual microbubbles form lines representing the arrangement of the microvasculature (Fig. 5). This method, microvascular imaging (MVI, Philips) has been applied in the breast where it reveals the neovascularity of malignancies better than unenhanced Doppler. All of these modes operate at very low powers (MI < 0.2 and sometimes as low as 0.02) and as well as not eliciting tissue harmonics, this has the major advantage that bubble destruction is minimized. In practical terms, using a very low MI means that working in real time is possible and this makes contrast studies much easier to perform since no special scanning techniques are required.

Applications in Oncology

The earliest oncological applications of microbubbles used conventional Doppler ultrasound in which the signal enhancement merely served to boost the Doppler signal intensity so that slower flow in smaller vessels could be detected. The limitations of Doppler remained, particularly the fact that bulk tissue movement is faster than blood flow in the microcirculation, precluding its detection. Thus, conventional Doppler with or without microbubble enhancement can only detect vessels down to arteriolar level. Nevertheless, studies in cancer of the breast, liver, and prostate showed that the neovascularization of malignancies was better detected after enhancement and that

(A)

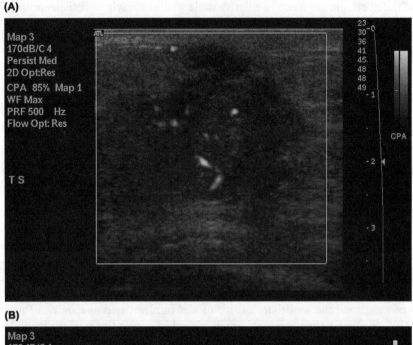

(B)

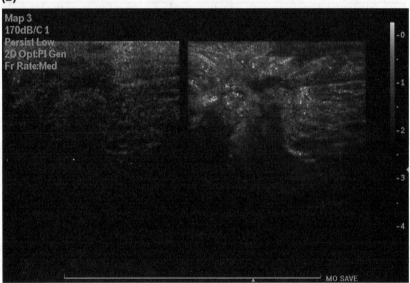

Figure 5 Microvascular imaging. In this mode, a low MI time sequence is cumulated over a period of time (in this example, 60 seconds) to display the motion tracks of microbubbles (Optison was used here) as they flow through the small vessels (**B**). The improved display of the neovasculature in this breast carcinoma compared with power Doppler (**A**) is striking. *Source*: MVI software, Philips Medical. (*See color insert for Fig. 5A.*)

this could improve both detection and differentiation of these tumors. Some of these early claims have not proved to be repeatable, perhaps because most of the early reports included only small numbers of patients. One application that seems to have stood the test of time is the value of enhanced Doppler in differentiating scar tissue from tumor recurrence (17). This is especially important in the breast where this important distinction may be very difficult to make clinically or with imaging methods. The demonstration that a suspicious mass is vascularized suggests that it is malignant and a biopsy should be performed, directed to the vascular portion of the lesion.

An analogous situation is the monitoring of residual tumor during interstitial ablation therapy (18). The liver is the very common target organ: ultrasound is generally used to guide placement of the probe (for RF, laser, or cryotherapy) and ablation is continued until no Doppler signals remain. Then enhancement with microbubbles may reveal persistent hypervascular regions that can be ablated immediately in the same session and the sensitivity of this approach is similar to that of enhanced CT (Fig. 6). Microbubbles allows the ablation session to be continued to completion without moving the patient to the CT scanner. This approach is particularly successful for hepatocellular carcinomas because they are usually hypervascular but is also effective for colo-rectal metastases.

For the most part however, simple Doppler techniques have been replaced by the nonlinear methods described above, and the assessment of the characterization of liver masses has proved to be a particularly useful application. Using SAE in the liver-specific phase, malignant tumors appear as defects surrounded by a colored mosaic pattern when the liver is scanned some five minutes after IV injection of a liver trophic agent such as Levovist. SAE has been shown to improve the conspicuity of liver metastases as well as to demonstrate new lesions not seen on conventional B-mode (19). It reveals subtle or isoechoic metastases and increases the sensitivity of ultrasound to the detection of metastatic disease. In a study of the specificity of SAE, a spectrum of benign and malignant focal liver lesions were assessed for SAE activity in the late phase after injection of Levovist. Metastases and hepatocellular carcinoma (HCC) showed no or low SAE signals while hemangiomas and focal nodular hyperplasia (FNH) had significantly higher scores.

In a multicenter prospective study using one of the tuned SAE modes (Agent Detection Imaging, ADI, Siemens), data from 142 patients was analyzed by blinded review (20). The reviewer's ability to distinguish benign from malignant masses improved significantly from about 80% on conventional scanning (using B-mode plus color Doppler) to around 90% with ADI. The contrast between the lesion and the surrounding liver was markedly higher for malignancies, which stood out as color defects, than for benign lesions (cysts excluded) (Fig. 7). All FNHs showed strong uptake, as did regions of irregular fatty deposition. Haemangiomas were variable: most showed at least moderate uptake but there were exceptions. On the other hand, while all cholangiocarcinomas and almost all metastases showed color negative regions (one each of melanoma, neuroendocrine and testicular tumor metastases showed some signals), a few HCCs did show moderate uptake and thus could not be distinguished from regenerating nodules which did show uptake. Surprisingly, the "hot" HCCs were not exclusively those that were well differentiated on histology, though the sampling error problem of percutaneous biopsies needs to be borne in mind in interpreting this finding.

Phase inversion mode scanning at high MI with Levovist increases the sensitivity of ultrasound in the detection of focal liver malignancies by improving their conspicuity (19–22). In a multicentre study of 123 patients, the sensitivity to liver metastases increased from 71% to 88% and more subcentimeter lesions were detected. These results were comparable to the sensitivity of contrast enhanced CT, which was used as the reference imaging modality, and PIM ultrasound detected some lesions that were not seen on CT, particularly subcentimeter lesions. The

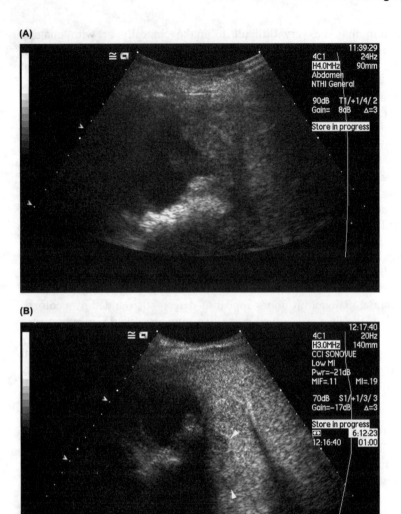

Figure 6 Contrast for interstitial ablation. In this patient with a liver metastasis from a colorectal primary that had previously been treated with radiofrequency ablation, the scan was requested because of rising markers. Beside the cavity there was an echogenic region, which was considered suspicious for tumor although it did not show signals on power Doppler (**A**) A contrast study (**B**) did not show any changes in this region but an echopoor region slightly deeper in the liver (*arrowheads*) that had not been noted on the baseline scan became increasingly obvious in the sinusoidal phase as the liver accumulated contrast (SonoVue was used with CCI, a pulse subtraction mode). This proved to be recurrent tumor on biopsy.

possibility that these were false positive for US was thought unlikely because in a subset of these patients, another reference investigation was available (MRI, intraoperative US, or laparotomy) and these showed yet more lesions than PIM US. Its role in hepatocellular carcinoma is unclear but in cholangiocarcinoma, a tumor that is notoriously difficult to define on ultrasound (presumably because of its infiltrating margins) stands out clearly against the enhancing liver (Fig. 8).

(A)

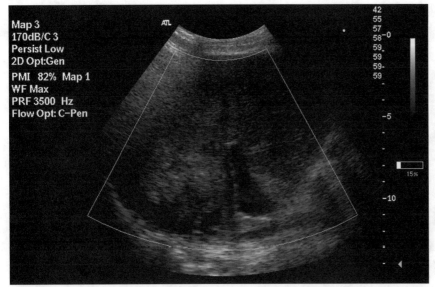

(B)

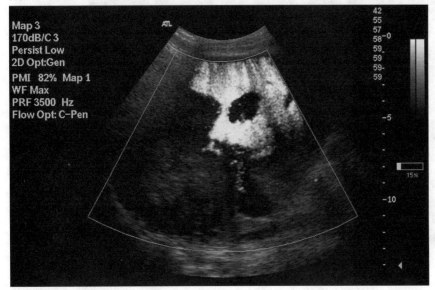

Figure 7 High MI detection of liver metastases. On this staging scan in a patient with a gastric carcinoma, the liver is suspiciously heterogeneous (**A**). In the late phase after administration of Levovist and using the ADI mode to detect the agent in healthy liver (**B**), large lesions are seen that were not obvious before. (*See color insert for Fig. 7B.*)

Low MI Modes in the Liver

The advantage of being able to work in real time using low MI modes with the phospholipid-perfluoro microbubble agents has enabled a three-phase approach to characterize liver masses. The same thinking is used in dynamic contrast CT and MRI but ultrasound has the added benefits of working in true real time and a study

(A)

(B)

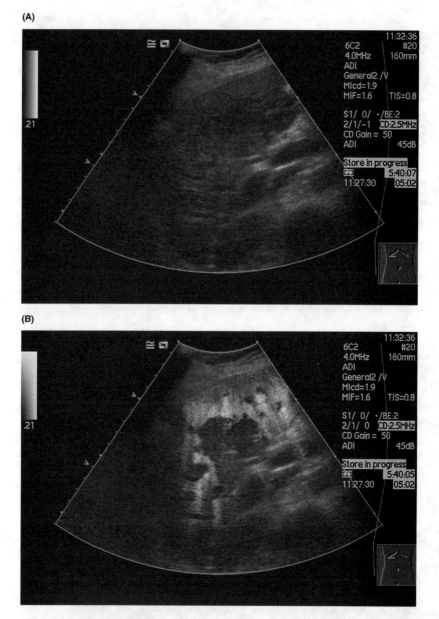

Figure 8 Contrast reveals cholangiocarcinoma. The liver appears slightly heterogeneous in this patient with a cholangiocarcinoma but no well-defined lesion is seen on the conventional scan (**A**), a common finding with this infiltrating tumor. In ADI mode after administration of a liver-trophic microbubble (Levovist), the normal liver is highlighted in color and the tumor is clearly revealed as an extensive color void (**B**). The discrepancy between the conventional and the contrast-enhanced scan is striking. (*See color insert for Fig. 8B.*)

can be repeated within a few minutes (because of the relatively short life of the agents) (Table 2) (23,24). In practice, the arterial and sinusoidal phases (at 15–30 seconds and 1–3 minutes, respectively) are the most useful (the times for US are earlier than for CT, perhaps because of the tight boluses achieved with the smaller volumes, typically a few mL, and the very high sensitivity to the microbubbles). The sinusoidal phase is a

Table 2 Vascularity of Liver Masses in Low MI Contrast Imaging

Metastases	Arterial	Portal	Sinusoidal	
Hypovascular	±	0	0	Marginal vessels
Hypervascular	++	0	0	Fill from margin
HCC	+++	0	0	Fill from margin
HA	+	0	+	Centripetal fill
FNH	+++	0	+	Central supply
RN	+	+	+	Normal liver
Fat	+	+	+	Normal liver

Abbreviations: HCC, hepato-cellular carcinoma; HA, hemangioma; FNH, focal nodular hyperplasia; RN, regenerating nodule in cirrhosis; fat, focal fatty change or sparing.

measure of the tissue's vascular volume, which is particularly high for the liver—since microbubbles are too large to cross the endothelium, there is no interstitial phase. The liver's arteries fill rapidly, at the same time as the adjacent kidney, and then the liver parenchyma, in general, progressively enhances over the next minute or so before gradually fading back to baseline. This pattern is shared by "lesions" that consist of normal liver such as focal fatty change and sparing and by regenerating nodules. The actual appearance on screen depends on the mode selected: In phase inversion modes, contrast shows as a brightening of the gray scale, while in CPS and VRI it shows as the appropriate tints (Figs. 9 and 10).

Vascular lesions have a variety of patterns of arterial supply, the peripheral arterial supply of vascular malignancies being typical (Fig. 11). Often these arteries are markedly tortuous and there may be several vascular poles. Hypovascular metastases are inconspicuous in this phase though circumferential vessels may be demonstrated in some cases. Vascular benign lesions may show a spectacular arterial supply, particularly FNH but here the supply is from a central artery (the changes may be so quick that they can be missed if the operator is not on the alert with the probe centered on the lesion). FNH then retains contrast and gradually disappears to blend with the liver except for the central scar, which may form a very obvious defect at this late stage, while malignancies, with their low vascular volume, remain echo-poor against the increasing signal from the liver sinusoids. This forms a general rule; lesions that are more prominent in the sinusoidal phase are suspicious of malignancy (cysts and abscesses exempted!) while those that disappear are likely to be benign.

Haemangiomas may show a pathognomonic pattern with early but subtle arterial filling that forms clumps at their periphery, followed by slow, centripetal fill-in, sometimes over several minutes. The fill-in may be complete, so that they eventually disappear, or may be partial, especially in larger lesions (presumably because of thrombotic or fibrotic regions). However many hemangiomas behave nonspecifically on these dynamic studies and in these cases the contrast study remains inconclusive.

While the necessary multicenter studies have not been completed, dynamic low MI contrast US shows strong promise in differentiating liver lesions. Whether the sinusoidal phase is equivalent to the liver-specific phase of agents like Levovist has not been studied in detail though many workers in the field suspect that this is lesions that were not apparent certainly on baseline and become obvious in the sinusoidal phase.

(A)

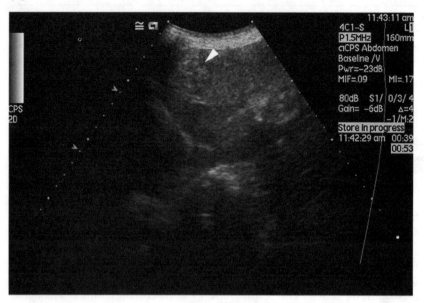

(B)

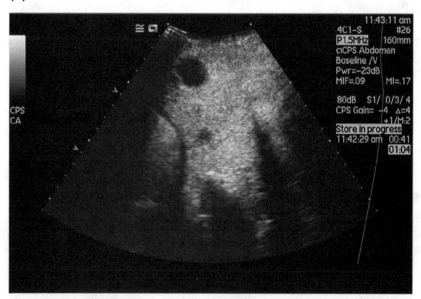

Figure 9 Low MI detection of liver metastases. A suspicious lesion in segment 2 (*arrowhead* in **A**) was found in this patient being staged for a gastric carcinoma. It was more clearly seen as a color defect after enhancement with SonoVue and using the low MI contrast pulse sequences mode (**B**). Scanning the remainder of the liver revealed three other lesions in segment 5 and 8 (*arrowheads* in **C**) that could not be detected on the simultaneous gray scale image (**D**). (*See color insert for Figs. 9B and C.*) (*Continued on facing page.*)

(C)

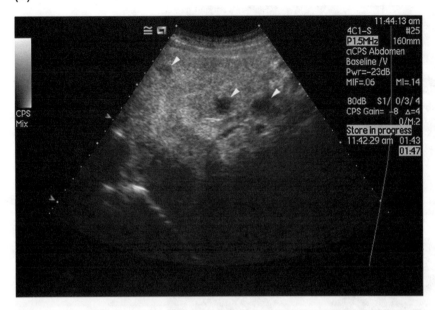

(D)

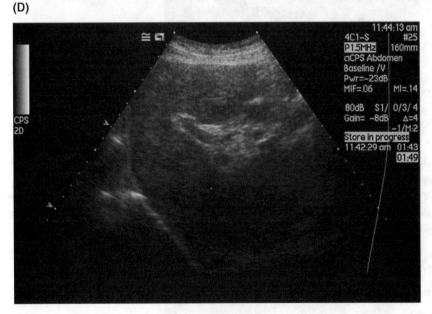

Figure 9C–D (*Continued*) (*See color insert for Figs. 9B and C.*)

Low MI Modes in Other Organs

The arterial supply to all organs is highlighted using the same low MI modes as in the liver but the three phases are not seen because of their simpler supply and lack of an equivalent to the sinusoidal phase. In the kidney, the neovascular supply to renal cell carcinomas is well demonstrated and collaterals can be detected. Transitional cell tumors have not been extensively reported. In the breast, impressive preliminary results have been reported but lower frequency transducers are optimal and had to

(A)

(B)

(C)

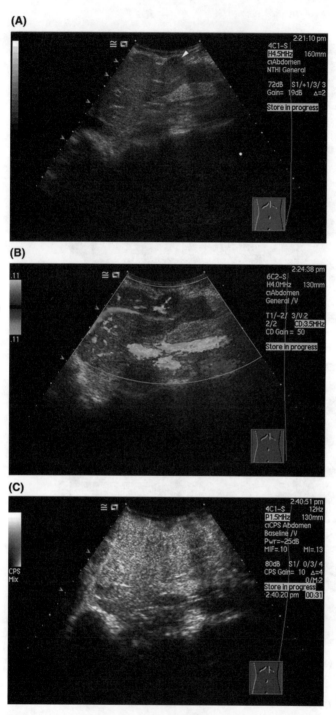

Figure 10 Regenerating nodule vs. hepatocellular carcinoma. The nodularity of the anterior surface of segment 3 in the liver of this cirrhotic patient (*arrowhead* in **A**) was considered suspicious for malignant transformation, especially as it was vascular on a color Doppler (**B**). SonoVue was administered and the suspicious regions showed complete filling at 30 seconds (**C**), suggesting that the tissue here was functioning as normal liver and therefore more likely to be regenerating nodules than hepatocellular carcinoma. (*See color insert for Figs. 10B and C.*)

be used (in fact, high frequency abdominal probes were used). This is because low **MI** multipulse modes have not yet been implemented on high frequency transducers and this has delayed progress in small parts applications as well as for intracavitary ovarian and prostate work, despite which some promising reports on improved

(A)

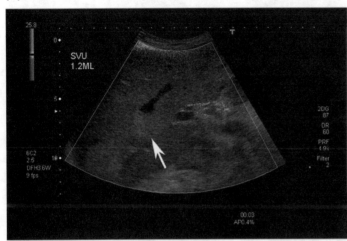

(B)

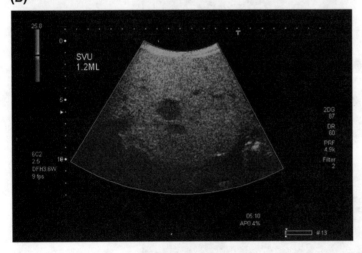

Figure 11 Hypervascular liver metastasis. The scan 3 seconds after injection of the contrast agent SonoVue (**A**) is effectively a baseline scan and shows an echogenic mass (*arrow*) typical of a colorectal cancer metastasis. This lesion rapidly accumulates contrast in the arterial phase so that it shows as an intense green color at 21 seconds (**B**), indicating that it is hypervascular. Thereafter, contrast washes out of the lesion rapidly at the same time as it continues to build in the liver, presumably by Kupffer cell uptake (**C** at 5 minute post injection). In this late or sinusoidal phase, additional lesions appear as color voids in **D** (**E** is the same as **D** but with the color layer switched off); these had not been noticed on the precontrast baseline scan. This microbubble mode, Vascular Recognition Imaging, depicts stationary or very slowly moving microbubbles in green (i.e., the microcirculation) and uses red and blue to indicate the direction of movement of flowing microbubbles in the macrocirculation. *Source*: Aplio scanner, Toshiba, Nasu, Japan. (*See color insert.*) (*Continued on next page.*)

(C)

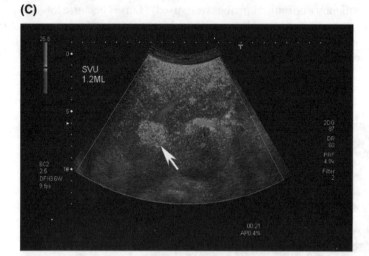

(D)

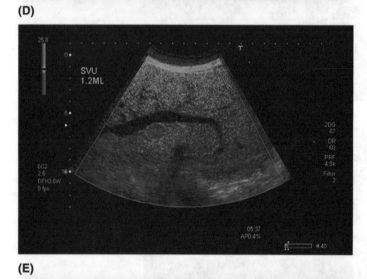

(E)

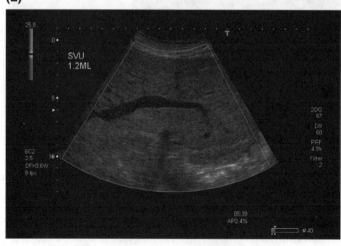

Figure 11C–E   (*Continued*) (*See color insert.*)

detection of prostatic carcinoma have been published, essentially using the tissue harmonic mode, which is not optimal (25).

Data are also lacking for the pancreas, adrenals, and bowel but in the spleen similar results to those achieved in the liver have been reported anecdotally—obviously the incidence of splenic malignancy is low. However, high MI SAE modes work well in the late phase for the spleen and this can be useful in determining whether a mass near the spleen is a splenunculus (SAE positive) or a malignant lymph node (SAE negative).

Functional Studies

The development of microbubbles as ultrasonic contrast agents offers the possibility of transit time studies with US for the first time. This can be performed by simply examining the passage of the contrast bolus or, in an approach unique to ultrasound, by actively destroying the agent in a plane or volume to create a negative bolus. Quantification depends on the finding that relative microbubble concentration is linearly related to Doppler signal intensity (10).

Following a bolus injection of microbubbles, their passage through a tissue of interest such as a tumor or organ can be quantified to generate transit time curves, as with nuclear medicine, CT, and MR; from these, functional information can be derived to yield indices such as bolus arrival time, time to peak intensity, area under the curve, wash in–wash out characteristics as well as more complex deconvolution indices. Since ultrasound contrast agents are confined to the vascular space (unlike CT and MR agents, which diffuse into the interstitial space) they may provide unique functional information not readily obtainable by other means.

An important application is the study of hepatic vascular transit times in which the hepatic veins are studied after a peripheral injection of a bolus of a microbubble. Early arrival of contrast is seen in malignancy (and also in cirrhosis) because of a shift in the liver's supply towards the hepatic artery. This technique has been shown to be a highly sensitive indicator of metastases (26). A prospective trial presently underway suggests that an early arrival predicts a high risk of developing liver metastases in patients with colo-rectal cancer who's livers were "clear" at staging: all 9/124 who had developed overt metastases at their one-year CT follow-up had early arrival times (<25 seconds) at the time of staging, and no patient cleared at staging and with a normal arrival time has developed overt liver metastases thus far. Presumably undetectable micrometastases were actually present in those patients with an early arrival time and this simple test could be used to select patients for intensive chemotherapy.

Time intensity curves can be drawn for an area of interest to document microbubble transit through, for example, a tumor bed (11). The indices (e.g., bolus arrival time) derived from them can be used to construct true functional images by displaying them on a pixel-by-pixel basis as an overlay on the gray-scale image. They are particularly promising for heterogeneous tissues such as tumors. These combined structural and functional maps hold great potential.

Active quantitation methods are based on creating a negative bolus by destroying the microbubbles in the scanned slice and observing its refill (so-called "reperfusion kinetics"). Intermittent high power ultrasound pulses are used to destroy microbubbles within the beam and the rate of replenishment in the field is measured. The reperfusion curve is a rising exponential described as

$$VI = VI_{max}(1 - e^{-\beta \times PI})$$

where VI is the video intensity, VI_{max} is the maximal video intensity (seen at long pulsing intervals), β is the constant describing the rate of rise of VI and PI is the pulsing interval. The initial upslope of this curve is proportional to microbubble speed as they refill the slice being insonated and VI_{max} relates to the fractional vascular volume. First developed as a way to estimate relative myocardial perfusion (27), the method has been applied to other tissues and is promising in tumors as a method to depict and measure their heterogeneous perfusion.

New Methods

Several novel ultrasonic imaging methods are currently being developed and evaluated in the laboratory and clinic.

Elastography

The stiffness (Young's modulus) of tissue has a much greater range than the bulk modulus that is used in B-mode imaging and tends to alter (usually increase) in pathology. It can be imaged by measuring the tissue's distortion (strain) under an applied stress (e.g., compression via the transducer). Known as elasticity imaging or elastography, the images produced have very high contrast and may significantly improve lesion detection within the breast, prostate and liver (28). Fast algorithms allow elastograms to be generated in real time (Fig. 12).

Vibro-acoustography is an interesting method for applying stress to a tissue deep within the body for elastography (29). Two ultrasound beams with slightly different frequencies in the kilohertz range are focused on a region in the tissue. The resulting interference causes the tissue to vibrate at a low frequency and this is detected by a microphone (hydrophone). By scanning the two beams across the tissue, an elastographic image is built up. This technique appears to be particularly adept at delineating calcium deposits within tissues, such as breast microcalcifications.

Acoustic Microscopy

Technical advances in transducer manufacture and in electronics are enabling the use of higher ultrasonic frequencies so that the use of 30 to 100 MHz probes is becoming realistic (30). These transducers usually rely on single element mechanical devices and are based on the polymer ferroelectric polyvinylidene fluoride (PVDF), which has a high bandwidth (>100%) but relatively poor sensitivity. The penetration through tissue is limited to a few millimeters but the spatial resolution is in the micron range, so the field is known as "acoustic microscopy." The eye is an important application for melanoma as well as nonmalignant conditions and the differentiation between benign pigmented skin lesions and melanoma seems possible using a number of acoustic tissue characteristics such as attenuation and impedance to produce images. Acoustic microscopy is also promising for the esophagus and stomach and could play a significant role in Barratt's esophagus to detect in situ dyplasia (31). A development of potentially far reaching benefit is the development of ultra-high frequency micro-transducers which is small enough to be inserted into tissue via a fine bore needle to obtain in situ histology.

Endoluminal US

The miniaturization of transducers has allowed interrogation of a wide variety of lumina (32). Small diameter probes can be inserted through needles and catheters.

(A)

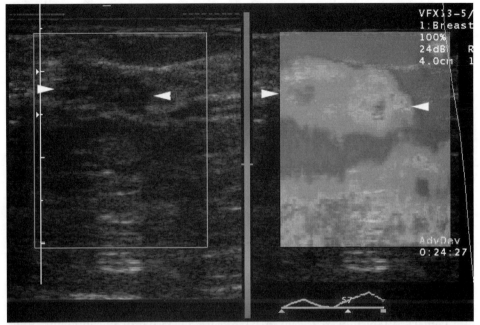

(B)

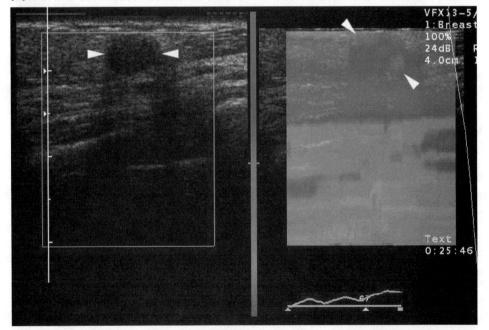

Figure 12 Elastograms of breast masses. The B-mode image on the left shows a small carci-noma (*arrowheads in* **A**, *left panel*) and its color-coded elastogram is larger (*arrowheads* in **A**, *right* panel), a typical finding with this technique. In comparison, fibroadenomas (*arrowheads in* **B**, *left*) appear approximately the same size and often show strain poles 180° apart (*arrow-heads in* **B**, *right*). *Source*: Images supplied by Dr WE Svensson; Elegra scanner and develop-mental software supplied by Siemens Medical, Issequa, Washington, U.S.A. (*See color insert.*)

Applications have been developed in the gastrointestinal tract, biliary system, uro-genital tract, and tracheobronchial tree making it difficult to access lesions to be fully characterized and biopsed. In the future, therapy may be administered via this route.

HIFU

HIFU or Focused Ultrasound Surgery, as a therapeutic technique is not a new concept but recent advances in probe design and alternate ultrasonic imaging methods make it likely to become a realistic clinical tool in the near future (33). HIFU uses a highly focused ultrasound beam to coagulate a well-defined volume of tissue by heating it to above 50°C. Maintenance of this temperature for one to seconds results in cell death, and a single US exposure destroys a cigar-shaped volume of tissue of 0.5 mL. The surrounding tissue is not damaged and there is a very sharp line of demarcation between coagulated and viable tissue. This completely non-invasive technique has been used to treat malignant tumors of the liver, prostate, and kidney and benign breast tumors via a percutaneous or transrectal approach without the need for general anesthesia (34). Although promising, HIFU is currently limited by the amount of tissue that can be coagulated by a single US exposure, the time required between exposures to allow local tissue cooling, the inability to treat through bone and problems of monitoring therapy in real-time. Technological advances promise to overcome many of these problems. Currently, HIFU tissue abla-tion damage is best observed using MRI which renders the treatment cumbersome and expensive. Since B-mode US cannot distinguish between coagulated and normal tissue, alternate ultrasonic imaging methods such as elastography, reflex transmission imaging and thermal imaging are likely candidates to depict the tissue damage. HIFU could also be deployed intraoperatively, e.g., in the treatment of liver metastases.

US Drug and Gene Delivery

Exposure to US causes a transient increase in cell membrane permeability, an effect known as sonoporation (35). Using this technique, tissues can be targeted to stimulate cellular uptake of a drug (e.g., a chemotherapeutic agent) or a gene. Sonoporation requires high acoustic powers (higher than that used in diagnosis and equivalent to those used in physiotherapy) but the power needed is markedly reduced when micro-bubbles are also present. A drug or gene can be incorporated in or on the surface of the microbubbles and tracked in the circulation with an imaging beam; when they are exposed to high power US, the microbubbles rupture, releasing the agent near the tar-get tissue (36). In the case of oncological drugs, this has the advantage of decreasing the dose of the drug needed, so reducing systemic side effects. Encouraging initial in vitro studies have demonstrated sonoporation without inducing cell death (37).

REFERENCES

1. Woo J. History of Ultrasound. 2002. http://www.ob-ultrasound.net/history.html.
2. Whittingham T. New and future directions in ultrasonic imaging. Brit J Radiol 1997; 70:S119–S132.
3. Whittingham T. An overview of digital technology in ultrasonic imaging. Eur Rad 1999; 9(suppl 3):S307–S311.
4. Desser T, Jeffrey R. Tissue harmonic imaging techniques: physical principles and clinical applications. Semin US CT MRI 2001; 22(suppl 1):1–10.

5. Entrekin R, Porter B, Sillesen, Hea. Real-time spatial compound imaging: application to breast, vascular and musculoskeletal ultrasound. Semin US CT MRI 2001; 22:50–64.

6. Johnson DD, Pretorius DH, Budorick NE, Jones MC, Lou KV, James GM, Nelson TR. Fetal lip and primary palate: three-dimensional versus two-dimensional US. Radiology 2000; 217:236–239.

7. Weismann C, Forstner R, Prokop E, Rettenbacher T. Three-dimensional targeting: a new three-dimensional ultrasound technique to evaluate needle position during breast biopsy. Ultrasound Obstet Gynecol 2000; 16:359–364.

8. Goldberg B, Raichlen J, Forsberg F, Ultrasound Contrast Agents. 2nd ed. London: Martin Dunitz, 2001.

9. Cosgrove D. Ultrasound contrast agents. In: Dawson, P, Cosgrove D, Grainger R, eds. Textbook of Contrast Media. Oxford: ISIS Medical Media, 1999:451–587.

10. Blomley, M, Eckersley, R, Cosgrove, D. Potential for Quantitation. In: Thomsen, H, Muller, R, Mattrey, R, eds. Trends in Contrast Media, Springer: Berlin 1999:343–353.

11. Eckersley R, Cosgrove D, Blomley M, Hashimoto H. Functional imaging of tissue response to bolus injection of ultrasound contrast agent. Proc IEEE Ultrasonics Symp 1988; 2:1779–1782.

12. Leighton T. The Acoustic Bubble. London: Academic Press, 1994

13. Forsberg F, Shi W. Physics of contrast microbubbles. In: Goldberg B, Raichen J, Forsberg F, eds. Ultrasound Contrast Agent. London: Martin Dunitz, 2001:15–24.

14. de Jong N. Physics of microbubble scattering. In: Nanda N, Schlief R, Goldberg B, eds. Advances in Echo Imaging Using Contrast Enhancement. Lancaster, England: Kluwer Academic, 1997:39–64.

15. Blomley MJ, Albrecht T, Cosgrove DO, et al. Improved imaging of liver metastases with stimulated acoustic emission in the late phase of enhancement with the US contrast agent SH U 508A: early experience. Radiology 1999; 210:409–416.

16. Hope-Simpson D, Chin C, Burns P. Pulse inversion doppler: a new method for detecting non-linear echoes from microbubble contrast agent. IEEE Transactions on Ultrasonics, Ferroelectrics and Frequency Control, 1999.

17. Kedar RP, Cosgrove D, McCready VR, Bamber JC, Carter ER. Microbubble contrast agent for color Doppler US: effect on breast masses. Work in progress. Radiology 1996; 198:679–686.

18. Solbiati L, Goldberg S, Ierace T, Dellanoce M, Livraghi T, Gazelle G. Radio-frequency ablation of hepatic metastases: postprocedural assessment with a US microbubble contrast agent—early experience. Radiology 1999; 211:643–649.

19. Blomley M, Albrecht T, Wilson S. Improved detection of metastatic liver lesions using pulse inversion harmonic imaging with Levovist: a multicentre study. Radiology 1999; 213(P):1685.

20. Bryant T, Blomley M, Albrecht T, et al. Liver phase uptake of a liver specific microbubble improves characterization of liver lesions: a prospective multi-center study. Radiology 2003. Submitted.

21. Harvey CJ, Blomley MJ, Eckersley RJ, Heckemann RA, Butler-Barnes J, Cosgrove DO. Pulse-inversion mode imaging of liver specific microbubbles: improved detection of sub-centimetre metastases [letter]. Lancet 2000; 355:807–808.

22. Quaia E, Bertolotto M, Forgacs B, Rimondini A, Locatelli M, Pozzi Mucelli R. Detection of liver metastases by pulse inversion imaging during Levovist late phase. Eur Radiol 2002; 13:475–483.

23. Wilson SR, Burns PN, Muradali D, Wilson JA, Lai X. Harmonic hepatic US with microbubble contrast agent: initial experience showing improved characterization of hemangioma, hepatocellular carcinoma and metastasis. Radiology 2000; 215:153–161.

24. Kim T, Choi B, Han J, et al. Hepatic tumors: contrast agent-enhancement patterns with pulse inversion harmonic US. Radiology 2000; 216:411–417.

25. Halpern EJ, Verkh L, Forsberg F, Gomella LG, Mattrey RF, Goldberg BB. Initial experience with contrast-enhanced sonography of the prostate. Am J Roentgenol 2000; 174:1575–1580.

26. Blomley MJ, Albrecht T, Cosgrove DO, et al. Liver vascular transit time analyzed with dynamic hepatic venography with bolus injections of an US contrast agent: early experience in seven patients with metastases [published erratum appears in Radiology 1999; 210(3):882]. Radiology 1998; 209:862–866.

27. Wei K, Jayaweera A, Firoozan S. Quantification of myocardial blood flow with ultrasound induced destruction of microbubbles administered as a constant venous infusion. Circulation 1998; 97:473–483.

28. Bamber J. Ultrasound elasticity imaging: definition and technology. Eur Radiol 1999; 9(suppl 3):S327–S330.

29. Fatemi M, Greenleaf J. Vibro-acoustography: an imaging modality based on ultrasound-stimulated emission. Proc Natl Acad Sci, 1999; 96:6603–6608.

30. Foster F, Pavlin C, Harasiewicz K. Advances in Ultrasound biomicroscopy. Ultrasound Med Biol 2000; 26:1–27.

31. Saijo Y, Tanaka M, Okawai H, Dunn F. The ultrasonic properties of gastric cancer tissues obtained with a scanning acoustic microscope system. Ultrasound Med Biol 1991; 17:709–714.

32. Liu J, Goldberg B. 2-D and 3-D endoluminal ultrasound. Ultrasound Med Biol 2000; 137–139.

33. ter Haar G. Intervention and therapy. Ultrasound Med Biol, 2000; 26(suppl 1):51–54.

34. Visioli AG, Rivens IH, ter Haar GR, Horwich A, Huddart RA, Moskovic E, Padhani A, Glees J. Preliminary results of a phase I dose escalation clinical trial using focused ultrasound in the treatment of localised tumours. Eur J Ultrasound 1999; 9:11–18.

35. Miller M. Gene transfection and drug delivery. Ultrasound Med Biol 2000; 26(suppl 1): 59–62.

36. Unger E. Targeting and delivery of drugs with contrast agents. In: Thomsen H, Muller R, Mattrey R, eds. Trends in Contrast Media. Medical Radiology. Berlin: Springer, 1999:405–412.

37. Brayman A, Coppage M, Vaidya S, Miller M. Transient poration and cell surface receptor removal from human lymphocytes in vitro by 1 MHz ultrasound. Ultrasound Med Biol 1999; 25:999–1008.

4

MR Lymphangiography: Technique

Anuradha Saokar and Mukesh Harisinghani
Division of Abdominal Imaging and Interventional Radiology, Department of Radiology, Massachusetts General Hospital, Boston, Massachusetts, U.S.A.

Jelle Barentsz
Department of Radiology, Radboud University Medical Center Nijimegen, Nijimegen, The Netherlands

---

A Note from the Editors

*T*he detection of metastases to lymph nodes is clinically important in the evaluation of virtually any type of primary tumor. Radiologists recognize the limitations of current morphological imaging techniques. Magnetic resonance (MR) lymphography using the intravenously administered contrast agent ferumoxtran-10 has emerged as a powerful new tool for the evaluation of nodal involvement. Much research attesting to its accuracy for nodal detection and characterization (including the detection of micrometastases) appears in the literature, although efficacy data related to changing patient management and altering clinical outcomes are generally lacking. The authors of this chapter are pioneers in the clinical evaluation of MR lymphography and herein discuss advanced aspects with an emphasis on the optimization of acquisition strategies.

INTRODUCTION

The determination of lymph node involvement (nodal staging) is mandatory when investigating patients with malignancy (1–3). Standard cross-sectional imaging techniques such as computed tomography (CT) and magnetic resonance imaging (MRI) apply unreliable indices such as nodal size and other morphological criteria to distinguish benign from malignant lymph nodes (4–6). This is principally because normal-sized nodes may contain microscopic metastatic disease and enlarged nodes can be reactive in nature; furthermore, it has been repeatedly shown that signal intensity on MR images as well as the presence of gadolinium enhancement is unreliable when trying to distinguish normal nodes from cancerous nodes (7,8).

Ferumoxtran-10 enhanced MRI (MR lymphangiography) has emerged as an extremely accurate tool to differentiate benign from malignant lymph nodes (9–11). This technique has been shown to accurately detect microscopic malignant deposits within normal-sized lymph nodes at a number of anatomical sites including the pelvis (9), axilla, head, and neck region. However, optimal MR scanning technique is critical to the successful interpretation of this novel imaging tool (12); in this chapter, we discuss strategies to optimize the technique of ferumoxtran-10–enhanced MR lymphangiography.

COMPOSITION AND MECHANISM OF ACTION OF FERUMOXTRAN-10

Ferumoxtran-10 is a reticulo-endothelial system–specific contrast agent consisting of ultra-small superparamagnetic iron oxide particles (USPIO) (13–17). Following intravenous administration, the lymphotropic nanoparticles enter the interstitial space and are transported via the lymphatics to draining lymph nodes (17). Benign, normally functioning lymph nodes contain macrophages. The ferumoxtran-10 particles are taken up by macrophages resulting in reduction in the signal intensity of nodal tissue due to the susceptibility effects of iron oxide particles. In malignant areas within lymph nodes, the macrophages are replaced by cancer cells and therefore there is lack of ferumoxtran-10 uptake in these areas resulting in an absence of signal intensity reduction (Fig. 1) (9).

TIMING OF CONTRAST ENHANCED IMAGING

The lyophilized iron oxide is reconstituted in normal saline and injected at a dose of 2.6 mg of iron per kilogram of body weight over a period of 20 to 25 minutes. Adequate nodal localization takes at least 24 hours. Hence, postcontrast imaging is performed 24 to 36 hours after ferumoxtran-10 administration. Scanning the patients before or after this optimal time window may result in inadequate accumulation of the contrast medium within benign lymph nodes, leading to their false characterization as malignant nodes (Fig. 2) (12).

MR IMAGING

Imaging Plane

Although axial imaging is often adequate, additional or alternative imaging planes may be warranted depending on the anatomic region that is being studied. For

(A)   **(B)**

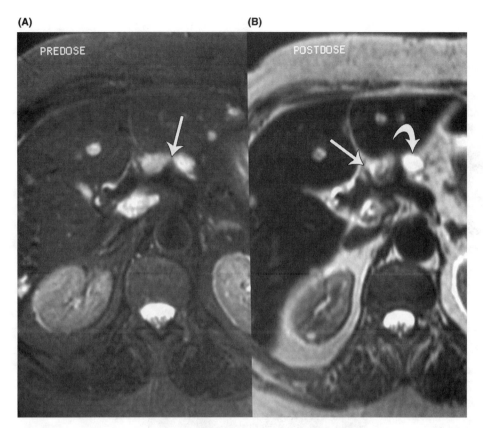

Figure 1 Malignant portal adenopathy in a patient with colon cancer. (**A**) Unenhanced T2-weighted image shows enlarged, hyperintense nodes (*arrow*) surrounding the portal vein. (**B**) Postferumoxtran-10 image shows a heterogeneous uptake (*arrow*) in medial nodes with the areas of darkening representing preserved nodal macrophages; the areas of retained hyperintensity correspond to tumor infiltration. The lateral node (*curved arrow*) is completely replaced with tumor. Note darkening of the liver because of contrast medium uptake by the reticuloendothelial system of the liver (Kupffer cells).

example, when evaluating pelvic nodes in patients with prostate cancer, additional imaging in an oblique plane parallel to the psoas muscle allows surgeons to precisely locate the lymph nodes in relation to the obturator nerve—an important surgical landmark (Fig. 3). Furthermore, this imaging plane enables the nodes to be optimally distinguished from vessels. Surgeons usually remove nodes from the so-called "obturator fossa," an area anterior and slightly posterior to the obturator nerve. An extended, more aggressive dissection is indicated when there is evidence on the postferumoxtran-10 MRI of nodal disease more than 2 cm posterior to the nerve.

Slice Thickness

Imaging with thin sections (3–4 mm) allows robust nodal detection and anatomical localization. Thin section imaging also improves nodal characterization by minimizing partial volume artifacts and aids in delineating hilar fat, a potential source for interpretation error (Fig. 4). High-spatial resolution imaging is useful for accurate

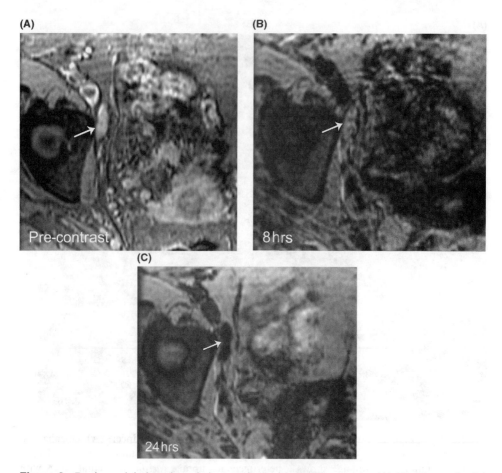

Figure 2 Benign pelvic lymph node in a patient with bladder cancer. (**A**) Unenhanced axial T2*-weighted MR image shows a hyperintense right external iliac node (*arrow*). (**B**) Axial MR image obtained early (8 hours) after administration of ferumoxtran-10 shows a slight, heterogeneous drop in signal intensity (*arrow*), which may be misinterpreted as malignant infiltration. (**C**) Delayed axial MR image obtained at the optimal 24-hours time point shows a homogeneous drop in signal intensity within the node (*arrow*). This finding indicates benignity, which was confirmed at surgery. *Source*: From Ref. 12.

characterization and detection of small metastatic foci within the nodes, and an in-plane resolution of at least 0.6×0.6 mm is advised.

Choice of Pulse Sequences

Ferumoxtran-10 shortens both T1 and T2* relaxation times. Shortening of T1 increases signal intensity and shortening of T2* decreases signal intensity in images that are appropriately weighted. Therefore, it is important to select a pulse sequence that is sensitive to either the T1 or the T2* effects of ferumoxtran-10. Choosing a pulse sequence sensitive to both can mask the presence of the contrast medium in lymph nodes. As the main emphasis is on lymph node characterization, the main sequence of choice is the T2*-weighted gradient-echo sequence. The sequence parameters for the T2*-gradient-echo sequence (appendix) are selected to enhance T2* sensitivity while concurrently

(A) (B)

(C) (D)

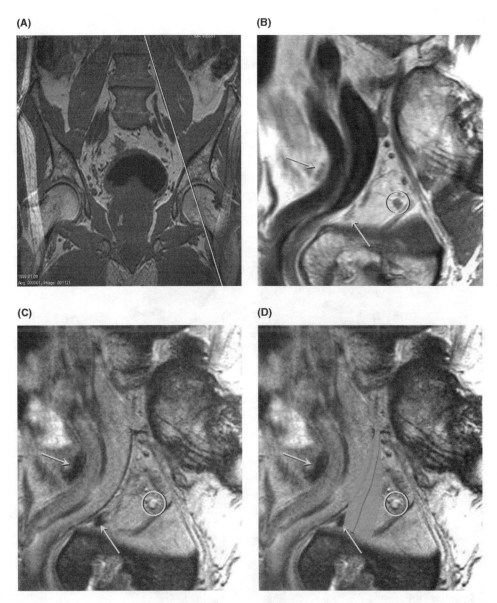

Figure 3 Oblique imaging for delineating the obturator fossa. (**A**) Coronal T1-weighted 3D-GRE MRI. The plane of Figure 3B (parallel to the psoas muscle) is indicated by the line. (**B**) T1-weighted SE MR image, obtained 24 hours postferumoxtran-10 (which is insensitive to iron oxide particles), shows normal size nodes (*arrows and circle*) of intermediate signal intensity. (**C**) T2*-weighted MEDIC MR image (which is sensitive to iron oxide) in the same plane shows low signal intensity in normal nodes (*arrows*), and high signal intensity in a 6 mm size metastatic node (*within circle*) in the internal iliac region. (**D**) The obturator fossa (*green*) around the obturator nerve (*solid green line*) is indicated. This is the routine area of node dissection in patient's prostate cancer. As the metastatic node is behind the obturator fossa (in the internal iliac region), the urologist should be informed about this finding preoperatively. (*See color insert for Fig. 3B.*)

(A)

(B)

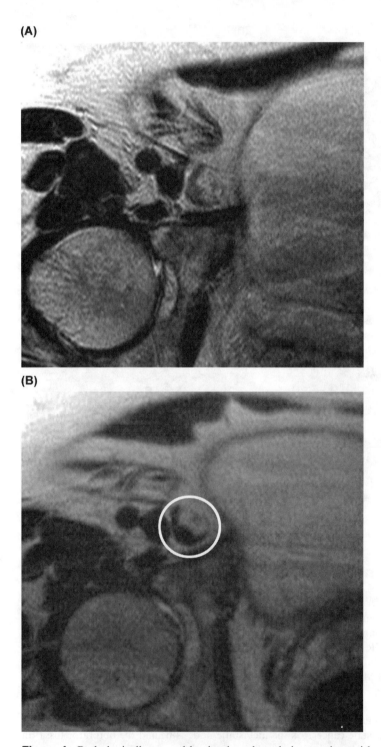

Figure 4 Pathologically proved benign lymph node in a patient with prostate cancer. Axial MR images, obtained with a 3 mm section thickness before (**A**) and after (**B**) administration of ferumoxtran-10 show a node (*circle*) with peripheral uptake of contrast material and a prominent central fatty hilum. Thin sections allow robust nodal characterization. *Source*: From Ref. 12.

limiting the influence of T1 effects (12). These include a lengthening repetition time (TR) or reducing flip angle to control T1 weighting and therefore heighten T2* effects. In addition, selecting a sufficiently long time-to-echo (TE) results in satisfactory signal intensity drop within benign nodes. A short TE can result in an inadequate signal intensity reduction leading to misinterpretation of a benign lymph node as being malignant (12).

In our practice, pre- and post-contrast scanning are done using the following sequences (appendix): two-dimensional (2D) axial T1-weighted gradient-echo, 2D axial T2-weighted fast spin echo and 2D axial T2*-weighted gradient-echo sequences (Fig. 5). In addition, post-contrast three-dimensional (3D) T1-weighted gradient-echo sequence can be performed for the surgical mapping of lymph nodes.

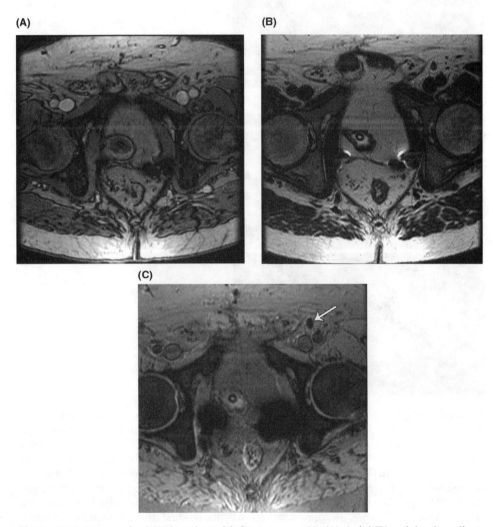

Figure 5 Sequences for MR imaging with ferumoxtran-10. (**A**) Axial T1-weighted gradient-echo, (**B**) T2*-weighted fast spin echo, and (**C**) T2*-weighted gradient-echo MR images, all obtained after administration of ferumoxtran-10, show a benign left inguinal lymph node (*arrow*). The node demonstrates homogeneous uptake of ferumoxtran-10 on the T2*-weighted gradient-echo image. Note the presence of artifacts from surgical clips that are greatest in Figure 5C due to greater susceptibility weighting. *Source*: From Ref. 12.

(A)

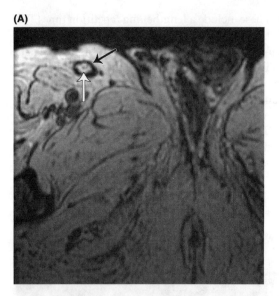

(B)

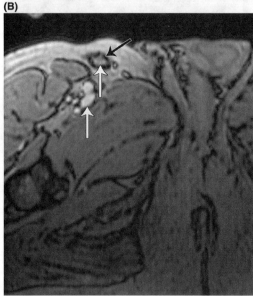

Figure 6 Fatty hilum of a lymph node at ferumoxtran-10 imaging of the pelvis. (**A**) Axial T2*-weighted gradient-echo MR image, obtained 24 hours after administration of ferumoxtran-10, shows a right inguinal node with peripheral decreased signal intensity (*black arrow*) and central high signal intensity (*white arrow*), an appearance that may be misinterpreted as representing a metastatic deposit. (**B**) Axial T1-weighted gradient-echo MR image shows that the central area of the node has high signal intensity (*top white arrow*), which indicates that this area represents the normal fatty hilum of the node. Note the enhancement of the femoral vessels (*bottom white arrow*) adjacent to the node, an appearance caused by the residual effect of circulating ferumoxtran-10. Peripheral decreased signal intensity (*black arrow*) in the node is seen but this effect is less reliable than on T2* sequence as shown in Figure 6A. *Source*: From Ref. 12.

Of the acquired sequences, T1- and T2-weighted sequences are used for nodal detection and anatomic localization. Additionally, the T1-weighted sequence helps to reduce false-positive interpretation by distinguishing fatty hilum from a metastatic node (Fig. 6). Postcontrast 3D T1-weighted gradient-echo sequence with a short TE can exploit the T1 enhancement properties of circulating Ferumoxtran-10 to delineate the vascular anatomy; mapping of the lymph nodes in relation to enhanced vessels on 3D rendering can be very useful to the operating surgeon (Fig. 7). The most crucial sequence for lymph node characterization is the $T2^*$-weighted gradient-echo sequence (12). Normal nodes show drop in signal intensity owing to the susceptibility effects of iron oxide reducing $T2^*$, while malignant lymph nodes will appear hyperintense.

Optimal TE for $T2^*$ Sequence

As imaging of normal lymph nodes with ferumoxtran-10 relies on signal intensity reductions due to susceptibility effects, choosing an appropriate TE value is important for making optimal diagnosis. Imaging with a very short TE may result in an

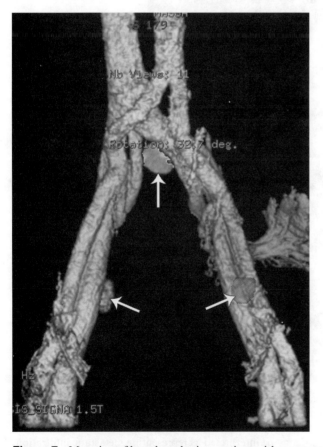

Figure 7   Mapping of lymph nodes in a patient with prostate cancer. Surface-shaded 3D-MR image showing the iliac vessels, distal aorta, and inferior vena cava, which are enhanced due to the effect of circulating ferumoxtran-10 on a T1-weighted 3D-GRE sequence. Malignant nodes are coded in red (*arrows*), thus showing their relationships to the major vessels; such renderings are useful for surgical planning. (*See color insert.*) *Source*: From Ref. 12.

(A)

(B)

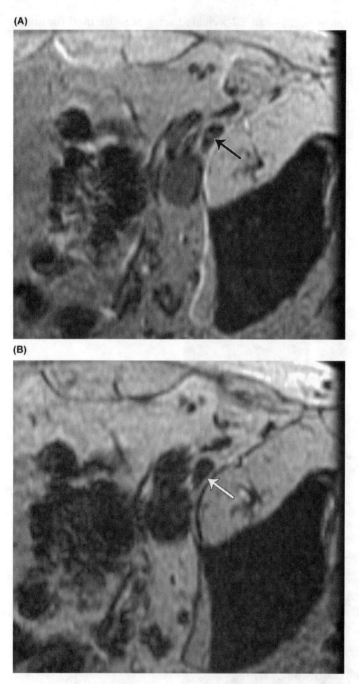

Figure 8 Optimal TE for imaging with ferumoxtran-10. Axial T2*-weighted MR imaging of the pelvis was performed in a patient with prostate cancer after administration of ferumoxtran-10. (**A**) Image obtained with a TE of 14 msec shows a left external iliac node with central heterogeneity (*arrow*), a finding that may be interpreted as representing metastatic infiltration. (**B**) Image obtained with a TE of 24 msec at the same time as Figure 8A above shows a more homogeneous drop in signal intensity (*arrow*). This finding indicates benignity, which was proven pathologically. *Source*: From Ref. 12.

inadequate signal drop resulting in erroneous interpretation. Figure 8 shows the differences in susceptibility with two different TE's in a benign lymph node.

Postferumoxtran-10 Imaging Only

A question often posed is whether it is necessary to image before and after ferumoxtran-10 administration. For "beginners," the best results will be obtained by comparing preferumoxtran-10 images with postferumoxtran-10 images. For more experienced users, the precontrast MRI can be replaced by postferumoxtran-10 sequences that are less sensitive to the susceptibility effects of iron oxide particles. For this purpose, a T1-weighted turbo spin-echo sequence can be used (Fig. 3B). If the same resolution and slice parameters are used, an insensitive image to iron can be compared with its corresponding sensitive $T2^*$ GRE image (Fig. 3C).

Quantitative Estimation of $T2^*$

In the clinic, lymph node characterization following ferumoxtran-10 administration is based on qualitative assessment of signal intensity changes within the nodes. The accuracy of this technique can be further improved by using quantitative methods to detect minimal malignant infiltration of small nodes. By performing a dual-echo $T2^*$-weighted gradient-echo sequence, it is possible to quantify ferumoxtran-10 uptake by calculating the $T2^*$ relaxation rate of the lymph node (12). However, an optimal $T2^*$ value that clearly differentiates between benign and malignant lymph nodes is yet to be determined.

CONCLUSIONS

Accurate nodal staging is important for deciding the choice of therapy and for predicting patient prognosis. MR lymphangiography using the intravenously administered contrast agent ferumoxtran-10, has emerged as a powerful new tool for the evaluation of nodal involvement. Accurate image interpretation of ferumoxtran-10–enhanced MR lymphangiography demands that careful attention be paid to the contrast administration and MR scanning technique.

APPENDIX

Typical Pulse Sequence Parameters

Pulse sequence parameters for the 1.5-T Horizon imager (GE Medical Systems, Milwaukee, Wisconsin, U.S.A.) are as follows:

1. T2-weighted fast spin-echo sequence: repetition time (TR) = 4500 to 5500 msec, time-to-echo (TE) = 80 to 100 msec, flip angle = 90°, three signals acquired, section thickness = 3 mm, gap = 0 mm, 256 × 256 matrix, and field of view = 22 to 30 cm.
2. $T2^*$-weighted gradient-echo sequence: TR = 300 to 400 msec, TE = 24 msec, flip angle = 20°, two signals acquired, section thickness = 3 mm, gap = 0 mm, 160 × 256 matrix, and field of view = 22 to 30 cm.

3. 2D T1-weighted gradient-echo sequence: TR = 175 msec, TE = 1.8 msec, flip angle = 80°, two signals acquired, section thickness = 4 mm, gap = 0 mm, 128 × 256 matrix, and field of view = 22 to 30 cm.

4. 3D T1-weighted gradient-echo sequence: TR = 4.5 to 5.5 msec, TE = 1.4 msec, flip angle = 15°, two signals acquired, section thickness = 5 mm, gap = 0 mm, 256 × 256 matrix, and field of view = 24 to 32 cm.

Pulse sequence parameters for the 1.5-T Magnetom Symphony imager (Siemens Medical Solutions, Erlangen, Germany) are as follows:

1. High spatial resolution 3D T1-weighted magnetization-prepared rapid gradient-echo (MP-RAGE) sequence: TR = 1540 msec, TE = 3.93 msec, TI = 800 msec, flip angle = 8°, one signal acquired, section thickness = 1 mm, gap = 0 mm, 256 × 256 matrix, extrapolated to 512 × 512, and field of view = 300 mm.

2. T1-weighted turbo spin-echo sequence: TR = 1800 to 2000 msec, TE = 15 msec, ETL 3, flip angle = 180°, two signals acquired, section thickness = 3 mm, gap = 0 mm, 512 × 384 matrix, and field of view = 285 mm. Images are obtained in the axial and oblique plane parallel to the iliac vessels.

3. 2D T2*-weighted fast low-angle shot (FLASH) or T2*-weighted multiecho data image combination (MEDIC) sequences: TR = 800 to 1500 msec, TE_{eff} = 18 msec, flip angle = 30°, two signals acquired, section thickness = 3 mm, matrix 512 × 512, and field of view 285 mm. Images are obtained in the same planes as the T1-weighted turbo spin-echo sequences.

REFERENCES

1. Kamura T, Tsukamoto N, Tsuruchi N, et al. Multivariate analysis of the histopathologic prognostic factors of cervical cancer in patients undergoing radical hysterectomy. Cancer 1992; 69:181–186.
2. Pollack A, Horwitz EM, Movsas B. Treatment of prostate cancer with regional lymph node (N1) metastasis. Semin Radiat Oncol 2003; 13:121–129.
3. Monig SP, Baldus SE, Zirbes TK, et al. Lymph node size and metastatic infiltration in colon cancer. Ann Surg Oncol 1999; 6:579–581.
4. Atula TS, Varpula MJ, Kurki TJ, Klemi PJ, Grenman R. Assessment of cervical lymph node status in head and neck cancer patients: palpation, computed tomography and low field magnetic resonance imaging compared with ultrasound-guided fine-needle aspiration cytology. Eur J Radiol 1997; 25:152–161.
5. Hilton S, Herr HW, Teitcher JB, Begg CB, Castellino RA. CT detection of retroperitoneal lymph node metastases in patients with clinical stage I testicular nonseminomatous germ cell cancer: assessment of size and distribution criteria. Am J Roentgenol 1997; 169:521–525.
6. Kvistad KA, Rydland J, Smethurst HB, Lundgren S, Fjosne HE, Haraldseth O. Axillary lymph node metastases in breast cancer: preoperative detection with dynamic contrast-enhanced MRI. Eur Radiol 2000; 10:1464–1471.
7. Dooms GC, Hricak H, Moseley ME, Bottles K, Fisher M, Higgins CB. Characterization of lymphadenopathy by magnetic resonance relaxation times: preliminary results. Radiology 1985; 155:691–697.
8. Barentsz JO, Jager GJ, van Vierzen PB, et al. Staging urinary bladder cancer after transurethral biopsy: value of fast dynamic contrast-enhanced MR imaging. Radiology 1996; 201:185–193.

9. Harisinghani MG, Barentsz J, Hahn PF, et al. Noninvasive detection of clinically occult lymph-node metastases in prostate cancer. N Engl J Med 2003; 348:2491–2499.
10. Anzai Y, Piccoli CW, Outwater EK, et al. Evaluation of neck and body metastases to nodes with ferumoxtran 10-enhanced MR imaging: phase III safety and efficacy study. Radiology 2003; 228:777–788.
11. Deserno WM, Harisinghani MG, Taupitz M, et al. Urinary bladder cancer: preoperative nodal staging with ferumoxtran-10-enhanced MR imaging. Radiology 2004; 233:449–456.
12. Harisinghani MG, Dixon WT, Saksena MA, et al. MR lymphangiography: imaging strategies to optimize the imaging of lymph nodes with ferumoxtran-10. Radiographics 2004; 24:867–878.
13. Weissleder R, Elizondo G, Wittenberg J, Lee AS, Josephson L, Brady TJ. Ultrasmall superparamagnetic iron oxide: an intravenous contrast agent for assessing lymph nodes with MR imaging. Radiology 1990; 75:494–498.
14. Weissleder R, Elizondo G, Wittenberg J, Rabito CA, Bengele HH, Josephson L. Ultrasmall superparamagnetic iron oxide: characterization of a new class of contrast agents for MR imaging. Radiology 1990; 175:489–493.
15. Muhler A, Zhang X, Wang H, Lawaczeck R, Weinmann HJ. Investigation of mechanisms influencing the accumulation of ultrasmall superparamagnetic iron oxide particles in lymph nodes. Invest Radiol 1995; 30:98–103.
16. Rogers JM, Jung CW, Lewis J, Groman EV. Use of USPIO-induced magnetic susceptibility artifacts to identify sentinel lymph nodes and lymphatic drainage patterns. I. Dependence of artifact size with subcutaneous Combidex dose in rats. Magn Reson Imaging 1998; 16:917–923.
17. Bellin MF, Lebleu L, Meric JB. Evaluation of retroperitoneal and pelvic lymph node metastases with MRI and MR lymphangiography. Abdom Imaging 2003; 28:155–163.

5

Image Processing in Tumor Imaging

Jianhua Yao

Department of Diagnostic Radiology, Warren G. Magnusson Clinical Center, National Institutes of Health, Bethesda, Maryland, U.S.A.

A Note from the Editors

M edical image processing has become a major force in the imaging of cancer. Virtually all cancer imaging requires some level of image post-processing. Among the most critical postprocessing functions are: image segmentation in which tumors are localized either manually or semiautomatically; image measurement in which physical and physiologic properties of tumors are characterized and mapped onto anatomic images; image visualization in which tumors are displayed in ways that are intuitively easy to grasp; and image registration in which two or more images are fused so that different tumor properties can be combined into one view. Image fusion and computer-aided diagnosis/detection combine many of these methods to produce synthetic images that display multiple parameters and highlight abnormalities that may be otherwise difficult to detect. Image processing methods will undoubtedly continue to contribute to progress in cancer detection and management.

The development of medical imaging has progressed remarkably over the past few decades. Medical imaging such as radiography, fluoroscopy, computed tomography (CT), magnetic resonance imaging (MRI), positron emission tomography (PET), single photon emission computed tomography (SPECT), and ultrasonography (US) can be used for detection, localization, visualization, and characterization of tumors. Many new imaging techniques including angiography, perfusion, and dynamic contrast enhancement imaging have been developed to study tumors. Because the information provided by medical images is enormous and sometimes not very intuitive, image processing and analysis is performed to extract useful information from the images. Image processing and analysis is usually conducted after the acquisition of the images, thus it is also called "postprocessing."

Medical image processing techniques make use of engineering approaches derived from the fields of computer vision, computer graphics, and artificial intelligence research. This chapter presents concepts and techniques for medical image processing and analysis, especially for applications in tumor imaging. It is organized into five sections: image segmentation, image measurement and quantification, image display and visualization, image registration, and computer aided diagnosis/detection.

IMAGE SEGMENTATION

Image segmentation is a technique to classify image pixels into anatomic regions, such as bones, muscles, and blood vessels, or pathological regions, such as tumors, tissue deformities, or multiple sclerosis lesions (1). In some applications, the goal of image segmentation is to extract the boundaries of the structures of interest. Image segmentation usually serves as the preprocessing step for further image processing tasks such as feature extraction, image registration, and quantitative measurement.

Medical image segmentation methods can be classified into three categories according to the degree of required human interaction—manual segmentation, semiautomatic segmentation, and fully automatic segmentation. Manual segmentation involves manually drawing the boundaries of the structures of interest or painting the region of anatomic structures with different labels. In manual segmentation, human operators not only apply the presented image information but also make use of additional knowledge such as anatomy and complex, poorly understood, psychological cognitive abilities. Manual segmentation is labor intensive, difficult to reproduce, and also subject to individual operator bias. However, it is still widely used in clinical trials, especially where a lot of human knowledge and expertise is required to distinguish tissues. In semiautomatic methods, the operators usually need to provide an initial start point for the segmentation and/or manually adjust the outcome of the computer segmentation. Most of current research is targeted at semiautomatic segmentation with the intention of having as little human interaction as possible. In fully automatic methods, the computer determines the segmentation without any human interaction. Fully automatic methods generally incorporate human intelligence and prior knowledge in the algorithms. Fully automatic methods are desirable in processing large batch of images. Currently, fully automatic segmentation methods are mainly restricted to the research environment. Clinical applications of image segmentation usually require some sort of human interaction.

In this section, semiautomatic and fully automatic image segmentation techniques are emphasized. Popular image segmentation techniques include threshold-based techniques, region growing techniques, pixel classification techniques, and model-based techniques. However, a single segmentation technique is not capable of yielding acceptable results in all settings. Methods are often optimized to segment specific anatomic structures in specific medical imaging modalities, for example, colon polyps in CT colonography or brain tumors in brain MR.

Threshold-Based Methods

Thresholding is a simple and effective region segmentation method (2). In this method, the objects in the image are classified by comparing their intensities with one or more intensity thresholds. If the histogram of an image expresses a bimodal pattern, the object can be separated from the background in the image by a single threshold. If an image contains more than two types of regions, it may be segmented by applying several individual thresholds or by using a multi-thresholding technique. The values of thresholds are generally estimated by the prior knowledge or intensity histogram of the image. Thresholds can be either global or local. A local threshold is determined adaptively in a local region around a pixel. Figure 1 demonstrates the extraction of a lung region from a chest CT using threshold-based techniques. The lung region is filled with air and therefore has a low Hounsfield number (HU). Figure 1A is a chest CT image, and Figure 1C shows the segmented lung region. The threshold T = –500 HU was selected as the middle value between two modes on the histogram (Fig. 1B).

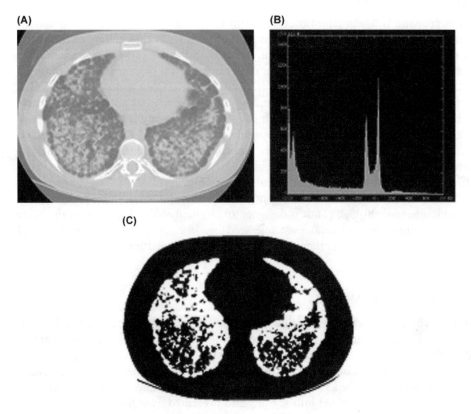

Figure 1   Threshold-based segmentation. (**A**) Lung CT image; (**B**) histogram; (**C**) segmented lung region. The threshold is –500 HU.

(A)   **(B)**

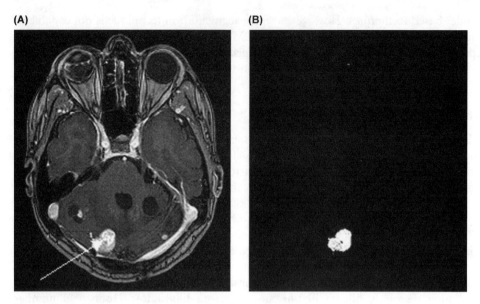

Figure 2   Region, growing segmentation. (**A**) Brain MR image; (**B**) segmented brain tumor. *Arrow* in (**A**) is pointing to the seed.

Region Growing Methods

Region growing is a segmentation method to extract a connected region of similar voxels from an image (3). Region growing starts with seeds that belong to the structure of interest. Neighbors of the seed are visited and those satisfying the similarity criteria are added to the region. The similarity criteria are determined by a range of pixel values or other features in the image. Seeds can be chosen manually or provided by an automatic seed-finding procedure. The procedure iterates until no more pixels can be added to the region. The advantage of region growing is that it is capable of correctly segmenting regions that have similar properties and generating connected region. Figure 2 demonstrates the segmentation of a brain tumor from a contrast-enhanced MRI image. A seed is placed inside the brain tumor and a region-growing technique is applied to extract the tumor region (Fig. 2B).

Watershed segmentation is a region-based technique combining region growing and image morphology (4). It is designed to segment multiple regions at the same time. It requires selection of at least one seed inside each object. A morphological watershed transformation is then applied to grow each seed into a region.

Pixel Classification Methods

Another type of segmentation methods is based on pixel classification. Pixels in an image can be represented in feature space using pixel attributes such as intensity and gradients. Supervised or unsupervised classifiers are employed to cluster pixels in the feature space. Basic classifiers include unsupervised methods such as fuzzy c-means, k-means, and supervised methods such as Bayes, and Neural Network (5). The pixel clusters are grouped into regions and presented as segmentation results.

Fuzzy c-mean clustering (FCM) is a popular pixel clustering technique in nonsupervised image segmentation for pixel classification, especially in multi-spectral

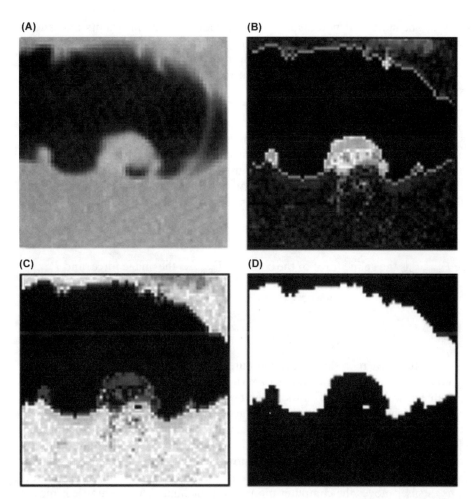

Figure 3 Fuzzy c-mean clustering in pixel classification-based segmentation. (**A**) CT–colonography image; (**B**) polyp tissue membership map; (**C**) nonpolyp tissue membership map; (**D**) lumen air membership map.

images such as MRI where T1-weighted, T2-weighted, and proton density–weighted images are available (6). In the FCM method, a set of tissue classes is first determined. Each pixel is then assigned membership values for the tissue classes according to its pixel attributes. The membership value of a certain class indicates the likelihood of the pixel belonging to that class. Figure 3 shows the FCM in CT–colonography. Three tissue classes, lumen air, polyp tissues, and nonpolyp tissues, are shown in Figures 3B, 3C and 3D, respectively. A threshold-based method can then be applied on the membership map to segment the region of interest.

Model-Based Segmentation

In model-based segmentation, a connected and continuous model is built for a specific anatomic structure. The model usually contains a priori knowledge of the structure to guide the segmentation. Some models incorporate prior statistical information drawn from a population of training datasets, such as the active appearance model (7). The statistical parameterization provides global constraints and allows the model to deform only in ways implied by the training sets.

In model-based segmentation, a rigid transformation (translation and rotation) is first determined for global alignment of the model with the image. Then a nonrigid transformation (such as elastic warping) is applied to maximize the similarity between the model and the corresponding region in the image. The resultant model is then the segmentation result, which represents the boundary of anatomic structures. The inherent continuity and smoothness of the models can compensate for noise, gaps, and other irregularities in the structure boundaries.

The active contour model is a widely used technique to segment structures in 2D images (8). In this technique, given an initial contour, several forces work together to drive the active contour to its destination. The forces that drive the active contour model can be expressed as

$$F = w_{in}F_{internal} + w_{im}F_{image} + w_{ex}F_{external} \tag{1}$$

where $F_{internal}$ is the spline force of the contour, F_{image} is the image force, and $F_{external}$ is the external force, and w_{in}, w_{im}, and w_{ex} are the respective weighting parameters. The internal force $F_{internal}$ can be written as

$$F_{internal} = \frac{1}{2}\int_0^1 (\alpha(s)|x'(s)|^2 + \beta(s)|x''(s)|^2)ds \tag{2}$$

where $x(s)$ is the curve representing the contour, $x'(s)$ is the first-order derivative of $x(s)$, and $x''(s)$ is the second-order derivative of $x(s)$. The first-order term makes the contour act like an elastic membrane, and the second-order term makes it act like a thin rigid plate. Figure 4 shows an application of the active contour model in colon polyp segmentation. The image force used in the model is the gradient of the membership function in FCM clustering described in the section entitled Pixel Classification Methods.

Another model-based technique is known as "live-wire" (9). This semiautomatic boundary tracing technique computes and selects optimal boundaries interactively as the user moves the computer mouse over the image. As the mouse is moved close to an object boundary, a live-wire boundary snaps to and wraps around the object of interest.

One limitation of the model-based segmentation is that the model might converge to the wrong boundaries. In some applications, the initial position of the model needs to be manually placed close enough to the desired boundary.

Relevance in Tumor Imaging

In tumor imaging researches, one major goal is to accurately locate the cancer. Some tumors can be distinguished from normal tissues by their image intensity so that a threshold-based or region growing technique can be employed. Some tumors can be identified by their shapes so that a model-based technique can be applied in tumor imaging. Some tumors may not have anatomic differences from normal tissues, but express differently in functional imaging such as PET and dynamic contrast-enhanced MRI (DCE MRI). In these cases, functional maps (discussed in the following section) are first generated, and the segmentation can be performed on those maps instead of original images.

Clinical acceptance of segmentation techniques depends on the ease of computation and the degree of user supervision. Interactive or semiautomatic methods are

(A)   (B)

(C)

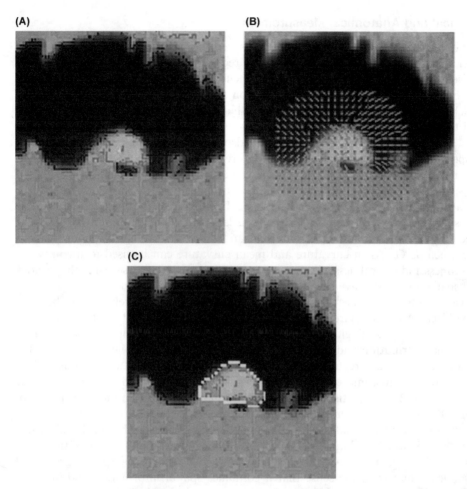

Figure 4 Model-based segmentation. (**A**) CT–colonography image; (**B**) image force map computed from Figure 3B; (**C**) segmented boundary of colon polyp.

likely to remain dominant in practice for some time, especially in applications where erroneous interpretations are unacceptable.

IMAGE MEASUREMENT AND QUANTIFICATION

Quantitative measurements are important for the analysis of medical images and the diagnosis of diseases. Performing the measurement directly on the image data provides a noninvasive way to get the physical and physiological properties of the anatomic structures. Sometimes image measurement is the primary goal of a clinical trial.

Measurement is usually performed after image segmentation to determine the properties of the segmented region. Quantitative measurements can be used to compare an individual patient to other patients or reference values. Measurements derived from a single patient may be compared over time, which is useful in tracking disease progression and monitoring treatment. Measurements of anatomic structures include physical properties such as size, shape, and density, and physiological attributes such as tissue perfusion and vascular permeability.

Physical and Anatomical Measurement

Size of a structure is the most intuitive measurement in many cases. Size of an object often tells the significance of a pathological region and is an important indication of a disease. Examples of size measurement include the longest diameter, which is the longest distance between any two points on the boundary; the effective diameter, which is the diameter of a circle having the same area as the region of interest; and the area/volume of a region.

Shape of an anatomic structure can also be quantified. The compactness of a shape can measure how closely a structure is related to a circle or a sphere. Compactness in 2D can be written as $C = P^2/4\pi A$, where P is the perimeter and A is the area of the shape. In 3D space, compactness can be written as $C = A^3/36\pi V^2$, where A is the surface area and V is the volume of the shape. In either case, the compactness of circle and sphere is one and that of other shapes is larger than one. Compactness has been used for quantifying mammographic calcification and breast tumors. Boundary curvatures such as Gaussian curvature and mean curvature can be used to quantify the curvedness and smoothness of a shape (11). Other shape properties such as shape index and spatial moments have been proposed to quantify anatomic shapes (12). Angular measurements often reflect the deformity of an object and the relationship between two objects. Angle measurement on bony structures is especially important for patho-anatomical analysis, diagnosis, and therapeutic planning in orthopedic diseases (13).

The distribution and statistics of pixel intensity within a region can reveal the smoothness, contrast, regularity, or homogeneity of tissues. Texture analysis such as statistical moments, and co-occurrence matrix provides ways to describe the tissue appearance (12). The statistical moments are computed based on the intensity histogram. The second moment of the histogram measures the intensity variance within the region, which correlates with the roughness perception. The third and fourth moments, skewness and kurtosis, reflect the asymmetry and uniformity of the intensity distribution. The co-occurrence matrix is also known as spatial gray level dependence matrix in the sense that it combines spatial information and intensity statistics (14). The inertia of the co-occurrence matrix characterizes the texture contrast of a region. The entropy of the matrix quantifies the level of randomness in the region. The angular second moment of the co-occurrence matrix can be used to describe the homogeneity of a region. Co-occurrence matrix was used in the analysis of prostate tumor and breast calcification (14,15).

Two examples of physical measurement application are bone mineral densitometry (BMD) and mammographic density measurement. BMD is a method to quantify the bone mass in the body (16). Osteoporosis is a common bone disease, which makes bone fragile and easy to fracture. Future risk of fracture can be predicted through a BMD measurement. Mammographic density measurement is a tool to measure the regions of brightness associated with fibroglandular tissues in the mammography, which is directly linked with the breast cancer risk. Mammographic density can be computed from the mammography using histogram analysis, or fractal analysis (17,18).

Functional and Physiological Quantification

In addition to the physical and anatomical measurements, functional and physiological measurements can be obtained from functional imaging modalities such as PET, functional MRI (fMRI), and DCE MRI. The functional quantifications are computed by applying pharmacokinetic or functional models to the original data, and generating parameter maps. The parameter maps are usually color-encoded and over-laid with the original images.

As an example of functional images, DCE MRI is a method to reveal the physiology of the microcirculation. DCE MRI measurement correlates well with tumor angiogenesis, which is the formation of new blood vessels that allow tumors to grow. After intravenous administration of Gd-DTPA, DCE MRI yields a description of the measured signal-time curves in terms of pharmacokinetic parameters. The signal-time curves are analyzed pixel-by-pixel to preserve the spatial information of MR images. A two-compartment pharmacokinetic model had been proposed to analyze DCE MRI data (19). In the model, two characteristic parameters, transfer rate $k21$ and amplitude A, are fit to characterize the tissue physiological properties. Transfer rate $k21$ is the rate for transfer of Gd-DTPA from the extracellular space to the plasma, which characterizes perfusion and vascular permeability of the lesion. The amplitude A reflects the degree of signal enhancement in a region. A tumor region is expected to have high $k21$ and A values. The two-compartment model has been successfully applied in analyzing breast tumors, brain tumors, and osteosarcoma. Another model characterizing the uptake slope in enhancing phase of Gd-DTPA in the cells has been used in the diagnosis of prostate tumors (20). Figure 5 shows color-encoded A parameter map (Fig. 5A) and $k21$ parameter map (Fig. 5B) of DCE MRI breast study, and take-off slope map (Fig. 5C) of a prostate study. The parameter maps are super-imposed on the original images.

Relevance to Tumor Imaging

Measurement of tumor volume and activity is an increasingly important goal in tumor imaging for studying structural changes over time and correlating anatomic information with functional activity and pathology.

Size measurement of a tumor is a common way to assess the tumor response to a treatment. During a tumor monitoring trial, a baseline study and several follow-up studies are obtained. The response is classified as one of following categories: (*i*) complete response (CR); (*ii*) partial response (PR); (*iii*) progressive disease (PD); and (*iv*) stable disease (SD). The longest diameter has been used in evaluating the solid tumors in response evaluation criteria in solid tumor (RECIST) (21). In RECIST, CR is defined as disappearance of all target lesions; PR is defined as at least a 30% decrease in the sum of longest diameter of target lesions; PD is defined as at least a 20% increase in the sum of longest diameter of target lesions; and the remaining cases are defined as SD.

Functional images such as dynamic MR can be used to study the tumor physiological activities, which are useful in differential diagnosis, therapy planning, and therapy follow-up.

IMAGE DISPLAY AND VISUALIZATION

Conventional films and light boxes can only convey 2D information. With the arrival of 3D images in biomedical field, it is desirable to visualize 3D volume information. Image processing and computer graphics techniques allow intuitive ways to display and visualize medical images. Common medical image display and visualization techniques include multi-planar reformatting (MPR), maximum intensity projection

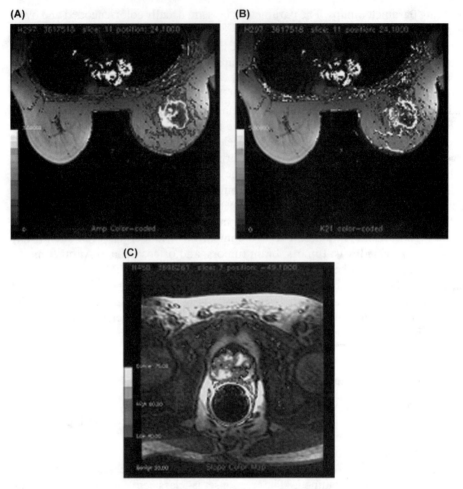

Figure 5 Functional parameter maps. (**A**) Amplitude map of breast study; (**B**) $k21$ map of breast study; (**C**) uptake slope map of prostate study. (*See color insert.*)

(MIP), surface rendering, and volume rendering. Virtual endoscope techniques based on volume rendering and surface rendering can be used to navigate the cavities inside human body.

MPR

3D tomographic images are usually acquired in transaxial plane. Coronal and sagittal views are desirable in some cases for a better perception of the image. MPR slices the 3D volume in different planes than the plane in which it was acquired. The three orthogonal views, axial, coronal, and sagittal, can be depicted in 3D space to demonstrate their spatial relationship. Figure 6 shows the axial, coronal, and sagittal views of a brain study. The reformatted image can also be on any arbitrary oblique plane in the volume space to visualize structures not on the orthogonal planes. In some cases, a curved section can be defined to render a curvilinear object such as the spinal canal (22).

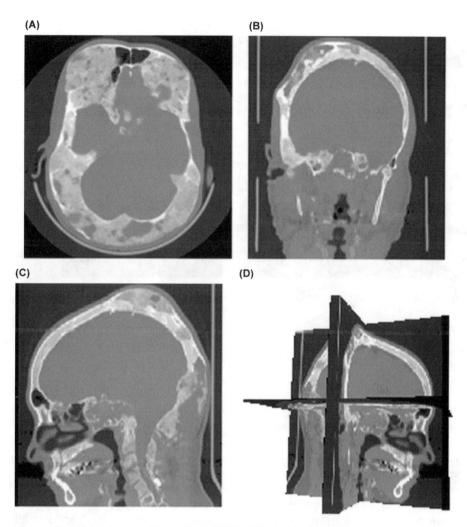

Figure 6   Multi-planar reformatting (MPR). (**A**) Axial view; (**B**) coronal view; (**C**) sagittal view; (**D**) combined view.

MIP

MPR yields 2D displays of cross-sections of a 3D image volume. To visualize the 3D volume, a camera model is necessary to capture the volume of an object in 3D space. The most common camera model consists of a source point (viewing point), a focal point (where the view is focused), and a viewing plane. The image seen from the viewing point through a 3D image volume is a volume visualization of the 3D volume.

The simplest volume visualization technique is the MIP (23). In this approach, the maximum intensity value along each ray of the projection is projected onto the viewing plane. The projection can be perspective or orthogonal. MIP is particularly useful for displaying vascular structures acquired using first pass intravenous contrast injections (arterial phase CT or MRI). MIP is generally presented as a movie where the projection plane is rotated around the center axis of the object and a MIP is generated at each angle. Figure 7 shows MIPs of the Circle of Willis in a MRA brain study.

(A)   **(B)**

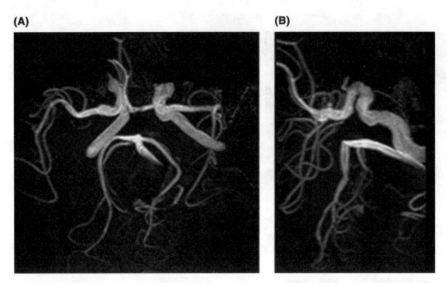

Figure 7 Maximum intensity projection of circle of Willis. (**A**) Anterior–posterior view; (**B**) lateral view.

Surface Rendering

The exterior surfaces of anatomic structures convey their size, shape, and relative location and orientation in 3D space. Surface rendering of structures can give physicians a 3D view, which cannot be easily obtained from 2D slices. Surface rendering is supported by computer graphics techniques, such as perspective projection, shading, and texture mapping.

Surface rendering first requires the extraction of the surfaces of the structures to be visualized. Surfaces are described in terms of a set of connected polygon patches or parametric surfaces such as B-spline surfaces and NURBS (24). Iso-surface extraction is a popular technique to extract the object boundaries (25). Given an iso-value (pixel intensity), an iso-surface is a surface that connects all points in the image having same intensity value as the iso-value. The advantage of iso-surface is at its detailed surface representation and that its generation can be automated. Iso-surface is sensitive to image noise and is only valid when the objects of interest are easily separable by their intensity. Another surface extraction technique is to first generate the 2D boundary contours of the object on each image slice and then tile the 2D contours to form a surface (26). The 2D contours can be generated using the segmentation techniques introduced in the section entitled Image Measurement and Quantification. The second technique generates a more accurate surface with much fewer triangles. Delaunay triangulation is another technique to construct a surface from boundary points (27). Figure 8 is a shaded surface display of a wrist.

Surface rendering is very effective in displaying the 3D shape of an anatomic structure. It requires relatively small amounts of data enabling interactive rendering on modern personal computers.

Volume Rendering

Surface rendering is very selective in extracting particular structures from the volume data. In cases where the anatomic structures of interest cannot be extracted with a

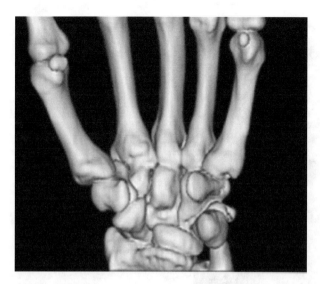

Figure 8 Surface rendering of a wrist.

unique iso-value, surface rendering may be difficult to use. In other cases, the interior structure of an object is the desired goal. Another technique for 3D image visualization is volume rendering. Volume rendering provides direct visualization of the 3D image volume without the need for prior surface segmentation, preserving the values and context of the original image data.

Volume rendering blends the image data weighted by a transfer function. The transfer function maps image intensity values into transparency values and colors. Popular transfer functions include ramp function and step function. Ray-casting approach is a widely used volume rendering technique (28). In this technique, every pixel on the viewing plane defines a ray connecting the viewing point and that pixel. Pixels in the 3D image volume and along the ray are integrated and blended to compute the final color and intensity of the corresponding pixel on the viewing plane. The most commonly used blending operation for volume rendering is

$$I_v = I_d \cdot (1 - T_d) + I_v \cdot T_d \tag{3}$$

where I_d and T_d are the data value and transparency of a point along the ray, I_v is the image value on the viewing plane. The blending operation is iterated along the ray from the viewing plane and the viewing point, and the image value on the viewing plane is updated at each iteration. Lighting and shading can also be provided to improve visual cues. Another volume rendering technique is based on texture mapping (29). In this technique, the volume is sliced into stacks of 2D texture maps parallel to the viewing plane, and the stack of texture maps is blended back-to-front to generate the volume rendered images. Texture mapping technique can exploit the capacity of texture hardware to accelerate the rendering, but rendering quality is poor since shading is difficult to apply.

Volume rendering conveys more information than surface rendering, but at the cost of increased rendering time. Volume rendering can be accelerated using specific hardware (30). A technique called shear-warp factorization can achieve interactive rendering rate by sacrificing a little image quality (29). Figure 9 is a volume rendering of the chest/abdominal region of a CT image.

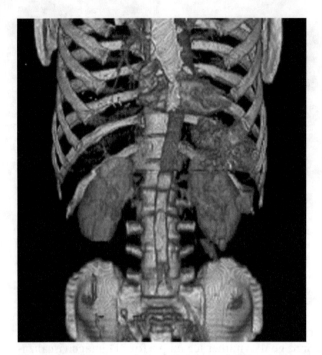

Figure 9   Volume rendering of chest and abdominal region. (*See color insert.*)

Virtual Endoscopy

Virtual endoscopy is a technique to simulate an endoscope passing through a hollow body passage such as the colon or trachea. In virtual endoscopy, a CT image is usually taken after inflating the passage with air (or using existing air). Then the viewing point is placed inside the passage in the image space. Volume rendering is employed to "see through" the air in the passage by setting certain transfer functions so that the air is totally transparent. A virtual flythrough is generated by moving the viewing point along the pathway. Virtual endoscopy can be used to non-invasively navigate tubular structures, which is useful for screening procedures. Applications of virtual endoscopy include virtual bronchoscopy and virtual colonoscopy. Figure 10 is a view from a virtual bronchoscopy.

Relevance to Tumor Imaging

Tumors are often buried deep inside the body and are usually hidden within normal tissues. 3D rendering techniques allow the visualization of the size and shape of the tumor from various directions, and more importantly, offer a visual perception of its spatial relation with surrounding regions. Figure 11 is a volume rendering of a kidney with tumors. The kidney is visualized semitransparently to allow visualization of opaque tumors within. The visual perception of the 3D location of tumors relative to the kidney is valuable in surgical planning, biopsy, and brachytherapy.

IMAGE REGISTRATION

More than one set of images is taken for diagnosis in many clinical applications. These images are usually acquired at different times or from different imaging

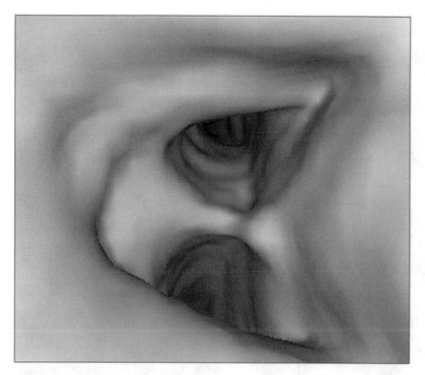

Figure 10 Virtual bronchoscopy.

modalities. In some cases, one patient's data is needed to compare with another patient's data or a standard reference. For different images to be analyzed together, they need to be registered within a common coordinate system.

Image registration is a technique to align two or more image volumes into the same geometric space. A rigid or nonrigid transformation is computed based on information from the images. Medical image registration can be classified based on the imaging modalities and the subjects involved in the registration. Registration between the same modalities, such as CT–CT, MR–MR is called "intramodal" registration; registration between different modalities, such as MR–PET is called "intermodal" registration. Registration between images of same patient at different times or from different modalities is "intrapatient" registration; and registration between images from different patients is "interpatient" registration. Inter-patient registration generally requires nonrigid transformation.

After image registration, information from multiple images can be fused into a single combined fusion image. The fusion can be accomplished by simply summing intensity values in two images, by imposing outlines from one view over the intensity of the other, or by encoding two images in different color channels. Image fusion provides a way to correlate different features of anatomic structures and functions from multiple images. Registration of images of the same patient at different times can be used to evaluate dynamic patterns of structural change during brain development, tumor growth, or degenerative disease processes.

Various image registration methods have been developed using different features to align two datasets, including point-, surface-, and intensity-based methods. Point- and surface-based methods make use of landmarks extracted from the images,

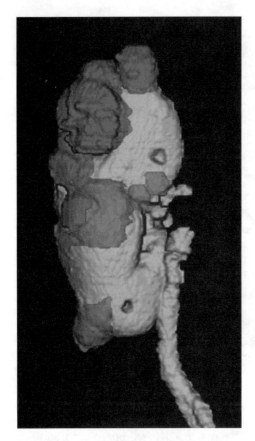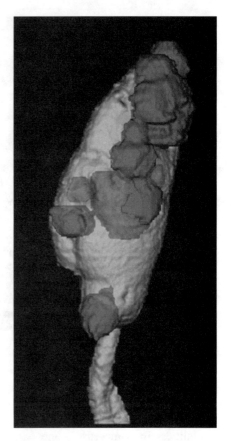

Figure 11 Volume rendering of a kidney with tumors. Darker regions are tumors. *Source*:
Courtesy of Ingmar Bitter. (*See color insert.*)

while intensity-based methods involve the optimization of a similarity measure of the
image intensities.

Point-Based Registration

Point-based registration involves determination of the coordinates of corresponding
landmark points in both images and estimation of a geometrical transformation
using these corresponding points (31). The landmark points may be either intrinsic
or extrinsic to the patient. Intrinsic points are derived from naturally occurring
features, for example, anatomic landmark points. Extrinsic points are derived
from artificially placed markers or fiducials. The landmark points should be
discernible in both images and the correspondence between landmark points should
be established.

Landmark points need to be accurately localized by an interactive identification
process or an automated algorithm. Optical or magnetic tracking devices are used to
localize the fiducial points in some applications such as image-guided therapy (32).

Point-based registration is computed by solving a least squared equation to
minimize the fiducial registration error, that is, the root-mean squared error of the
corresponding landmark points. The algorithm for direct computation of the
transformation involves alignment of centroids of the two point sets, followed by

transformation to minimize the sum of squared distance between the two point sets, which can be achieved by matrix manipulations using the singular value decomposition (SVD) method (33,34). The locations of three noncolinear point landmarks are sufficient to establish a rigid transformation (translation and rotation). The transformation that aligns the corresponding fiducial points is used to register the two images.

Point-based registration can usually achieve high accuracy, but requires the placement of markers or manual identification of anatomic landmarks. Point-based registration is mostly employed in image-guided surgery to register preoperative images with intraoperative images, where tracking devices are often used to localize manually placed fiducials (35).

Surface-Based Registration

Surface-based registration relies on the 3D boundary surfaces of anatomic structures presented in the images for alignment. Surface-based registration is similar to point-based registration except that much more information is involved and point correspondences are not available. The general approach is to search iteratively for the transformation that minimizes the distance between two surfaces, which are represented as triangular patches made up of large numbers of points. The methods to extract 3D surfaces from images were introduced in the section entitled Image Display and Visualization.

Several algorithms have been proposed to align two surfaces, including the "head and hat" algorithm, and the iterative closest point (ICP) technique (36,37). In the ICP technique, the surface from one dataset is the "data" shape X, and the surface from the other dataset is the "model" shape Y. The ICP technique is as follows:

(i) For every point $\{x_i\}$ in the "data" shape X, find its closest projective point $\{y_i\}$ on the "model" shape Y. N is the total number of points in the "data" shape.

(ii) Minimize the target registration error (TRE) between $\{x_i\}$ and $\{y_i\}$. Solve

$$\min \arg\left(\sum_i^N |Rx_i + t - y_i|^2\right) \tag{4}$$

to get an optimal transformation (R,t) to bring $\{x_i\}$ closer to $\{y_i\}$, here R is rotation and t is translation.

(iii) Update the point set $\{x_i\} = \{Rx_i + t\}$

(iv) Repeat step (1) to (3) until the average distance between $\{x_i\}$ and $\{y_i\}$ is smaller than a threshold value.

Instead of using points on the surface, some methods used the geometric features (such as ridge curves) on the surface for registration (38). Figure 11 demonstrates surface based registration using ICP techniques. The images are from two craniofacial CT studies of a patient with fibrous dysplasia, a bone disorder. The images were taken about one year apart. The exterior surface of the skull was extracted and registered. Then the CT volume is transformed using the obtained registration (39). The first row in Figure 12 shows the registration process of the skull surface. The second row in the figure shows the alignment process of one axial slice of the images. The two slice images are displayed in a checkerboard pattern with one image on odd numbered grids and the other on even numbered grids.

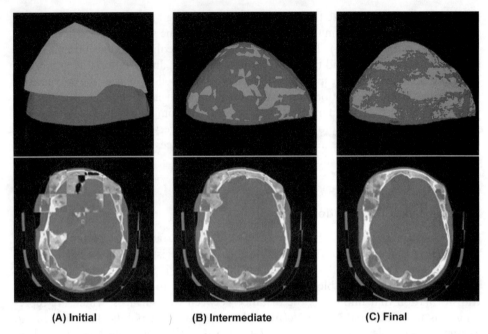

(A) Initial   **(B) Intermediate**   **(C) Final**

Figure 12 Surface-based registration of craniofacial CT images. (*Top row*) Registration process of skull surfaces. (*Bottom row*) Alignment process of CT images.

Surface-based registration uses more anatomic information than just a few landmarks in point-based registration, so it is more robust. However, constructing the surface from medical images is not trivial and frequently requires manual editing.

Intensity-Based Registration

Intensity-based registration involves computing a transformation between two datasets based on pixel or voxel intensity values. The premise of intensity-based registration is that if two images are well aligned, they will look similar to one another. More explicitly, if one image is resampled to the grid of the other image, the image intensities at each voxel should be similar. Several intensity similarity measures have been proposed to quantify the degree of similarity between two images, including normalized image subtraction, normalized cross correlation, entropy of difference image, gradient correlation, pattern intensity, gradient difference, and mutual information (40–42). Registration is achieved when the similarity measure reaches the global maximum. The maximization of similarity measure is a nonlinear optimization problem, which can be solved using standard mathematical approaches such as Powell's method, and Levenburg-Marquardt method (34).

Most intensity-based image registrations assume that there is a linear functional relationship between pixel values of two images. However, if two images are formed using very different beam energies or from different imaging modalities (inter-modality registration), a functional relationship between pixel values may not exist. "Mutual information" similarity measure was proposed to address this problem, which came from the information theory (42). The measure is based on the similarity of probability distributions (intensity histograms), which does not assume linear intensity functional relationship. The mutual information measure

(*S*) is given by

$$S = \frac{\sum_{x,y} p_{1,2}(x,y) \log p_{1,2(x,y)}}{p_1(x)p_2(y)} \tag{5}$$

where $p_1(x)$ and $p_2(y)$ are probability distributions in respective images, $p_{1,2(x,\,y)}$ is the joint probability distribution, and x and y are intensity values. Mutual information has been found very effective in multimodal image registration between modalities such as MR, PET, and CT.

Intensity-based registration has the advantage that the entire image volume is used in establishing the correspondence. The methods can be automatic but are usually very slow because of large amount of information involved in the computation.

Nonrigid Registration

Nonlinear spatial transformations are often needed for interpatient registration and intrapatient registration over time. The registration needs to reflect the variability in the anatomic features between different individuals and changes with time, including differences in shape and size as well as differences in internal density distribution.

One class of nonrigid registration is based on the deformation field computed from landmarks identified within the images. The process is accomplished in two steps—global matching achieved by alignment of landmarks, followed by local deformation based on viscous fluid, piecewise affine transformation, or optical flow (43–45).

Another class of nonrigid registration is based on statistical models derived from a population of patients. In this method, a statistical model consisting of an average instance and its statistical variability is first computed from training datasets (7,46). The registration is accomplished by a statistical optimization of the state of the statistical model. The average instance is warped within its statistical range to match the structure of interest. The statistical model serves as a common reference for the registration. Once both images are registered to the statistical model, the transformation between them can be derived.

2D–3D Registration

2D–3D registration is a special category of image registration where 3D images such as CT, MR are brought into alignment with 2D images such as X-ray fluoroscopy, ultrasound images, and video images. CT and MR images are frequently used in clinical diagnosis and surgical planning, but their use as interventional imaging modalities has been limited because of the expense and space within the operating room. Common modalities for guiding surgical interventions are X-ray fluoroscopes or ultrasound devices. These images are acquired in real time, but only present 2D information. A number of important anatomical features cannot be visualized well in 2D images, such as relative 3D location and orientation of anatomic structures. One method to provide 3D information during the intervention is to register and fuse preoperative 3D images with 2D intraoperative images (47).

In typical 2D–3D registration, the 3D images are projected to the 2D planes where the 2D images are taken. The projection images are then compared with 2D images to evaluate the alignment. The position and orientation of the 3D image volume is then updated until its projections reach optimal match with the 2D images.

Similar to 3D–3D registrations, landmark points, surfaces, and pixel intensities can be used for the 2D–3D registration (48).

Relevance to Tumor Imaging

One task in tumor imaging is to evaluate the tumor growth and monitor treatment. Two images acquired over time need to be registered before they can be used for quantitative comparison.

Tumors are often distinguished by their unique physiological properties such as vascular permeability. Functional imaging modalities such as PET and DCE MRI are used to study tumor physiology. However, these functional images are usually lower in resolution and do not display anatomy well. High-resolution images such as CT are needed to view the structures. The registration between functional images and structural images will present both functional activity and anatomic structure in the same view.

In some dynamic imaging studies, where multiple sequences of images need to be taken at different phases of the contrast injection, the patient might move between image sequences. This movement might compromise the accuracy of image analysis. The registration between different sequences of images in the same study can offset the patient movement, which is also called motion correction. Image subtraction may be applied after the motion correction to show the change of contrast agents in the tissues.

COMPUTER-AIDED DIAGNOSIS/DETECTION

Computer-aided diagnosis/detection (CAD) can be defined as a diagnosis made by radiologists using the output of a computerized image analysis as an aid. The computer system acts as a "second reader" by screening the studies and pointing out abnormalities. The final judgment is made by a radiologist. CAD can help improve sensitivity by detecting lesions that might be missed by radiologists.

Figure 13 is the block diagram of a CAD system. A typical CAD system has two phases: training phase and diagnosis phase. In the training phase, a set of training data is first collected. Then radiologist's diagnostic knowledge is applied to analyze the training data and to derive diagnosis rules. In the diagnosis phase, clinical images are taken as input. An image segmentation step is then performed to extract structures of interest. Shape and density features of the structures are computed. A set of features is then selected and fed into a classifier. By using the diagnosis rules obtained in the training phase, the classifier distinguishes actual lesions from false lesions, and hopefully, malignant lesions from benign lesions. The preliminary diagnosis is then reported prior to a final diagnosis.

Features for classification include those traditionally used by radiologists and higher-order features, which may not be very intuitive. Potential features include shape features such as circularity, spherelarity, compactness, irregularity, and elongation, or density features such as contrast, roughness, and texture attributes. Different diagnostic tasks require different sets of useful features. Feature selection techniques, such as forward stepwise methods and genetic algorithms, are applied in the training phase to choose useful feature sets (49). Several classifiers have been proposed for different applications, including linear discriminant analysis, Bayesian methods, artificial neural network, and support vector machine (50).

The quality of a CAD system can be characterized by the sensitivity and specificity of the diagnosis. Sensitivity refers to the fraction of diseased cases

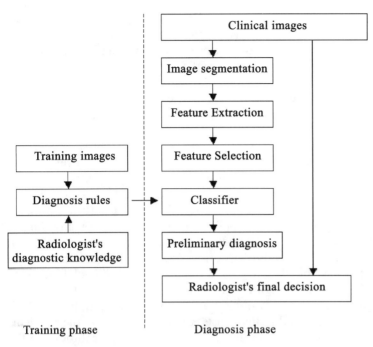

Figure 13 Block diagram of computer-aided diagnosis.

correctly identified as positive in the system (true positive fraction, TPF). Specificity refers to the fraction of disease-free cases correctly identified as negative. "Receiver operating characteristic" (ROC) curves are used to describe the relationship between sensitivity and specificity. The ROC curves show the true-positive fraction (TPF = sensitivity) versus the false-positive fraction (FPF = 1 – specificity). In addition to ROC curves, Free-response ROC (FROC) curves (TPF versus false positive per images) were proposed to more accurately represent the number of false positive detections (51). The area under the ROC and FROC curve is a measure of the quality of a CAD system. There is a trade-off between specificity and sensitivity. A successful CAD system should detect as many true lesions as possible meanwhile rejecting as many false positives as possible.

The applications of CAD include the detection of breast microcalcification and mass, pulmonary nodule, and colon polyps. CAD systems are especially useful for the screening of diseases, where a large volume of low incidence examinations need to be screened rapidly. Several companies are currently developing commercial CAD software in mammography, chest radiography and chest CT. R2 Technology Inc's ImageChecker CAD system has received FDA approval for clinical use.

CAD involves all other aspects of image processing techniques. For instance, image segmentation and registration are necessary for feature extraction, and image visualization and measurement are essential for clinical presentation.

DISCUSSION AND CONCLUSION

Medical imaging has become an essential component in many fields of biomedical research and clinical practice. For example, radiologists identify and quantify tumors from MRI and CT images, and neuroscientists detect regional metabolic brain activity from PET and MRI images. Analysis of medical images requires sophisticated image processing techniques. In this chapter, we described several medical image processing fields and emphasized their relevance to tumor imaging researches. The purpose of image segmentation is to localize the tumor regions; image measurement is to quantify the tumor properties; image visualization is to provide intuitive ways to present the tumor; image registration is to fuse two images so that different tumor properties can be combined in one view; finally, CAD could be used in the clinical diagnosis/detection of tumors.

There are quite a few medical image processing and analysis software packages available, both for clinical practices and research activities. Major medical imaging device companies routinely provide high-level image processing workstations to be sold with their imaging equipment. A number of open source or freeware image processing suites are also available. For example, MIPAV is a free software package developed at NIH (52). It is a Java-based application, which can run on any computer platform. MIPAV incorporates a lot of advanced image processing techniques in its package. Insight Segmentation and Registration Toolkit (ITK) is an open-source software package developed by several groups organized by National Library of Medicine. It includes cutting-edge segmentation and registration algorithms.

Medical image processing is a multidisciplinary application area, which involves radiologists, scientists, and technologists. Clinicians recognize the problems and applications during their daily clinical practice. Scientists find solutions to the problems and customize existing tools or develop new tools for the applications. Technologists use the image processing tools to process the clinical images. Radiologists apply the image processing outcome in the diagnosis.

Medical image processing has evolved into an established discipline. It is a very active and fast-growing field. Image processing techniques have already shown great potential in detecting and analyzing tumors in clinical images and this trend will undoubtedly continue into the future.

ACKNOWLEDGMENTS

The author thanks Betty Wise and Ingmar Bitter for providing some of the images in this chapter.

REFERENCES

1. Rogowska J. Overview and fundamentals of medical image segmentation. In: Bankman IN, ed. Handbook of Medical Imaging, Processing and Analysis, Academic Press, 2000.
2. Rosenfeld A, Kak AC. Digital image processing. Academic Press, 1982.
3. Adams R, Bischof L. Seeded region growing. IEEE Trans Pattern Anal Mach Intell 1994; 16:641–647.
4. Vince L, Soille P. Watersheds in digital spaces: an efficient algorithm based on immersion simulations. IEEE Trans Pattern Anal Mach Intell 1991; 13(6):583–598.
5. Dawant BM, Zijdenbos AP. Image segmentation. In: Sonka, M and Fitzpatrick, JM, eds. Handbook of Medical Imaging. Medical Image Processing and Analysis. Vol. 2. SPIE, 2000.
6. Xu C, Pham DL, Prince J. Finding the brain cortex using fuzzy segmentation, isosurface, and deformable surface models. The XVth International Conference on Information Processing in Medical Imaging (IPMI), 1997.

7. Cootes TF, Beeston C, et al. A Unified Framework for Atlas Matching Using Active Appearance Models. IPMI, Springer, 1999.
8. Kass M, Witkin A, Terzopoulos D. Snakes: active contour models. Int J Comput Vision 1988:321–331.
9. Barrett WA, Mortensen EN. Interactive live-wire boundary extraction. Med Image Anal 1996; 1(4):331–341.
10. Rangayyan RM, El-Faramawy NM, Desautels JE, Alim OA. Measures of acutance and shape classification of breast tumors. IEEE Trans Med Imaging 1997; 16:799–810.
11. Weisstein EW. CRC Concise Encyclopedia of Mathematics. 2nd ed. Chapman & Hall, 2003.
12. Bankman IN, Spisz TS, Pavlopoulos S. Two-Dimensional Shape and Texture Quantification. In: Bankman IN, ed. Handbook of Medical Imaging, Processing and Analysis. Academic Press, 2000:215–230.
13. Richolt JA, Hata N, et al. Three-dimensional bone angle quantification. In: Bankman IN, ed. Handbook of Medical Imaging, Processing and Analysis. Academic Press, 2000.
14. Basset O, Sun Z, Mestas JL, Gimenez G. Texture analysis of ultrasonic images of the prostate by means of co-occurrence matrices. Ultrason Imaging 1993; 15:218–237.
15. Thiele DL, Kimme-Smith C, Johnson TD, McCombs M, Bassett LW. Using tissue texture surrounding calcification clusters to predict benign versus malignant outcomes. Med Physics 1996; 23:549–555.
16. Grampp S, Genant H, et al. Comparison of noninvasive bone mineral measurements in assessing age-related loss, fracture discrimination, and diagnostic classification. J Bone Miner Res 1997; 12:697–711.
17. Yaffe MJ, Byng JW, Boyd NF. Quantitative image analysis for estimation of breast cancer risk. In: Bankman IN, ed. Handbook of Medical Imaging, Processing and Analysis. Academic Press: 2000:323–340.
18. Chen CC, Daponte JS, Fox MD. Fractal feature analysis and classification in medical imaging. IEEE Trans Med Imaging 1989; 8:183–189.
19. Brix G, Semmler W, et al. Pharmocokinetic parameters in CNS Gd-DTPA enhanced MR Imaging. J Comput Assist Tomogr 1991; 15(4):621–628.
20. Alexander JO, Choyke P, Yao J. Evaluation of prostate cancer with dynamic contrast enhanced MRI for the diagnosis of prostate cancer: a comparison of analytic techniques. Toronto, canada: ISMRM, 2003.
21. Therasse P, Arbuck SG, Eisenhauer EA, et al. New guidelines to evaluate the response to treatment in solid tumors. J Natl Cancer Inst 2000; 92(3):205–216.
22. Robb R. Three-Dimensional Biomedical Imaging—Principles and Practice. New York: VCH Publishers, 1994.
23. Schroeder W, Martin K, Lorensen B. The Visualization Toolkit. Prentice Hall, 1998.
24. Gueziec A. Extracting surface models of the anatomy from medical images. In: Sonka M, Fitzpatrick JM, eds. Handbook of Medical Imaging. Medical Image Processing and Analysis. Vol. 2. SPIE, 2000.
25. Lorensen W, Cline H. Marching cubes: a high resolution 3D surface construction algorithm. Comput Graph 1987; 21:163–169.
26. Meyers D, Skinner S, Sloan K. Surfaces from contours. ACM Trans Graph 1992; 11(3):228–258.
27. Boissonnat JD, Geiger B. Three dimensional reconstruction of complex shapes based on the Delaunay triangulation. Le Chesnay, France: Inst Nat Recherche Inf Autom (INRIA), 1992.
28. Levoy M. Efficient ray tracing of volume data. SIGGRAPH, 1993.
29. Lacroute P. Fast volume rendering using a shear-warp factorization of the viewing transformation. Computer Science. StanfordCalifornia1995.
30. LaRose D. Iterative X-ray/CT registration using accelerated volume rendering. Robotics Institute. Pittsburgh, PA: Carnegie Mellon University, 2001:150.

31. Maurer CR, Aboutanos GB, et al. Registration of 3-D images using weighted geometrical features. IEEE Trans Med Imaging 1996; 15(6):836–849.

32. Ulrich Wiesel AL, Martin Boerner, Hagen Skibbe. ROBODOC(R) at BGU Frankfurt—experiences with the pinless system. Computer Assisted Orthopaedic Surgery (CAOS)/ USA. Pittsburgh: Shadyside Hospital, 1999.

33. Arun KS, Huang TS, Blostein SD. Least-squares fitting of two 3-D point sets. IEEE Trans Pattern Anal Mach Intell 1987; 9(5):698–700.

34. Press WH, Teukolsky SA, et al. Numerical Recipes in C. 2nd ed. Cambridge University Press, 1992.

35. Yao J, Taylor RH, et al. A progressive cut refinement scheme for revision total hip replacement surgery using c-arm fluoroscopy. Medical Image Computing and Computer Assisted Intervention—MICCAI '99. Cambridge, UK: Springer, 1999.

36. Pelizzari CA, Chen G, et al. Accurate three-dimensional registration of CT, PET, and/or MR images of the brain. J Comput Assist Tomogr 1989; 13:20–26.

37. Besl PJ, McKay ND. A method for registration of 3-D shapes. IEEE Trans Pattern Anal Mach Intell 1992; 14(2):239–256.

38. Subsol G, Thirion JP, Ayache N. In: A general scheme for automatically building 3D morphometric anatomical atlas: application to a skull atlas. France: INRIA, 1995.

39. Butman J, Yao J, et al. Dynamic remodeling of bone in fibrous dysplasia on series craniofacial CT. ASNR, Washington, D.C., 2003.

40. Van Den Elsen P, Pol E, et al. Grey value correlation techniques used for automatic matching of CT and MR volume images of the head. Medical Imaging. SPIE, 1994.

41. Studholme C, Hill D, Hawkes D. Multiresolution voxel similarity measures for MR-PET registration. IPMI 1995, 1995.

42. Wells W, Viola P, et al. Multi-modal volume registration by maximization of mutual information. Med Image Anal 1996; 1:35–51.

43. Haller J, Christensen GE, et al. Hippocampal MR imaging morphometry by means of general pattern matching. Radiology 1996; 199:787–791.

44. Christensen G. Consistent linear-elastic transformations for image matching. Information Processing in Medical Imaging 1999.

45. Joshi SC, Miller MI. Landmark matching via large deformation diffeomorphisms. IEEE Trans Image Proc 2000; 9(8):1357–1370.

46. Chen M, Kanade T, et al. 3-D Deformable registration of medical images using a statistical atlas. Pittsburgh, PA: Carnegie Mellon University, 1998.

47. Yao J, Taylor R. Deformable registration between a statistical bone density atlas and X-ray images. International CAOS 2002.

48. Penney GP, Weese J, et al. A comparison of similarity measures for use in 2D/3D medical image registration. IEEE Trans Med Imaging 1998; 17(4):586–595.

49. Jain A, Zongker D. Feature selection: evaluation, application, and small sample performance. IEEE Trans Pattern Anal Mach Intell 1997; 19(2):153–158.

50. Giger ML, Huo Z, et al. Computer-aided diagnosis in mammography. In: Sonka M, Fitzpatrick JM, eds. Handbook of Medical Imaging, Volume 2. Medical Image Processing and Analysis. SPIE, 2000.

51. Bowyer KW. Validation of medical image analysis techniques. In: Sonka M, Fitzpatrick JM, eds. Handbook of Medical Imaging, Vol. 2. Medical Image Processing and Analysis. SPIE, 2000.

52. McAuliffe M, Lalonde F, et al. Medical Image Processing, Analysis & Visualization in Clinical Research. IEEE Computer-Based Medical Systems (CBMS), 2001:381–386.

6
Advances in Radiotherapy Planning

Cynthia Ménard, Deborah Citrin, and Kevin Camphausen
Radiation Oncology Branch, CCR, NCI, NIH, DHHS, Bethesda, Maryland, U.S.A.

James Deye and Norman C. Coleman
Radiation Oncology Sciences Program, NCI, NIH, DHHS, Bethesda, Maryland, U.S.A.

Robert C. Susil
Department of Biomedical Engineering, Johns Hopkins University Schoool of Medicine, Baltimore, Maryland, U.S.A.

A Note from the Editors

*R*adiotherapy has traditionally made use of only the most basic image guidance. Recent advances, however, have made radiotherapy the most advanced form of image guided therapy. New dosimetry software enables three-dimensional conformal therapy to be performed with external beam or with brachytherapy. Fiducial markers, which are implanted prior to therapy, allow real-time motion correction to minimize non-target therapy. Recent advances in magnetic resonance imaging (MRI) and computed tomography (CT) guided brachytherapy promise to improve the delivery of high dose rate therapy to the desired target while significantly reducing side effects caused by undesired damage to normal tissue.

INTRODUCTION

Radiation therapy is a leading example for the use of image guidance in localized cancer therapy. Since the discovery of the therapeutic benefits of ionizing radiation more than 100 years ago, great technical advances have been made in the field. A desired radiation dose profile can now be delivered with exceptional precision to targets defined by the radiation oncologist. Advances in imaging technologies result in a more accurate delineation of the target for radiation treatments, whereby clinicians can safely decrease the margin of normal tissue included in radiation treatment fields to account for target uncertainty. Decreasing the margins, and in effect the amount of normal tissue treated, allows for dose escalation and the potential for higher rates of cure with equivalent or reduced normal tissue complications. With technical advances in radiation delivery, defining the target, moreover, the dose required for tumor cure has become a predominant area of uncertainty.

Radiation therapy planning and delivery is a rapidly evolving field, clearly driven by advances in computer and imaging technology. It is the objective of this chapter to elucidate general concepts of radiation therapy, describe modern techniques in treatment planning, and identify opportune areas for imaging contributions in radiation therapy.

EXTERNAL BEAM PHOTON THERAPY (TELETHERAPY)

Teletherapy means therapy at a distance, and constitutes the primary noninvasive treatment modality in radiation oncology. Linear accelerators are designed to deliver high-energy photon treatments to a fixed point in three-dimensional (3D) space known as the isocenter. In most cases, the patient is positioned such that the target volume is located at the isocenter. The design of the linear accelerator and treatment room includes a gantry, which can rotate 360° around the isocenter in an axial direction, a table that can angle the patient in a plane parallel to the floor of the treatment room, and a collimator rotating 360° perpendicular to the track of the beam (1). Combining table movements with gantry angulation, results in near total freedom of rotation around the isocenter, allowing for an infinite combination of beam arrangements (Fig. 1). Modern linear accelerators can achieve very high levels of precision in targeting the isocenter (2). The isocenter is projected by lasers, which are visible on the patient's skin. As more beams are added to a treatment plan, the ability to conform to the target while lowering dose to surrounding normal tissue increases, with the high-dose region limited to the intersection of the beams.

Conformal Radiation Therapy

Treatment plans based on two-dimensional (2D) multislice images sets, such as computed tomography (CT) images, allow for 3D conformal radiation therapy (3D-CRT). With this technology, organs and targets are defined within 3D space, and the dosimetrist can generate digitally reconstructed radiographs (DRRs) from CT datasets with important target and nontarget volumes, projected at near infinite variations of patient and machine positions. These DRRs, also known as "beam's eye views" (As they are constructed from the perspective of the treatment beam projected through the patient), allow more rapid determination of optimal treatment angle, and simplify the use of complex beam arrangements (Fig. 2). They also provide a reference against which

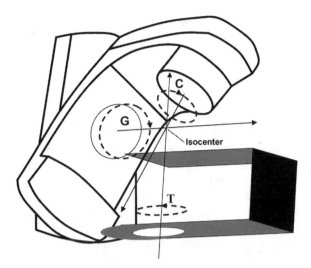

Figure 1   Linear accelerator geometry. The collimator (**C**), gantry (**G**), and table (**T**) rotational axes intersect at the mechanical isocenter. The table surface translates in three dimensions (superior-inferior, anterior-posterior, and right-left) to permit alignment of the mechanical and patient isocenter.

radiographic films ("portal" films), generated from a given treatment beam can be compared. "Conformation" of a given beam to the target is achieved with the aid of a multileaf collimator (MLC). This device consists of two panels of multiple opposing lead "leaves," which enter the path of the radiation beam to block the radiation in their

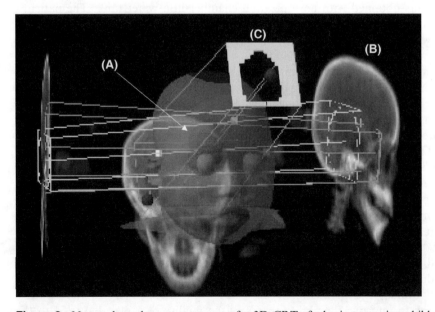

Figure 2   Noncoplanar beam arrangement for 3D-CRT of a brain tumor in a child. Note that radiation beams travel above and behind the eyes to converge on the target (**A**). DRRs (**B**) from a projected beam position can be compared with digital radiographs (portal films) obtained at the time of treatment. MLC (**C**) conforms to the shape of the target for a given beam orientation.

shadow. The shape of the "unblocked" beam can, therefore, closely conform to the shape of the target (Fig. 2).

Intensity-Modulated Radiation Therapy

Although 3D-CRT can precisely conform to a given target volume, it cannot readily create convex high-dose regions, nor can it ultimately control the profile of high-dose within the target. This can only be achieved with intensity modulation of treatment beams, which results in highly conformal treatments with a near perfect match between the high-dose area and the complex shape of the target (3).

The computer-driven movements of the MLC leaves can be adjusted to allow for longer or shorter durations in the path of the beam, and as a result, modulate the intensity of the radiation profile for a given beam orientation. In dynamic intensity-modulated radiation therapy (IMRT), the MLC leaves are moved while the beam is in the "on" position. In static IMRT ("step and shoot"), the beam is turned "off" while the leaves are moving, and turned on again when each new MLC leaf configuration is achieved. As more beams are added to the treatment plan, each with the appropriate modulation, the ability to shape the dose around the target improves (4). The result of IMRT is a highly conformal high-dose region with rapid dose fall-off that can "bend" into areas of convexity in the target, adhere closely to complex borders, and shape the high-dose profile within the target as desired (Fig. 3A) (3).

Radiation Dosimetry

Absorbed radiation dose is defined in Gray (Gy), which describes the amount of energy (Joule) absorbed in a mass of tissue (kg) (5,6). Dose calculations in patients have been conventionally based on empirical models, and derived from physical dose measurements obtained with an ionization chamber in a water tank. The patient's radiation absorption and scattering characteristics are then assumed to approximate that of a water tank, and corrections are applied to account for differences in shape and tissue densities (such as bone and air), which impact on the attenuation of the photon beam. These two variables can be measured directly from the patient's CT scan. More sophisticated calculation engines are now being investigated and integrated in treatment planning systems, including Monte Carlo techniques. Monte Carlo calculations use statistical sampling techniques and measured photon interaction cross-sections to obtain a probabilistic approximation of dose. They require high computational power, as high accuracy calculations require the tracking of as many as 10^8 incident photons (7).

Calculated dose profiles in a given treatment plan are displayed on the corresponding planning CT images with isodose lines that connect all points on the image that encompass a specified dose. These isodoses appear similar to a topographical map, with gradations of dose represented by higher and lower isodose lines. Such a presentation allows the clinician to readily choose a plan that treats the intended target and protects normal structures. One limitation of the standard isodose presentation is that it is typically in a single plane, thus multiple slices must be reviewed to completely evaluate the plan (Fig. 3A).

Efforts to improve the ability to assess the quality of a plan have led to the development of the dose–volume histogram (DVH) (8). The histogram graphically depicts both dose and volume information for normal organs or target structures of interest. The creation of a DVH begins with the planning software dividing each

(A)

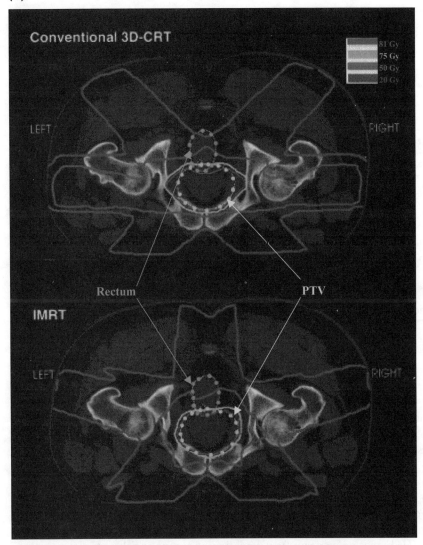

Figure 3 (A) Dose distributions of treatment plans designed for a patient with prostate cancer. Note the improved conformality of the PTV coverage by the 75 and 81 Gy isodose lines in the IMRT plan. Also, note that the 50 Gy isodose line avoids the femoral heads in the IMRT plan. **(B)** DVH of the CTV, rectal wall, bladder wall, and femoral heads displayed for the treatment plans shown in Figure 3A. *Source:* From Ref. 78. (*Continued on next page.*)

volume into multiple equal subvolumes (voxels) and the total dose into equal increments. The software then determines how many voxels of a specified organ receive each level of dose. In a cumulative DVH, the percent volume of a structure is plotted against each incremental dose. This allows the clinician an opportunity to evaluate an anatomical structure in its entirety, with better ability to determine if there is adequate coverage of the target and sparing of normal tissues. Cumulative DVHs can also allow a clinician to compare various plans more readily by comparing the DVHs for each anatomical structure of interest (Fig. 3B).

(B)

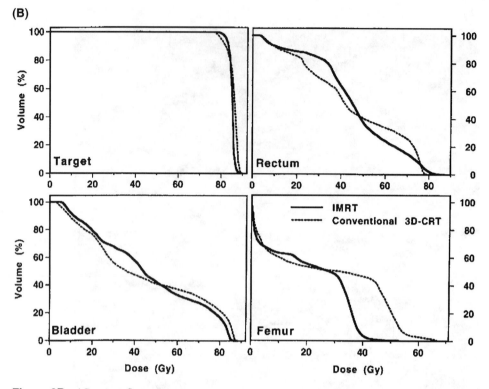

Figure 3B (*Continued*)

The widespread availability of treatment planning software with DVH capability has led to significant improvements in the ability to predict the probability of a normal-tissue complication, and has allowed clinicians to adjust treatment fields to reduce the probability of morbidity and complications (9,10). For example, extensive data exists regarding a correlation between the percentage of lung receiving radiation more than 20 Gy and the likelihood of life-threatening radiation pneumonitis (11). Clinicians continue to investigate the possibility of extending the predictive value of DVHs to tumor-control probability (12). Note, however, that the potential predictive value of DVHs hinges on an accurate delineation of organs at risk or target structures of interest, and precise day-to-day setup reproducibility.

Inverse Planning

The ability to deliver highly conformal treatment relies on the ability to determine the optimal combination of beams, arcs, and modulation for each individual case. With the advent of technologies such as IMRT, in which an infinite combination of beams or arcs can be combined with an infinite variety of modulation patterns, inverse planning has become essential.

Radiation treatment planning has traditionally utilized "forward planning," a method by which beam arrangements and modification devices are chosen based on clinical experience. Optimization of the dose distribution is made with sequential adjustments of the beam angle field sizes and the modification devices, until a clinically acceptable dose distribution is accomplished. This trial and error technique can generate clinically acceptable treatment plans for simple beam arrangements; however, with increasing number of beams and modulating capabilities, it is unrealistic to expect an optimal plan to be generated in a reasonable timeframe or in a consistent manner using iterative "forward planning."

Advancements in computer planning technology have led to the development of "inverse planning," in which a computerized algorithm determines the optimal modulation pattern. Desired dose goals for target tissues and dose constraints for nontarget tissues are defined by the clinician along with the relative importance of each dose goal or constraint, and the tolerance for higher or lower doses within each organ or tissue. The computerized algorithm is then used to determine the optimal method for delivering this dose within the constraints that have been defined. Although the planning solutions derived in this manner are not typically intuitive, the result of inverse treatment planning is an optimized, highly conformal treatment plan produced in a time-efficient manner, which takes into account the relative importance of the normal and target tissues within the treatment field (13).

Delivery

Immobilization

To accurately deliver treatments to the intended target, the patient must be immobilized in a comfortable and reproducible position. Immobilization of the trunk and extremities is often accomplished with the aid of vacuum-molded bags of polystyrene beads or polyurethane foam molds which can be customized to each patient. Masks of thermal plastic materials, which become compliant when heated can be applied to the head and neck, and secured to the treatment couch or head holder to ensure reproducibility of neck flexion and head position.

Once immobilized with one of these aids, the table and patient position can be adjusted such that the surface marks previously drawn on the patient at the time of treatment planning "line up" with the laser projection of the isocenter in the treatment room. This technique assumes that the anatomical target is in a constant relationship to the surface reference marks, which can often lead to inaccuracies. Thus, additional techniques are required to improve the accuracy of isocenter targeting.

Verification and Localization

At the outset and through a course of radiotherapy, plain radiographs of all treatment fields are obtained on the treatment unit to verify the location of the isocenter in reference to bony landmarks and to compare against planning DRRs. These radiographs can now be generated digitally, and verified by the clinician prior to delivery of the treatment. Although this step improves the setup accuracy achieved with surface marks alone (14,15), it does not account for internal organ motion. Motion of organs and targets in relation to bony structures is an unavoidable effect of respiration, peristalsis, and weight loss during and between treatments (16). Several techniques have recently been developed to account for interfraction and intrafraction organ motion.

CT portal images or "cone beam CT" is a new technology being evaluated as a mechanism for providing portal images with soft-tissue contrast (17,18). These images can be generated with therapeutic megavoltage (MV) X rays, or with diagnostic kilovoltage X rays from a conventional system mounted at 90 degrees to the

(A)   **(B)**

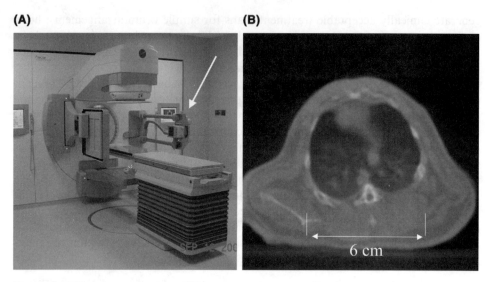

Figure 4 Kilovoltage cone-beam CT system for image-guided radiation therapy. This system (**A**) employs a conventional X-ray source (*arrow*) and state-of-the-art flat-panel detector technology to generate a series (300–600) projection radiographs over 360°. The projections are used to reconstruct a 3D representation of the patient's internal anatomy while in treatment position. This technology has been adapted to the Elekta Synergy RP system. Performance is demonstrated in a small animal with a single axial slice through the reconstructed dataset displayed at lung windows (**B**). *Source*: Courtesy of D. Jaffray, Princess Margaret Hospital, Toronto.

treatment unit on the gantry (Fig. 4) (19). MV CT requires only minor adjustments to the linear accelerators, but results in CT images of a much lower soft-tissue and spatial resolution within a clinically acceptable dose range (20). The benefit of CT imaging is a much more accurate depiction of soft-tissue target location on the treatment unit. Although promising, this imaging technology remains investigational.

Alternatively, transabdominal ultrasound can be utilized in target positioning. The prostate gland is an example of a target that moves significantly between treatments. Changes in bladder and rectal filling can alter the location of the prostate by as much as 2 to 4 mm on a daily basis with occasional displacements of up to 20 mm (21). Daily ultrasound-guided positioning has led to greater certainty of the location of the prostate gland. The location of the treatment field can therefore be adjusted on a daily basis to account for any organ motion. This positioning system is reproducible, noninvasive, and effective for daily localization of the prostate gland (22).

Another option to localize targets at the time of therapy includes the placement of radiopaque markers or "seeds" in the soft-tissue target prior to planning and treatment (23,24). These markers can be readily visualized on planning CT images, DRRs, and portal radiographs. The optimal location of the markers in relation to the isocenter can therefore be known, verified, and adjusted prior to treatment.

Gating Techniques

Movement of organs during a treatment, or intrafraction motion, poses a significant problem for diseases such as lung cancer, where respiration can result in a substantial displacement of tumors. Giraud et al. found a mean displacement of 3 to 4 cm with maximal inspiration and expiration in lung tumors, with a maximal displacement of 7 cm (25). Additional margins of healthy lung are often treated to ensure coverage of the tumor during respiration. This results in higher risks of treatment-related complications, such as pneumonitis.

The simplest method of correcting for respiratory variation is to teach patients "quiet breathing" techniques or breath holding that results in minimal diaphragmatic movement (26–28). Unfortunately, many patients receiving therapy for lung cancer are unable to hold their breath for prolonged periods of time. Another method is respiratory gating. Various gating technologies exist, but typically, a respiratory sensor is placed on the patient, which relays information to the treatment machine. Sensors of respiration include sensors of abdominal wall tension, light-emitting diodes (29), temperature-sensitive thermocouple devices placed in the nostril (30), and infrared sensors (31). The treatment is delivered at defined intervals during the patient's respiratory cycle. The planning CT scan and localization films must also be obtained in the same phase of respiration. Respiratory gating can also been used in treating tumors below the diaphragm, such as liver tumors (32).

Verification of Dose Delivery

Verification of the dose delivered to a patient presents a difficult challenge. As mentioned previously, predicted dose can be calculated with mathematical models that take into account a number of patient and radiation-beam variables. Techniques exist for measuring radiation dose actually delivered to a point on the body surface or in the body cavity, but are impractical for daily use. These include diodes and thermoluminescence dosimeters (TLDs) (33). TLDs are crystalline solids that trap electrons in an excited state after exposure to ionizing radiation. Heating of TLDs following exposure to radiation, results in a luminescence that can be translated to a radiation dose.

Small implantable dosimetry devices are in development and undergoing early clinical trials (34). These devices measure the radiation delivered to a substrate, and relay this information to an electromagnetic sensor placed outside the patient. Much like fiducial markers, they must be surgically implanted prior to treatment, and may migrate during the course of therapy, confounding measurements if they are placed near an area of rapid fall-off in dose. Nonetheless, this technology may help elucidate the relationship between predicted and actual dose delivered for a given patient through a course of therapy, although it will be limited to a few dose points.

"STEREOTACTIC" FORMS OF TELETHERAPY

Stereotaxis is the technique used to localize a target within surrounding normal tissue using a localization device equipped with a fixed fiducial system. These treatment technologies vary in the immobilization device, fiducial system, and dose delivery, but share a common theme of highly conformal therapy delivered to an immobilized target localized with sophisticated imaging. Stereotactic localization is frequently used with single fraction (stereotactic radiosurgery) or fractionated external beam radiation therapy (stereotactic radiotherapy). "Gamma knife" units have numerous radioactive cobalt sources in a hemispherical helmet, aligned so that the sources are all directed at the center of the sphere (35). Sources can be blocked or collimated to produce the desired dose distribution. Alternatively, linear accelerators can be modified to deliver stereotactic treatments, typically with the use of mounted, small multileaf collimators and gantry arc rotations around the isocenter (36).

For most intracranial stereotactic treatments, a rigid headframe is fixed to the patient's skull. The headframe typically includes an attachable fiducial device, which is used to define a coordinate system for target location in reference to the headframe. This fiducial system allows the translation of 2D CT or magnetic resonance imaging (MRI) data into a 3D volume that can be localized in reference to the headframe, and treatments planned in reference to the headframe. During treatment delivery, the headframe is fixed to the treatment table, ensuring the accuracy of alignment and preventing interfraction movement. This system allows for highly accurate delivery, in the order of 1 to 2 mm (36).

Various other forms of stereotactic therapies are in development, including Cyberknife^{TM}, which is a frameless robotic linear accelerator delivery system designed to deliver arcs (37,38). A single treatment with this device can include hundreds or thousands of beams delivered with multiple isocenters, allowing a high degree of conformality with rapid fall-off of dose beyond the target tissue. The system mandates accurate target localization, typically accomplished with implanted fiducial markers.

BRACHYTHERAPY

Brachytherapy, or short-distance therapy, places a small radioactive source inside or in close proximity to the tumor. By virtue of the inverse square law, whereby dose decreases exponentially as the distance from a source increases, a steep dose gradient is achieved, resulting in a highly conformal high-dose region. As such, brachytherapy requires a high level of accuracy and precision in source placement. Permanent seed brachytherapy, which is commonly performed for localized prostate cancer, uses radioactive sources that are permanently implanted in the target volume and deliver doses through the course of their radioactive life. In temporary brachytherapy, source(s) are fed, or "afterloaded" into needles, catheters, or hollow tubes that have been placed in or near the tumor. When the desired dose has been delivered, the source(s) are retracted and the tubes removed from the patient. Brachytherapy can also be classified according to the rate with which dose is delivered, with high-dose rate (HDR) brachytherapy defined as 200 cGy/min or more.

Planning for brachytherapy is simpler than for external beam therapy. The dosimetry is dictated by the photon energies emitted from the radioactive source, and is primarily calculated with the inverse square law (39). However, as the source of radiation is physically closer to the intended target, the location of the target in relation to the source at the time of delivery is more accurate. Planning systems can now perform image-based inverse planning for brachytherapy (40–42). Only two variables (source position and source strength) need to be optimized using computer programs designed to achieve conformal dose to a planning target volume. With HDR brachytherapy, a single high-intensity ^{192}Ir source can be placed at a variety of positions (dwell position) for a desired length of time (dwell time) within each needle, catheter, or applicator tube (Fig. 5). It is important to accurately identify the location of these tubes,

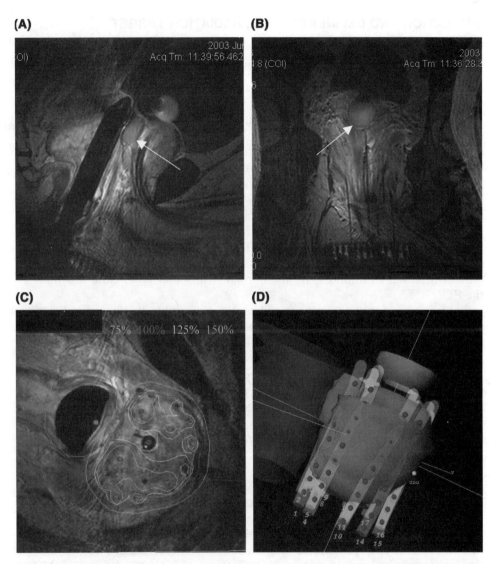

Figure 5 MRI-guided HDR brachytherapy for prostate cancer. (**A**) Sagittal, (**B**) coronal, and (**C**) axial images of the prostate gland after placement of 17 brachytherapy catheters under MRI guidance. Note a well-visualized urachal cyst (*arrow*) that was not perforated during the procedure. Isodose curves (**C**) displayed on axial images demonstrate that the prostate target (*red*) is encompassed by 100% or more of the prescribed dose. (**D**) 3D rendering of the spatial relationship between structures of interest and brachytherapy catheters and source positions (*red: prostate target, fuchsia: urachal cyst, blue: foley catheter balloon, and pink: rectum and endorectal coil*).

as well as the precise location of the first dwell position, as all dwell positions are determined from this reference. There are a number of X-ray and CT "markers" that can be placed inside the tubes during image acquisition, and which help identify the location of the first dwell position on the image. A small, but growing number of commercial brachytherapy devices are now MRI compatible, but no MRI "markers" have yet been developed (Fig. 5).

SIMULATION AND DELINEATING THE RADIATION TARGET

Target Volumes

Compared to the level of precision and accuracy that can be achieved in radiation delivery, target volume delineation remains one of the most important areas of uncertainty and error. The physician must first outline on the planning CT scan a gross tumor volume (GTV), corresponding to any gross tumor that can be felt on physical examination, or visualized with imaging. Following this, a margin of variable size must be added to this volume to define the clinical target volume (CTV). CTV should include those tissues suspected to contain microscopic tumor cells that are not visualized with current imaging techniques. It is estimated depending on histological subtype and anatomical location. Advances in imaging microscopic disease in situ would significantly improve our ability to define the CTV. Finally, a margin that accounts for setup uncertainty and organ motion must be added to the CTV to generate a planning target volume (PTV) (43). By convention, radiation treatment portals are designed with the goal to entirely cover the PTV, deliver a uniform dose distribution to it, and spare the normal tissues that lie in close proximity to the PTV.

Definitions for target volumes will continue to evolve as imaging and delivery techniques improve. The "rule" for dose uniformity within the PTV has been largely a matter of tradition and convention. More recently, there have been suggestions that nonuniformity within the PTV, specifically regions of increased dose, may actually increase the local control. The ability of IMRT to deliver nonuniform dose patterns by design, introduces the concept of "dose sculpting" (44). New terms, such as biological target volume (BTV), have been introduced to describe biological properties of tumors. The BTV could be imaged with novel techniques, reflecting the radiosensitivity of a given tumor subvolume (44).

Computed Tomography

Before computed tomography (CT) was available, target volumes were defined based on surface anatomy, bony anatomy, and intraluminal contrast. Given the uncertainty of the size of tumors, and the location of organs and tumors in relation to bony anatomy, large margins of normal tissues were included to account for these uncertainties and to prevent marginal misses. As CT became available, soft-tissue tumor volumes were localized with more certainty, and they were often translated manually onto the plain films used to set treatment fields. A significant amount of uncertainty remained regarding the location of the target within these constraints (45).

The standard of care for radiation treatment simulation is now CT based. A CT simulator consists of a large bore CT (to accommodate various patient positions and sizes), a flat patient table resembling the linear accelerator treatment tables, triangulation lasers projecting to an isocenter, and specialized software to accomplish virtual planning of potential beam arrangements. CT markers are placed on the patient's body surface at the level of reflection of the triangulation lasers, which are intersecting at the isocenter. This information can then be sent to a treatment planning system for dose calculations.

The distinct advantages of CT simulation include a 3D data set, accuracy of spatial reference, surface contour information, and measurements of the electron density of tissues. Hounsfield units, the CT intensity unit for a given pixel, are directly proportional to tissue electron density, and in effect are also proportional to tissue attenuation and scattering of the photon beam (46). Although vascular and bowel contrast is often helpful in normal tissue and tumor target delineation, it is seldom utilized in CT simulation for fear of invalidating the electron density information derived from Hounsfield units (47). If the benefit of contrast enhancement to delineate the target is deemed important, no inhomogeneity corrections based on CT density are applied to the dosimetric calculation.

Magnetic Resonance Imaging

Magnetic resonance imaging (MRI) offers a 3D dataset, arbitrary imaging planes, and unparalleled soft-tissue contrast, making it the modality of choice for imaging the vast majority of soft-tissue tumors. Because of its greater soft-tissue contrast, MRI has been shown to provide more consistent target delineation than CT for a variety of sites (48–50) and integration of magnetic resonance (MR) images has been shown to reduce interphysician variation, resulting in more reproducible plans (51). Most treatment planning systems permit "fusion" (i.e., deformable registration) of images acquired in MRI scanners with the CT planning images to aid in target delineation. This step has the potential for registration errors and is time consuming.

Performing radiation treatment planning based directly on MRI images, or MRI simulation, could circumvent this step. MRI scanners could be adapted for simulation by adding triangulation lasers and modifying the patient table to be flat. However, there are a number of challenges that must be overcome to perform radiation treatment planning based solely on MRI images. These challenges are the subject of active research and include, (i) the generation of DRRs for treatment verification, (ii) the correction of spatial distortions due to nonuniform magnetic field gradients, (iii) an adaptation of the planning software for tissue inhomogeneity correction, (iv) reproducible immobilization within the constraints of magnet bore size, (v) an imaging field of view which encompasses the entire surface of the patient, and (vi) addressing motion artifacts due to the long scan times.

As previously described, DRRs are required to verify patient setup relative to bony landmarks, on the treatment table. Various approaches have been proposed to generate DRRs from MRI images including automated techniques using a defined range of intensity values on T1-weighted images and manual segmentation of the bones (52). Because the MR dataset does not contain density information, the material within the specified upper/lower threshold can be assigned pseudodensities. This allows dosimetrists to generate MR-based DRRs of the skull. Further research and development are required to adapt current treatment planning software to this technique and extend it to other body sites.

Spatial distortions on MR images are chiefly the result of nonlinear magnetic field gradients (which, ideally should produce magnetic fields that vary linearly with position). In principle, this deviation from linearity is knowable for each scanner architecture and can be accurately corrected. All commercial systems allow users to apply 2D geometric correction algorithms to the image sets (Fig. 6). Correction for error in the third dimension (slice select), is achievable but not readily available on most MRI scanners at this time (53). Note that the magnitude of spatial distortion is directly proportional to the distance from the scanner isocenter, and if not corrected, may introduce a significant error in the spatial allocation of a radiation isocenter, based on surface references which are always located at a radial distance

(A)

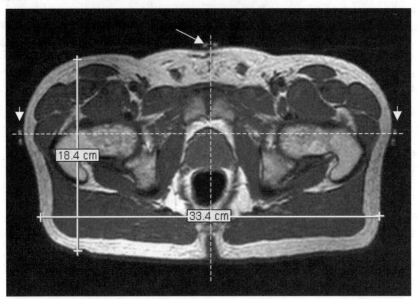

(B)

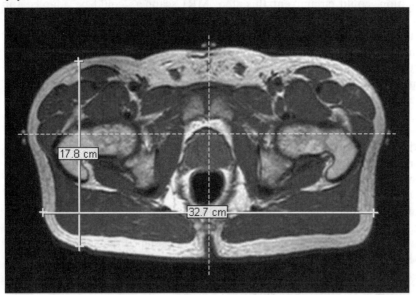

Figure 6 Axial MR simulation images. The isocenter is placed at the level of the prostate gland, and fiducial markers (*arrow*) are placed on the skin at the point of reflection of the triangulation lasers. (**A**) Uncorrected and (**B**) corrected images for gradient nonlinearity show a small difference in the projected location of the isocenter (*dashed line intersection*) and in skin contour measurements.

from the scanner isocenter. This is less of a problem for brachytherapy planning as catheters and tumors are positioned at the scanner isocenter.

Minor patient-induced distortions, such as susceptibility and chemical shift distortions, are not easily corrected. However, early studies have confirmed that the magnitude of radiation dosimetric error introduced by spatial distortion after geometric corrections are applied to MR images, is minimal and comparable to those obtained with CT planning (54,55). Again, more studies are needed to confirm the dosimetry accuracy of MRI simulation and to identify those body sites especially prone to susceptibility and chemical shift distortions.

Unlike CT Hounsfield units, MR images do not contain information related to the electron density of tissues. Attenuation correction for inhomogeneities in tissue electron density is not easily applied to treatment plans generated solely from MR images. However, the electron density of soft tissues is almost identical to that of water, and there is only minimal change in the attenuation of high-energy X rays through bone. The major sources of dosimetric error related to beam attenuation are the lungs and air cavities. Segmenting air cavities and the lungs on MR images, and manually assigning them densities, can easily circumvent majority of the problems (52). In the balance, one must judge whether improvements gained in target delineation accuracy with MRI supersede the small dosimetric error introduced by a lack of attenuation correction for electron density.

In the vast majority of cylindrical high-field MRI systems, patients are placed inside a 60-cm diameter bore. This severely constrains patient position and immobilization, which must be identical between simulation and treatment. Open magnets offer more freedom of positioning and patient size at the cost of much lower magnetic field strengths, and consequently, a lower image quality. Moreover, immobilization devices must be MRI compatible. With careful planning and adaptation, these constrains are easily surmountable for the majority of patients and treatment sites.

The problem of motion artefact is not unique to MRI, and is the subject of much research in radiation delivery as detailed previously. MRI scan times often closely resemble radiation treatment times and may well be better suited for treatment planning than CT "snapshots in time." Moreover, similar or identical solutions to target motion can be applied to both image acquisition and radiation delivery, such as respiratory gating (56). For abdominal images, drugs like glucagon can be administered to temporarily inhibit peristalsis and improve image quality (57). Finally, anatomical movies that can measure the magnitude of organ or target motion for a given patient over time can be acquired with MRI, allowing for a smaller and more accurate margin allocation around the CTV (58).

Beyond its evident advantages in anatomical imaging, MRI promises to be a leading imaging modality in the field of biological imaging. It is beyond the scope of this chapter to review all the emerging techniques in this field. However, a few concepts are especially germane to radiation treatment planning and should be emphasized. First, any MRI technique, from anatomical to molecular, that aids in improving tumor definition stands to significantly improve the quality of radiation treatment. Promising advances in tumor delineation within the prostate gland with magnetic resonance spectroscopic imaging (MRSI) (59) is a good example, whereby clinicians may now preferentially target a predominant tumor nodule for delivery of higher doses (60). Second, imaging techniques, which help to characterize physiological or biological properties of tumors and their subvolumes, may be used to generate a radiosensitivity map, and as such the dose required for tumor cure. For example, this may include maps of hypoxia (61), tumor cell proliferation (62), and angiogenesis (63). Third, MRI examinations can be safely repeated at various intervals throughout a course of radiotherapy and may play a key role in the dynamic adaptation of radiation treatment plans as a tumor responds to therapy.

(A)

(B)

(C)

(D)

(E)

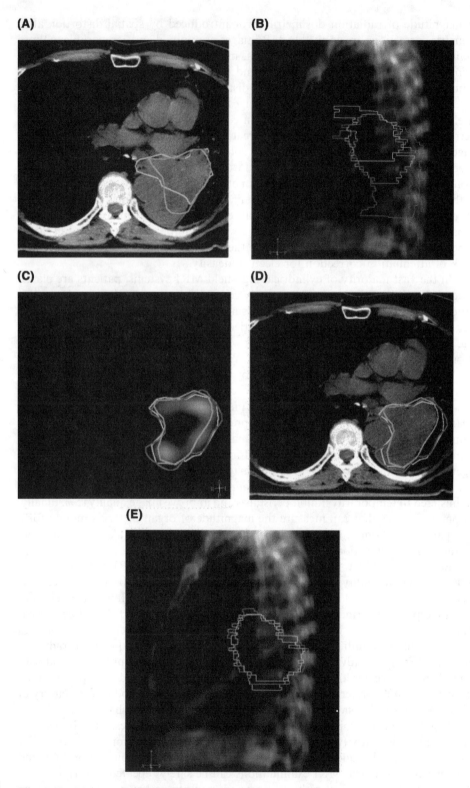

Figure 7 *(Caption on facing page)*

Positron-Emission Tomography

Radiation treatment plans cannot be solely based on positron-emission tomography (PET) (or SPECT) images, which lack key anatomical information such as surface contour and normal tissue definition. However, when registered to CT planning images, they stand to significantly impact the accuracy of target delineation. The main advantage of PET is its unparalleled sensitivity to detect microscopic disease otherwise not visualized. This, in theory, should translate to more accurate definitions of the CTV for radiation treatment planning.

There is mounting evidence that PET imaging with fluordeoxyglucose (FDG), a metabolic tracer with remarkable sensitivity and specificity to tumor uptake across many histological types, can have a profound impact on radiation treatment planning. Both retrospective and prospective studies, most of which were preformed in patients with lung cancer, show that FDG-PET images often influence the radiation treatment fields. Such studies identify patients with micrometastatic disease who are unlikely to benefit from intense local therapy, or directly impact the design of the radiation treatment planning by altering the target volume. FDG-PET has been demonstrated to significantly reduce interobserver variability in defining the GTV (64), and has shown value in treatment planning for lung (65), anal canal (66), cervical (67), and brain tumors (Fig. 7) (68).

Beyond tumor delineation, PET imaging can map out normal tissue functions (e.g., lung perfusion), and identify those normal tissues outside the PTV that must be spared from irradiation to preserve their function (69). Some emerging PET tracers can also measure radiobiological tumor functions, such as hypoxia (70), proliferation (71), and apoptosis (72), thereby allowing us to further define the dose required to achieve cure in a given patient.

PET information can be integrated to CT planning images by deformable registration of the image sets based on multimodality surface markers (73), or with dedicated, treatment planning, combination PET/CT scanners which result in a moreaccurate, and less time consuming coregistration (74). Much like MRIscanners, PET/CT scanners can be adapted for simulation by adding triangulation lasers and a flat patient table. However, the bore of the current combined systems is much smaller than for dedicated CT simulators, limiting patient size and position with this approach.

BIOLOGICAL IMAGING AND THE FUTURE OF RADIATION ONCOLOGY

Given that radiotherapy is a unique modality where dose delivery is precisely guided by anatomical images, and response is dictated by the radiobiology of the tissues, imaging and biology can and must be studied in concert. Imaging research in radiation oncology

---

Figure 7 (*Facing page*) Case example where the addition of FDG-hybrid PET data reduced observer variability in localization of the GTV. (**A**) A CT image showing the areas localized by three different observers using CT only. (**B**) Substantial discordance as to the location of the inferior extent can be seen on the lateral DRR displaying the GTVs based on CT. (**C**) FDG-hybrid PET image of the same region, showing the areas localized by each observer using registered PET and CT information. (**D**) The coregistered CT image showing the same areas as in (**C**). (**E**) The lateral DRR displaying GTV CT/FDG demonstrates a more consistent volume and better agreement, particularly at the inferior extent. *Source*: From Ref. 64.

stands to contribute greatly to advances in diagnostic and molecular imaging. Such research is likely to be focused on areas that stand to have an impact on the accuracy of radiation delivery, and include improvements in tumor delineation and characterization with novel biological imaging techniques, the development of imaging systems that can accommodate various patient positions and have an accurate spatial reference, and technical strategies for addressing organ motion through the course of an image acquisition. Furthermore, invasive interventional brachytherapy procedures can be performed under image guidance (75) and tissue can be acquired during these procedures with accurate image registration of biopsy sites (76). Such tissue acquisition provides much needed histopathological and molecular validation to biological imaging techniques currently in development. These same interventional and biological images can then serve for radiation treatment planning, with exceptional dose reference.

The field of biological imaging promises to bridge the gap between physics and biology in radiation oncology (77). The concept of radiation dose will invariably evolve from energy deposited in tissue (Gy) to more relevant bioeffects of radiotherapy, including events triggered at the molecular level. Ideally, radiobiology models should be applied and integrated into treatment planning, a difficult task at present given the tremendous patient and tumor variability. With biological reference images for individual patients, bioeffective treatment planning may well become a reality.

CONCLUSION

The current level of accuracy and precision in radiation treatment delivery is predominantly limited by our ability to localize tumors and normal tissues by conventional imaging techniques at the planning stages and during radiation delivery. Increasing the conformality of treatments should allow for dose escalation and a higher likelihood of tumor cure with decreased normal tissue injury. Modern radiation delivery mandates the integration of novel imaging techniques, and close collaboration with diagnosticians, imaging scientists, and biologists.

REFERENCES

1. Washington CM, Leaver DT. Principles and Practice of Radiation Therapy. Vol. 1. St. Louis: Mosby, 2003.
2. Wyman DR, Ostapiak OZ, Gamble LM. Analysis of mechanical sources of patient alignment errors in radiation therapy. Med Phys 2002; 29:2698–2704.
3. Leibel SA, Fuks Z, Zelefsky MJ, et al. Intensity-modulated radiotherapy. Cancer J 2002; 8:164–176.
4. Verhey LJ. Comparison of three-dimensional conformal radiation therapy and intensity-modulated radiation therapy systems. Semin Radiat Oncol 1999; 9:78–98.
5. ICRU Report 51: quantities and units in radiation protection dosimetry. Bethesda: International Commision on Radiation Units and Measurements, 1993.
6. Johns H, Cunningham, JR. The Physics of Radiology. Baltimore: Williams & Wilkins, 1978.
7. Nahum AE. Condensed-history Monte-Carlo simulation for charged particles: what can it do for us? Radiat Environ Biophys 1999; 38:163–173.
8. Drzymala RE, Mohan R, Brewster L, et al. Dose-volume histograms. Int J Radiat Oncol Biol Phys 1991; 21:71–78.
9. Koper PC, Stroom JC, van Putten WL, et al. Acute morbidity reduction using 3DCRT for prostate carcinoma: a randomized study. Int J Radiat Oncol Biol Phys 1999; 43:727–734.

10. Teh BS, Mai WY, Uhl BM, et al. Intensity-modulated radiation therapy (IMRT) for prostate cancer with the use of a rectal balloon for prostate immobilization: acute toxicity and dose-volume analysis. Int J Radiat Oncol Biol Phys 2001; 49:705–712.

11. Graham MV, Purdy JA, Emami B, et al. Clinical dose-volume histogram analysis for pneumonitis after 3D treatment for non-small cell lung cancer (NSCLC). Int J Radiat Oncol Biol Phys 1999; 45:323–329.

12. Willner J, Baier K, Caragiani E, Tschammler A, Flentje M. Dose, volume, and tumor control prediction in primary radiotherapy of non-small-cell lung cancer. Int J Radiat Oncol Biol Phys 2002; 52:382–389.

13. Verhey LJ. Issues in optimization for planning of intensity-modulated radiation therapy. Semin Radiat Oncol 2002; 12:210–218.

14. Creutzberg CL, Visser AG, De Porre PM, Meerwaldt JH, Althof VG, Levendag PC. Accuracy of patient positioning in mantle field irradiation. Radiother Oncol 1992; 23:257–264.

15. Creutzberg CL, Althof VG, Huizenga H, Visser AG, Levendag PC. Quality assurance using portal imaging: the accuracy of patient positioning in irradiation of breast cancer. Int J Radiat Oncol Biol Phys 1993; 25:529–539.

16. Jaffray DA, Yan D, Wong JW. Managing geometric uncertainty in conformal intensity modulated radiation therapy. Semin Radiat Oncol 1999; 9:4–19.

17. Seppi EJ, Munro P, Johnsen SW, et al. Megavoltage cone-beam computed tomography using a high-efficiency image receptor. Int J Radiat Oncol Biol Phys 2003; 55:793–803.

18. Sidhu K, Ford EC, Spirou S, et al. Optimization of conformal thoracic radiotherapy using cone-beam CT imaging for treatment verification. Int J Radiat Oncol Biol Phys 2003; 55:757–767.

19. Jaffray DA, Siewerdsen JH, Wong JW, Martinez AA. Flat-panel cone-beam computed tomography for image-guided radiation therapy. Int J Radiat Oncol Biol Phys 2002; 53:1337–1349.

20. Loose S, Leszczynski KW. On few-view tomographic reconstruction with megavoltage photon beams. Med Phys 2001; 28:1679–1688.

21. Langen KM, Jones DT. Organ motion and its management. Int J Radiat Oncol Biol Phys 2001; 50:265–278.

22. Serago CF, Chungbin SJ, Buskirk SJ, Ezzell GA, Collie AC, Vora SA. Initial experience with ultrasound localization for positioning prostate cancer patients for external beam radiotherapy. Int J Radiat Oncol Biol Phys 2002; 53:1130–1138.

23. Crook JM, Raymond Y, Salhani D, Yang H, Esche B. Prostate motion during standard radiotherapy as assessed by fiducial markers. Radiother Oncol 1995; 37:35–42.

24. Balter JM, Lam KL, Sandler HM, Littles JF, Bree RL, Ten Haken RK. Automated localization of the prostate at the time of treatment using implanted radiopaque markers: technical feasibility. Int J Radiat Oncol Biol Phys 1995; 33:1281–1286.

25. Giraud P, De Rycke Y, Dubray B, et al. Conformal radiotherapy (CRT) planning for lung cancer: analysis of intrathoracic organ motion during extreme phases of breathing. Int J Radiat Oncol Biol Phys 2001; 51:1081–1092.

26. Mah D, Hanley J, Rosenzweig KE, et al. Technical aspects of the deep inspiration breath-hold technique in the treatment of thoracic cancer. Int J Radiat Oncol Biol Phys 2000; 48:1175–1185.

27. Rosenzweig KE, Hanley J, Mah D, et al. The deep inspiration breath-hold technique in the treatment of inoperable non-small-cell lung cancer. Int J Radiat Oncol Biol Phys 2000; 48:81–87.

28. Wong JW, Sharpe MB, Jaffray, et al. The use of active breathing control (ABC) to reduce margin for breathing motion. Int J Radiat Oncol Biol Phys 1999; 44:911–919.

29. Minohara S, Kanai T, Endo M, Noda K, Kanazawa M. Respiratory gated irradiation system for heavy-ion radiotherapy. Int J Radiat Oncol Biol Phys 2000; 47:1097–1103.

30. Kubo HD, Hill BC. Respiration gated radiotherapy treatment: a technical study. Phys Med Biol 1996; 41:83–91.

31. Mageras GS, Yorke E, Rosenzweig K, et al. Fluoroscopic evaluation of diaphragmatic motion reduction with a respiratory gated radiotherapy system. J Appl Clin Med Phys 2001; 2:191–200.

32. Wagman R, Yorke E, Ford E, et al. Respiratory gating for liver tumors: use in dose escalation. Int J Radiat Oncol Biol Phys 2003; 55:659–668.

33. Essers M, Mijnheer BJ. In vivo dosimetry during external photon beam radiotherapy. Int J Radiat Oncol Biol Phys 1999; 43:245–259.

34. Scarantino C. In vivo dosimetery during external beam radiotherapy utilizing an implantable telemetric and dosimetric device, ACRO 13th Annual Meeting, Phoenix, Arizona, 2003.

35. Yamamoto M. Gamma knife radiosurgery: technology, applications, and future directions. Neurosurg Clin North Am 1999; 10:181–202.

36. Hartmann GH, Bauer-Kirpes B, Serago CF, Lorenz WJ. Precision and accuracy of stereotactic convergent beam irradiations from a linear accelerator. Int J Radiat Oncol Biol Phys 1994; 28:481–492.

37. King CR, Lehmann J, Adler JR, Hai J. Cyberknife radiotherapy for localized prostate cancer: rationale and technical feasibility. Technol Cancer Res Treat 2003; 2:25–30.

38. Ponsky LE, Crownover RL, Rosen MJ, et al. Initial evaluation of Cyberknife technology for extracorporeal renal tissue ablation. Urology 2003; 61:498–501.

39. Crownover RL, Wilkinson DA, Weinhous MS. The radiobiology and physics of brachytherapy. Hematol Oncol Clin North Am 1999; 13:477–487.

40. Lessard E, Hsu IC, Pouliot J. Inverse planning for interstitial gynecologic template brachytherapy: truly anatomy-based planning. Int J Radiat Oncol Biol Phys 2002; 54:1243–1251.

41. Lachance B, Beliveau-Nadeau D, Lassard E, et al. Early clinical experience with anatomy-based inverse planning dose optimization for high-dose-rate boost of the prostate. Int J Radiat Oncol Biol Phys 2002; 54:86–100.

42. Lessard E, Pouliot J. Inverse planning anatomy-based dose optimization for HDR-brachytherapy of the prostate using fast simulated annealing algorithm and dedicated objective function. Med Phys 2001; 28:773–779.

43. ICRU Report 62, prescribing, recording and reporting photon beam therapy (Supplement to ICRU Report 50). Bethesda: international commission on radiation units and measurements, 1999.

44. Ling CC, Humm J, Larson S, et al. Towards multidimensional radiotherapy (MD-CRT): biological imaging and biological conformality. Int J Radiat Oncol Biol Phys 2000; 47:551–560.

45. Flickinger JC, Deutsch M. Manual reconstruction of tumor volumes from CT scans for radiotherapy planning. Radiother Oncol 1989; 14:151–158.

46. Guan H, Yin FF, Kim JH. Accuracy of inhomogeneity correction in photon radiotherapy from CT scans with different settings. Phys Med Biol 2002; 47:N223–N231.

47. Williams G, Tobler M, Gaffney D, Moeller J, Leavitt DD. Dose calculation errors due to inaccurate representation of heterogeneity correction obtained from computerized tomography. Med Dosim 2002; 27:275–278.

48. Potter R, Heil B, Schneider L, Lenzen H, al-Dandashi C, Schnepper E. Sagittal and coronal planes from MRI for treatment planning in tumors of brain, head and neck: MRI assisted simulation. Radiother Oncol 1992; 23:127–130.

49. Ten Haken RK, Thornton AF Jr, Sandler HM, et al. A quantitative assessment of the addition of MRI to CT-based, 3-D treatment planning of brain tumors. Radiother Oncol 1992; 25:121–133.

50. Milosevic M, Voruganti S, Blend R, et al. Magnetic resonance imaging (MRI) for localization of the prostatic apex: comparison to computed tomography (CT) and urethrography. Radiother Oncol 1998; 47:277–284.

51. Debois M, Oyen R, Maes F, et al. The contribution of magnetic resonance imaging to the three-dimensional treatment planning of localized prostate cancer. Int J Radiat Oncol Biol Phys 1999; 45:857–865.

52. Ramsey CR, Oliver AL. Magnetic resonance imaging based digitally reconstructed radiographs, virtual simulation, and three-dimensional treatment planning for brain neoplasms. Med Phys 1998; 25:1928–1934.

53. Liu H. An efficient geometric image distortion correction method for a biplanar planar gradient coil. Magma 2000; 10:75–79.

54. Mah D, Steckner M, Palacio E, Mitra R, Richardson T, Hanks GE. Characteristics and quality assurance of a dedicated open 0.23 T MRI for radiation therapy simulation. Med Phys 2002; 29:2541–2547.

55. Mah D, Steckner M, Hanlon A, et al. MRI simulation: effect of gradient distortions on three-dimensional prostate cancer plans. Int J Radiat Oncol Biol Phys 2002; 53:757–765.

56. Amoore JN, Ridgway JP. A system for cardiac and respiratory gating of a magnetic resonance imager. Clin Phys Physiol Meas 1989; 10:283–286.

57. Marti-Bonmati L, Graells M, Ronchera-Oms CL. Reduction of peristaltic artifacts on magnetic resonance imaging of the abdomen: a comparative evaluation of three drugs. Abdom Imaging 1996; 21:309–313.

58. Mah D, Freedman G, Milestone B, et al. Measurement of intrafractional prostate motion using magnetic resonance imaging. Int J Radiat Oncol Biol Phys 2002; 54:568–575.

59. Kurhanewicz J, Vigneron DB, Hricak H, Narayan P, Carroll P, Nelson SJ. Three dimensional H-1 MR spectroscopic imaging of the in situ human prostate with high (0.24–0.7-cm3) spatial resolution. Radiology 1996; 198:795–805.

60. Zaider M, Zelefsky MJ, Lee EK, et al. Treatment planning for prostate implants using magnetic-resonance spectroscopy imaging. Int J Radiat Oncol Biol Phys 2000; 47:1085–1096.

61. Howe FA, Robinson SP, McIntyre DJ, Stubbs M, Griffiths JR. Issues in flow and oxygenation dependent contrast (FLOOD) imaging of tumours. NMR Biomed 2001; 14:497–506.

62. Konouchi H, Asaumi J, Yanagi Y, et al. Evaluation of tumor proliferation using dynamic contrast enhanced-MRI of oral cavity and oropharyngeal squamous cell carcinoma. Oral Oncol 2003; 39:290–295.

63. Knopp MV, Giesel FL, Marcos H, von Tengg-Kobligk H, Choyke P. Dynamic contrast-enhanced magnetic resonance imaging in oncology. Top Magn Reson Imaging 2001; 12:301–308.

64. Caldwell CB, Mah K, Ung YC, et al. Observer variation in contouring gross tumor volume in patients with poorly defined non-small-cell lung tumors on CT: the impact of 18FDG-hybrid PET fusion. Int J Radiat Oncol Biol Phys 2001; 51:923–931.

65. Mah K, Caldwell CB, Ung YC, et al. The impact of (18)FDG-PET on target and critical organs in CT-based treatment planning of patients with poorly defined non-small-cell lung carcinoma: a prospective study. Int J Radiat Oncol Biol Phys 2002; 52:339–350.

66. Ung YC, Ehrlich LE, Ganguli SN. 18FDG Hybrid PET and CT fusion improves target volume definition in treatment planning for carcinomas of the anal canal. Int J Radiat Oncol Biol Phys 2001; 50:1416.

67. Mutic S, Malyapa RS, Grigsby PW, et al. PET-guided IMRT for cervical carcinoma with positive para-aortic lymph nodes-a dose-escalation treatment planning study. Int J Radiat Oncol Biol Phys 2003; 55:28–35.

68. Rajasekar D, Datta NR, Gupta RK, Pradhan PK, Ayyagari S. Multimodality image fusion in dose escalation studies of brain tumors. J Appl Clin Med Phys 2003; 4:8–16.

69. Seppenwoolde Y, Engelsman M, De Jaeger K, et al. Optimizing radiation treatment plans for lung cancer using lung perfusion information. Radiother Oncol 2002; 63:165–177.

70. Chao KS, Bosch WR, Mutic S, et al. A novel approach to overcome hypoxic tumor resistance: Cu-ATSM-guided intensity-modulated radiation therapy. Int J Radiat Oncol Biol Phys 2001; 49:1171–1182.

71. Wagner M, Seitz U, Buck A, et al. 3′-[18F]fluoro-3′-deoxythymidine ([18F]-FLT) as positron emission tomography tracer for imaging proliferation in a murine B-Cell lymphoma model and in the human disease. Cancer Res 2003; 63:2681–2687.

72. Kemerink GJ, Boersma HH, Thimister PW, et al. Biodistribution and dosimetry of 99mTc-BTAP-annexin-V in humans. Eur J Nucl Med 2001; 28:1373–1378.
73. Forster GJ, Laumann C, Nickel O, Kann P, Rieker O, Bartenstein P. SPET/CT image co-registration in the abdomen with a simple and cost-effective tool. Eur J Nucl Med Mol Imaging 2003; 30:32–39.
74. Lardinois D, Weder W, Hany TF, et al. Staging of non-small-cell lung cancer with integrated positron-emission tomography and computed tomography. N Engl J Med 2003; 348:2500–2507.
75. D'Amico AV, Cormack RA, Tempany CM. MRI-guided diagnosis and treatment of prostate cancer. N Engl J Med 2001; 344:776–777.
76. Susil RC, Camphausen K, Choyke P, et al. MRI-guided transperineal prostate interventions in a standard 1.5T magnet. Magnetic resonance in medicine submitted for publication.
77. Coleman CN. Linking radiation oncology and imaging through molecular biology (or now that therapy and diagnosis have separated, it's time to get together again!). Radiology 2003; 228:29–35.
78. Zelefsky MJ, Fuks Z, Happersett L, et al. Clinical experience with intensity modulated radiation therapy (IMRT) in prostate cancer. Radiother Oncol 2000; 55(3):241–249.

7

Clinical PET in Oncology

Gary J. R. Cook
Department of Nuclear Medicine, Royal Marsden Hospital, Sutton, Surrey, U.K.

Wai Lup Wong
Paul Strickland Scanner Centre, Mount Vernon Hospital, Northwood, Middlesex, U.K.

A Note from the Editors

---

*T**his is a general "must read" clinical chapter covering the usage of FDG-PET for the management of patients with cancer. Both authors are clinicians with radiological and nuclear medicine training and they use FDG-PET in their practices. Medical image processing has become a major force in the imaging of cancer. They discuss FDG-PET in the clinical settings of the common problems faced by radiologists on a daily basis which include tissue characterization, staging, response assessment and evaluation of residual disease. The images in this section are up to date with full use of CT-PET technology.*

Functional imaging with positron emission tomography (PET) has recently taken on an increasingly important role in the management of patients with cancer, reflecting a growing need to evaluate disease status, not only at the time of diagnosis and staging, but also at regular intervals during follow-up. In most countries of the world, PET imaging has limited availability, and close liaison between cancer clinicians and imagers is essential if optimum utilization is to be achieved. As with all imaging techniques the choice of PET as an option is dependent on many factors, which include the information being sought, the availability and the accuracy of PET imaging, and local expertise. At a time of increasing demand for imaging resources and increasing health-care costs, economic factors increasingly influence decisions regarding the usage of PET in a given clinical situation. PET creates tomographic images that represent metabolic activity of underlying tissue processes. Major developments that have enabled the successful clinical implementation of this technique include radio-pharmaceuticals that resemble endogenous biological compounds, quantification of tracer distribution, volume data acquisition, whole-body tomographic imaging, and most recently simultaneously acquired CT data. This chapter cannot adequately cover these areas, and readers are invited to review the many specialist texts that cover the areas of hardware, tracers, provide organ-by-organ reviews, and discuss economic considerations. Instead, we intend to review ^{18}F-fluoro-2-deoxy-D-glucose [^{18}FDG] PET from the standpoint of clinical usage evaluating its use for diagnosing cancer, for staging patients with cancer, for prognostication, to evaluate residual disease, and to detect recurrence. For the sake of brevity, each of these themes will be discussed in greater depth for one or two of the commonest cancers to provide readers with an idea on the principles of ^{18}FDG PET use in clinical practice.

PRINCIPLES OF PET

PET is a functional imaging modality that employs radiotracers to exploit altered metabolic and biochemical function in vivo. Until the early 1990s, because of a limited axial field of view within the scanner, the technique was reserved almost exclusively for neuropsychiatric and cardiac research. With the advent of a simple change in scanner design, which allowed passage of the scanning couch through the gantry, it became possible to perform whole-body PET. Subsequently oncological imaging has become the predominant clinical and research application. Recognizing its value, the expenses of ^{18}FDG PET clinical studies are now reimbursed by health-care providers in many countries. This, together with the establishment of PET tracer distribution networks, has seen an enormous increase in the use of ^{18}FDG PET to such an extent that it is now almost inconceivable for a cancer center not to have access to PET imaging.

It has been known for many years that many malignant tumors demonstrate enhanced glycolytic activity (1). Following the early work of Sokoloff with ^{14}C-labeled deoxyglucose, the radiopharmaceutical ^{18}FDG has become the most commonly used clinical PET tracer in oncology (2). Like glucose, deoxyglucose enters cancer cells via membrane glucose transporters, particularly Glut-1, and its overexpression, which is commonly seen in malignant cells, results in increased tracer uptake (3). Both glucose and deoxyglucose undergo phosphorylation by the enzyme hexokinase, which is also overexpressed in cancers. While glucose then undergoes further enzymatic reactions, deoxyglucose remains effectively trapped in the

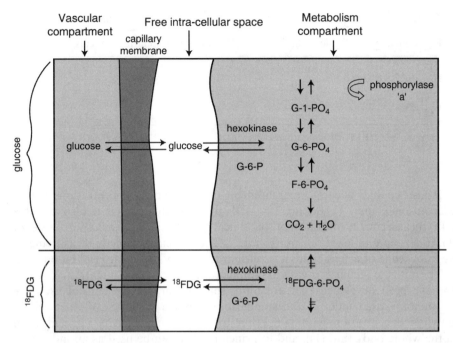

Figure 1   Three-compartment model of glucose and FDG kinetics. Glucose and FDG enter the cell and are phosphorylated by hexokinase to glucose-6-phosphate (G-6-P) and FDG-6-phosphate (FDG-6-P), respectively. Whilst glucose-6-phosphate can undergo further enzymatic reactions, FDG-6-phosphate is effectively trapped as there is little dephosphorylation by glucose-6-phosphatase (G-6-P) in most tissues and tumors.

intracellular compartment, a reason why this tracer is advantageous for imaging (Fig. 1). The [18]FDG signal, however, also depends on a variety of other factors including blood flow and delivery, the state of tissue hypoxia as well as the number of viable tumor cells present. Furthermore, increased uptake of [18]FDG can be seen following radiotherapy, due to activated inflammatory cells (4), and in granulomatous disorders (5).

A major advantage of PET is that many biological elements, including carbon, nitrogen, and oxygen, have positron emitting radionuclides, allowing substitution of a radionuclide atom for a non-radioactive atom within biological compounds of interest. New PET radiopharmaceuticals are being developed that may have more specific roles such as functional oncological imaging with ^{18}F-fluorothymidine (a tracer for cellular proliferation) and ^{11}C-methionine (a tracer for amino acid transport). Unfortunately, most positron emitting radionuclides have very short half-lives (Table 1) and are thus difficult to use even where there is a cyclotron available close to an imaging facility. ^{18}F-fluorine has a half-life of approximately two hours, allowing sufficient time for radiolabeling of ligands and subsequent transfer to distant scanning facilities. It is for this reason that [18]FDG-labeled biological tracers are favored in PET applications.

PET has an advantage over conventional single photon nuclear medicine imaging in that using PET it is relatively easy to measure the effects of attenuation of photons within the body and to accurately make corrections for this. Attenuation correction improves image quality for qualitative interpretation of clinical

Table 1 Common Clinical PET Radionuclides and Radiopharmaceuticals

Radionuclide	Physical half-life	Example radiopharmaceuticals
^{18}F	110 min	^{18}FDG ^{18}FLT
^{11}C	20 min	^{11}C-methionine ^{11}C-choline
^{13}N	10 min	^{13}N-ammonia
^{15}O	2 min	^{15}O-water

Abbreviations: ^{18}FLT, ^{18}F-fluorothymidine; ^{18}FDG, ^{18}F-fluoro-2-deoxy-D-glucose.

scans. It also enables accurate measurement of radioactive concentrations within tissue in absolute units (MBq mL^{-1}). With dynamic imaging, it is also possible to make measurements of rates of biological processes, e.g., metabolic rate of ^{18}FDG, in absolute units of mL min^{-1} mL^{-1}. These accurate kinetic measurements require knowledge of arterial activity concentrations, and hence arterial blood sampling. To mitigate against invasive sampling simplified semi-quantitative parameters have been developed that are more suitable for routine clinical use. The most commonly used index is the standardized uptake value (SUV) that relates the activity concentration within a lesion to the average activity concentration within the whole body [Eq. (1)], and in principle SUV can be used as an index that can be compared between different patients or to record changes in tumor activity over time to monitor therapy. There has been some controversy over the best method to measure SUV and whether corrections are required to allow for effects of different levels of plasma glucose, different body size and composition, and for the partial volume effect (6). Undoubtedly, there are some limitations in the use of SUV but in routine clinical practice, it serves as a simple, robust, and reproducible parameter that is effective for monitoring change. For more complex research applications, kinetic analyses using Patlak graphical analysis or nonlinear regression and compartmental modeling might be more appropriate but at the expense of complexity and invasiveness (7).

$$SUV = \frac{\text{activity in ROI (MBq)/vol (mL)}}{\text{injected activity (MBq)/patient wt (g)}} \tag{1}$$

where SUV is the standarized uptake value, ROI is the region of interest.

Metabolic abnormalities usually precede morphological changes in malignant tumors. Diagnosis with PET relies primarily on the detection of disordered metabolic function rather than derangement of morphology, and as a result PET is more sensitive than CT and MR for detection of cancer. Lack of anatomical localization of foci of abnormal metabolism limits the value of PET for planning treatment (8). Software registration techniques have been developed to combine ^{18}FDG PET to CT and MR (9). However, these methods are labor intensive, and unless registration of data sets is planned prospectively results are often suboptimal. Combined PET/CT scanners are now commercially available that enable accurate and seamless fusion of functional and anatomical information from PET and CT performed consecutively but within the same scanner gantry (Fig. 2). The CT data can also be used to correct the PET scan for attenuation effects thereby speeding up patient throughput such that whole-body imaging is now possible in less than 30 minutes.

(A)

(B)

(C)

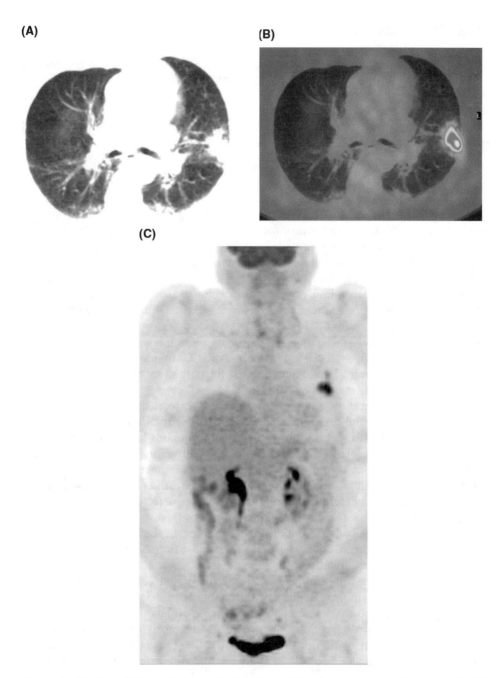

Figure 2 Equivocal biopsy findings. (**A**) A patient with a lung parenchymal lesion on the left side. CT guided percutaneous biopsy did not provide a definitive result. (**B**) FDG PET–CT showed intense uptake within the lesion consistent with malignancy. (**C**) FDG PET (projection image) showed no other sites of active disease. Subsequent surgery confirmed NSCLC (T2, N0, M0). (*See color insert for Fig. 2B.*)

DIAGNOSING CANCER

The establishment of the diagnosis of malignancy remains firmly within the domain of clinical evaluation, complemented by biopsy techniques which may require imaging guidance. From time to time characterization of a lesion may be difficult to achieve by these means with intrapulmonary lesions being a particular problem. Other areas that present problems include the indeterminate adrenal mass, pleural effusions, and pancreatic and thyroid lesions.

Pulmonary Nodules

Bronchoscopic biopsy and CT complemented by CT guided fine needle aspiration cytology (FNAC) are the mainstays for evaluating lung parenchymal lesions, and they are valuable when they provide a definitive result. But the probability of achieving this can be less than 50% for benign lesions. Another disadvantage of FNAC is the risk of pneumothorax which may require admission to the hospital for chest drainage. Depending on the study being considered, the sensitivity of [18]FDG PET for detecting malignant lesions is between 83% and 100% with a specificity of between 83% and 90% (Fig. 2) (10). A specific situation where [18]FDG PET has proved useful for characterizing the nature of a lesion is in patients with proven potentially curable non-small cell lung cancer (NSCLC) in one lung with an indeterminate lesion in the contra-lateral lung because the pathology of the latter lesion can profoundly influence management (10,11).

Abscesses and granulomas including those due to sarcoidosis, tuberculosis, anthracite inhalation, and fungus can all mimic malignant lesions in the lung. False negative results with [18]FDG PET are very unusual for lesions larger than 1 cm in size although bronchoalveolar carcinoma, highly differentiated neuroendocrine carcinoma, and adenocarcinoma especially within a scar have all been reported to cause confusion (11). Improvements in CT techniques are likely to increase the number of sub-centimeter indeterminate pulmonary nodules detected. These lesions pose a diagnostic dilemma because only a small minority of them are malignant and they cannot be readily biopsied by percutaneous techniques. In the literature the smallest malignant lesion identified with [18]FDG PET was a 6 mm NSCLC. The majority of lesions studied were relatively large, and as such the reliability of [18]FDG PET for characterizing sub-centimeter lesions remains unclear (10). With financial restraints,[18]FDG PET in most centers will probably be restricted to those parenchymal lung lesions which are not accessible to bronchoscopic or percutaneous biopsy, where these techniques have failed to provide a diagnosis or in patients where a percutaneous biopsy with its attendant risk of a pneumothorax is relatively contra-indicated, such as those with severely compromised respiratory function.

Adrenal Lesions

On survey of the literature,[18]FDG PET was used to distinguish between malignant and benign adrenal lesions in four studies with a total of 161 lesions in 142 patients. There were 55 true positive results, 47 true negative results, four false positive results, and no false negative results (12–15). In the prospective study of 33 adrenal masses in 27 patients with proven lung cancer FDG PET had a sensitivity of 100% and a specificity of 80% (15). Recently promising results have been obtained when chemical shift MRI has been used to characterize adrenal lesions on the basis of their fat content. There are currently no studies available which compare FDG PET to chemical shift MR.

Pleural Effusions

The ability of [18]FDG PET to characterize the nature of pleural effusions is less clear. Encouraging results were obtained in a preliminary report on the ability of [18]FDG PET to distinguish between malignant and benign pleural effusions (16). However, in a subsequent study which included 25 NSCLC patients who had pleural effusion on staging CT,[18]FDG had a sensitivity of 95% and a specificity of only 67% (17). Nevertheless, both studies showed [18]FDG PET to be more accurate than cytological evaluation and as accurate as thoracoscopic biopsy. False positive results will probably limit the utility of [18]FDG PET to provide a definitive diagnosis but it may be able to complement thoracoscopy by highlighting areas most likely to provide a positive biopsy. The ability of a negative [18]FDG PET to exclude malignancy is unknown because of the small number of benign effusions studied so far.

Other Common Clinical Problem Areas

MR and biopsy are the techniques of choice for the diagnosis of primary brain and spinal cord tumors. In some patients,[18]FDG PET can provide additional important information about grade of tumor which can have significant diagnostic and therapeutic implications (18). In some patients,[18]FDG PET can complement MRI for delineating the full extent of disease at the primary site. In select patients, where there is uncertainty on anatomical imaging and also a relative contra-indication to biopsy, it can be useful for distinguishing between benign and malignant lesions (19). The major shortcoming of [18]FDG PET in brain application is the intrinsic high background activity of the cerebral cortex and other gray matter structures and lower anatomical resolution compared to MRI. This limits its use as a method for detecting low-grade tumors, and it is not an adequate screening modality for the detection of intracranial metastatic disease by itself.

[18]FDG PET cannot replace CT but instead is complementary to CT in the evaluation of pancreatic lesions particularly when malignancy is being suspected and where CT has failed to identify a discrete mass or in patients in whom biopsy is not definitive. There are a small number of studies in the literature that suggest that [18]FDG PET can be of value for characterizing pancreatic masses (20) when there is a need to distinguish between chronic pancreatitis and malignancy. False positive lesions include acute pancreatitis and cholangitis, and false negative findings can occur in patients who are diabetic and hyperglycemic at the time of [18]FDG PET scan, in well differentiated neuroendocrine as well as some cystic neoplasms.

Initial enthusiasm for using [18]FDG PET for characterizing *thyroid and parotid gland* lesions has not been substantiated by subsequent results. Both malignant and benign lesions in these glands can be equally avid for [18]FDG (21,22). Conventional methods of assessment remain the mainstay for characterizing and staging thyroid and parotid gland malignancies.[18]FDG PET also appears to be of limited use for detecting sarcomatous change in neurofibromas, as neurofibromas can themselves be avid for [18]FDG (23).[18]FDG PET is recommended for localizing the site of the primary tumor in patients presenting with squamous cell lymph node metastases in the neck without an obvious primary tumor in the mucosa of the aerodigestive tract (Fig. 3).

(A)

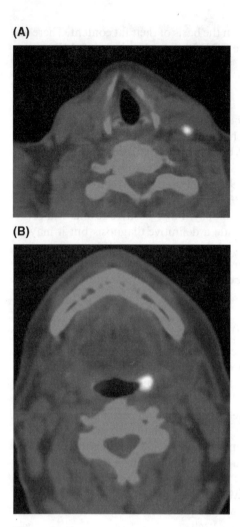

(B)

Figure 3   Squamous carcinoma of unknown primary origin in the head and neck region. This patient presented with a left level III squamous cell carcinoma lymph node metastasis. No primary tumor was evident on CT, MRI and EUA which included multiple biopsies and bilateral tonsillectomies. (**A**) Fused FDG PET–CT through the neck. FDG PET scan confirmed high uptake in the level III node. (**B**) Fused FDG PET also shows increased uptake in the left tonsillar fossa inferiorly, indicating the site of the primary tumor which was confirmed by subsequent repeat EUA and biopsies. (*See color insert.*)

STAGING CANCERS

Accurate delineation of disease extent is a major requirement in the management of cancer patients as disease extent not only influences prognosis but also dictates the treatment plan. Clinical assessment complemented by imaging is adequate for delineating disease at the primary site in the majority of patients. Nodal disease and visceral metastases however cannot be detected reliably and consistently even with state-of-the-art CT scanners, MR machines, and ultrasound. Identification of tumor within lymph nodes with these techniques is largely based on the assumption that enlarged nodes contain tumor. But normal sized nodes can contain tumor, and enlarged nodes can be due to reactive hyperplasia. The characterization of abnormalities, especially when small, may pose significant clinical challenge, and foci of disease in unexpected sites that cause minimal anatomical distortion present a further problem in detection. On review of the literature it is clear that [18]FDG PET is a valuable adjunctive technique for staging the majority of cancers (20). Clinically, however, it is most relevant in those cancers where there is a high risk of nodal or distant metastases or a combination of both. However, as noted above [18]FDG PET cannot replace CT and MR as a screening tool for brain metastases.

Lung Cancer

For NSCLC as many as 60% of patients can have bony metastases at presentation, with up to 40% having no symptoms whatsoever. In those patients being considered for thoracotomy the prevalence of mediastinal nodal disease may be as high as 60% (24,25). Curative surgical resection is the treatment of choice for the early stages of NSCLC. Mediastinal nodal disease is usually an indication for radiotherapy instead of surgical resection, and the presence of distant metastases also precludes lung tumor resection (Fig. 4). In a prospective co-operative study of 155 NSCLC patients which compared the ability of CT and MR for detecting mediastinal nodal metastases at 642 nodal stations, CT and MR had sensitivities of 52% and 48%, and specificities of 69% and 64%, respectively (26). This is in comparison to a meta-analysis of FDG PET which included 14 studies and 514 patients and CT with 29 studies and 2226 patients, where FDG PET had a mean sensitivity and specificity of 79% and 91% in contrast to CT with a sensitivity of 60% and specificity of 77% (27). The authors concluded that the superiority of [18]FDG PET over CT was independent of performance index or clinical context (27). Where [18]FDG PET fits into the investigation algorithm of staging the mediastinum in NSCLC is still a topic for debate. Researchers have proposed that pre-operative patients with no abnormal uptake beyond hilar nodes on [18]FDG PET should proceed directly to tumor resection, provided that there are no other contra-indications, as these patients have only a small chance of harboring mediastinal or distant visceral metastases (8,28). Proponents of this approach accept that [18]FDG PET is not absolutely accurate in excluding mediastinal disease. However, extrapolating from CT data, they argue that given [18]FDG PET can achieve a specificity of at least 90% for detecting mediastinal metastases, there should be no significant difference in survival when using [18]FDG PET compared with invasive staging (29). The incidence of false positive [18]FDG PET observations in the mediastinum is an important and consistent finding which emerges from all the studies, in up to 20% of patients (8). As such an isolated abnormal [18]FDG PET uptake in the mediastinum should not necessarily exclude surgery. Such a finding requires further investigation by mediastinoscopy with [18]FDG PET improving the sensitivity of mediastinoscopy (30).

There is convincing evidence that [18]FDG PET can more accurately detect bony metastases in patients with NSCLC (30,31). A retrospective review of 110 consecutive NSCLC patients found that the accuracy of [18]FDG PET was 96% compared with 66% when using radionuclide bone scanning (24). Both techniques had a high sensitivity of 90% but [18]FDG PET was more specific, 98% compared with 68% in concordance with other similar studies in the literature (24,32,33). The main cause of uncertainty with [18]FDG PET was its inability to distinguish between uptake in bone and adjacent soft tissue which should be resolved with PET–CT (24).

(A)   **(B)**

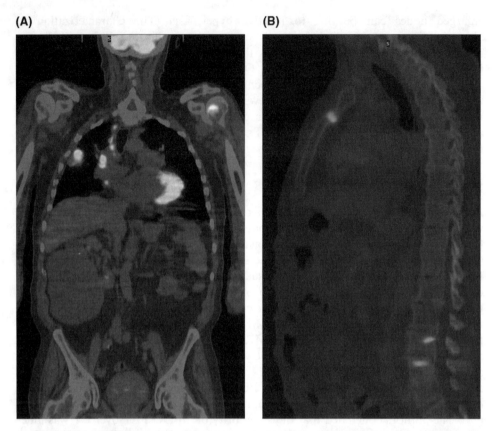

Figure 4 Staging lung cancer. (**A**) A patient with a lung parenchymal lesion. It was not possible to establish a histological diagnosis with CT guided percutaneous biopsy. (**B**) FDG PET CT showed intense uptake within the pulmonary lesion consistent with malignancy. It suggested disease within ipsilateral hilar and right paratracheal nodes, corresponding to normal sized nodes on CT and also a deposit within the left proximal humerus. Deposits were also seen within the sternum and in the fourth and fifth lumbar vertebral bodies. (*See color insert.*)

In a study of 102 pre-operative NSCLC patients,[18]FDG PET resulted in a different clinical stage in 62 patients: it lowered disease stage in 20 and raised it in 42 (8). These findings are in line with a study of 96 patients, with suspected or proven NSCLC, where the addition of [18]FDG PET to conventional workup prevented unnecessary surgery in one of five patients. In a survey of 167 patients, the highest yield of unexpected metastases was observed in stage III patients. The authors recommended that [18]FDG PET should form part of the assessment prior to radical radiotherapy (34). The value of [18]FDG PET in radiotherapy patients is supported by three further series where [18]FDG PET resulted in significant alterations in radiotherapy treatment plans, and in one study this translated into a lower early mortality rate (35–37).

It can be seen that [18]FDG PET is undoubtedly of value for the initial assessment of patients with NSCLC. For the clinician however, where it most cost effectively fits into the investigation algorithm of this group of patients is less clear (38–40).

Other Malignancies

For the preoperative staging of *esophageal cancer* [18]FDG PET has proved to be useful and is used by many as a routine. The significant contribution of [18]FDG PET to the detection of lymph nodes, liver, and bone metastases has been shown in several studies, resulting in alterations in treatment in a significant proportion of patients (41).

Sentinel node dissection is at present the method of choice for assessing the extent of lymph node involvement in patients with primary cutaneous malignant *melanoma* (42). In those patients where this cannot be done, especially in those with a high risk of nodal metastases and also in patients at high risk of visceral metastases, [18]FDG PET can be contributory (42,43). The sensitivity and the specificity of [18]FDG PET vary according to the clinical stage and anatomical location of the melanoma lesions.

With regard to [18]FDG PET for the staging of musculoskeletal tumors and germ cell tumors, preliminary results appear promising (44–47). The great variety of *musculoskeletal neoplasms* makes it difficult to make definitive general statements about using [18]FDG PET. However, [18]FDG PET has been shown to be able to differentiate low from high-grade sarcomas, and it has been stated that biopsy of [18]FDG avid areas enables optimal characterization of lesions. Limitations of [18]FDG PET include the differentiation of low-grade neoplasms from benign lesions and the probably lower sensitivity for detecting osteosclerotic bone metastases. In the primary staging of *germ cell* tumors, [18]FDG PET has a high specificity provided enlarged nodes are visible on CT scanning. It seems unlikely that [18]FDG PET will contribute to the initial clinical staging of stage I tumors and thus will be unlikely to identify patients who do/do not require adjuvant chemotherapy. Furthermore, it appears that [18]FDG PET is more sensitive to the more aggressive histological types of testicular cancer (choriocarcinoma, yolk cell tumors, and embryonal carcinoma) and less sensitive to the presence of better differentiated teratoma variants.

Currently, [18]FDG PET is not recommended for the staging of all *head and neck*, breast, ovarian, bladder, prostate, and pancreatic cancer patients. With these cancers, it nevertheless can be of value in select patients. For example, PET–CT or CT/MR carefully correlated with [18]FDG PET is of use for more precisely delineating extent of macroscopic disease at the primary site in extensive maxillary antral carcinomas and also in upper aerodigestive tract malignancies, where sub-mucosal extension is a feature such as with post-cricoid and endotracheal carcinomas (48). In addition, [18]FDG PET can also be of value in assessing indeterminate lymph nodes or visceral lesions that cannot be characterized following conventional staging. Specifically, in head and neck squamous cell carcinoma [18]FDG PET can influence the treatment plan in those patients with a high risk of nodal disease, e.g., T3/4 supraglottic carcinoma and equivocal nodal findings in the contra-lateral neck on conventional assessment. [18]FDG PET is also valuable in those patients with a low risk of nodal disease, e.g., T1 lip carcinoma and possible disease in the ipsilateral neck.

There is limited data to show that [18]FDG PET can detect unsuspected peritoneal deposits in *ovarian cancer* (49). When used in this setting, careful correlation with diagnostic CT or the CT component of the PET–CT is often required to distinguish [18]FDG activity within bowel from peritoneal deposits. With regard to pancreatic cancer, [18]FDG PET may detect metastatic sites not suspected following CT staging (50).

[18]FDG PET is of limited value for the staging of *prostate cancer*. It cannot consistently and reliably delineate the extent of disease at the primary site because [18]FDG activity within tumor can be obscured by [18]FDG activity within the bladder,

especially when the tumor is small and activity within the bladder is high and also because [18]FDG uptake in foci of cancer and benign hyperplasia can overlap substantially. Furthermore, for the detection of sclerotic metastases radionuclide bone scanning remains superior to [18]FDG PET (51).

Lymphoma

There is substantial evidence to show that in the staging of non-Hodgkin's lymphoma (NHL) and Hodgkin's lymphoma (HL) there is a good concordance between [18]FDG PET and whole-body CT (20). Moreover, [18]FDG PET can detect more sites of disease compared with conventional assessment (52–54). However, in the majority of patients, conventional assessment including whole-body CT is all that is necessary for planning treatment. [18]FDG PET is relevant in the subgroup of patients where there is a clinical need for clarification between localized disease and disseminated disease. Included in this group are those patients where there is a clinical suspicion of disseminated disease that cannot be confirmed by conventional techniques or when imaging suggests widespread disease that is not apparent clinically (48). [18]FDG PET however cannot consistently detect foci of low-grade NHL and foci of mucosal associated lymphoid tissue (MALT) lymphoma (55,56). Other issues which occasionally occur when [18]FDG PET is used for staging of lymphoma include physiological uptake in bowel which mimics mesenteric nodal disease and distinguishing between sarcoidosis and lymphoma as both pathologies can result in intense abnormal [18]FDG PET uptake in lymph nodes.

PROGNOSTICATION

A number of small studies have suggested that degree of [18]FDG PET uptake at the primary site can act as an independent prognostic indicator. In one series of *NSCLC* patients, regardless of clinical stage at presentation, patients with avid primary tumors which had an SUV(maximum) of greater than 10 survived approximately 13 months less compared with those with an SUV(maximum) of less than 10, and those with an SUV(maximum) of greater than 10 and an associated large morphologically lesion had a median survival of less than six months (57). In another similar NSCLC study, a cut-off SUV(maximum) of 7 had the best discriminative value for outcome in the group of 125 patients, as a whole, and also within the surgical cohort. Patients with resected tumor of less than 3 cm had an expected two year survival of 86% if the SUV(maximum) was below 7 and 60% if above 7. The SUV(maximum) was above 7 in nearly all resected tumors larger than 3 cm, and patients in this group had an expected two year survival of 43% (58). Uptake of [18]FDG PET at the primary site has also been found to be a prognostic marker in *head and neck SCC* with in general the higher the SUV(maximum) the poorer the outcome (59–61).

CANCER RECURRENCE

Early detection of small volume recurrent disease is a particular problem with morphological imaging techniques. Challenges include the differentiation of posttreatment changes from recurrent disease, identification of recurrence when biochemical tumor markers are elevated but no disease is identified on conventional imaging, and for the exclusion of distant metastatic disease when curative resection of recurrent tumor is being planned.

Colorectal Cancer

An area where [18]FDG PET has proven to be particularly effective is in the evaluation of recurrence of colorectal cancer. It can be extraordinarily difficult using morphological features to exclude recurrent tumor in the pelvis following surgery or surgery with radiotherapy, as normal tissue planes are disrupted and distorted. High accuracy for recurrent tumor detection has been reported for [18]FDG PET (62). It has however been noted that increased uptake of [18]FDG by macrophages and activated inflammatory cells occurs as a consequence of radiotherapy, which can be present for up to six months following radiotherapy; so a positive scan during this early period needs to be interpreted with some caution particularly in patients with normal tumor markers, however, a negative scan result can be reassuring. There is increasing evidence that [18]FDG PET can play a complementary role in the evaluation of extent of recurrent disease before surgical resection. Although the sensitivity for hepatic metastases measuring less than 1 cm is limited, overall it performs better than CT alone in this situation (63). To date there have not been comparisons with MRI using liver specific contrast agents or adequate studies comparing [18]FDG PET with multidetector CT. In up to 67% of patients with rising carcino-embryonic antigen levels and no disease identified on conventional imaging, [18]FDG PET can detect a definitive site of recurrence (64,65). In colorectal cancer patients with recurrent disease where surgical resection is planned, [18]FDG PET is not only helpful in evaluating the area of suspected disease but it will also detect unexpected sites of disease in 29% to 69% of cases, leading to a change in management in up to 29% of cases (Fig. 5) (62,64,66).

Other Malignancies

[18]FDG PET is valuable for the evaluation of recurrent *head and neck tumors* (67). High sensitivity and specificity have been recorded for the use of [18]FDG PET in this circumstance. However, there are a number of normal variants for the uptake of [18]FDG in the head and neck that present potential pitfalls with false positive interpretation, particularly when normal symmetrical uptake is lost. For example, lymphatic tissue in Waldeyer's ring often shows moderate uptake of [18]FDG. Apparent increased uptake is seen on the untreated side after tonsillectomy, soft palatal resection, and also radiotherapy to the head and neck, and this should not be mistaken for pathology. It is in this circumstance, that careful correlation with the clinical history and also co-registered PET and MRI or CT imaging is especially helpful (9). False positive uptake has been observed within the early period after radiotherapy due to the inherent inflammatory reaction, but this usually subsides by four to six months (67). Other tumors where [18]FDG PET has proven a useful tool in detecting recurrence include *lung cancer, lymphoma, and testicular tumors* (20).

Detection of recurrent *brain tumors* is a challenging problem for CT/MRI as it can be difficult to differentiate tumor from post-treatment gliosis. The use of [18]FDG PET alone in this situation may not be optimal as it may be difficult to detect recurrent tumor against the background of normal cortical activity. The degree of [18]FDG uptake correlates well with the grade of recurrence and may be helpful in directing

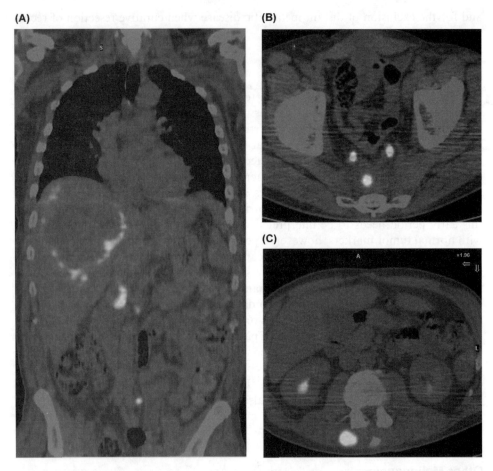

Figure 5 Pre-surgical evaluation: a patient with relapse of rectal cancer and an isolated liver metastasis on conventional assessment. Resection of the liver metastasis was planned. (**A**) FDG PET–CT confirmed the presence of the liver metastasis. It also showed unexpected disease within normal sized nodes in the retroperitonium. (**B**) FDG PET–CT showed that there was residual active disease within fibrosis in the pelvis. (**C**) Additionally, a deposit within erector spinae muscle is seen. The patient's management was changed from surgery to palliative treatment. (*See color insert.*)

biopsies to the most active area of tumor. Some investigators advocate the use of ^{11}C-methionine PET in addition to [18]FDG. The relatively low uptake of ^{11}C-methionine into normal brain cortex allows better definition of tumor extent than with [18]FDG alone (68).

ASSESSMENT OF RESIDUAL DISEASE

Lymphoma

A commonly asked question at the end of therapy is the extent of active disease in a residual tumor mass. For example, in patients with lymphoma, a radiologically detectable residual abnormality following therapy occurs in up to 88% of patients, more likely when the initial disease is bulky, the precise incidence depending on presenting histology (Fig. 6). With CT, which is conventionally used to assess response to treatment in lymphoma, it can be impossible to distinguish between active disease and fibrosis and because of this some patients unnecessarily receive radiotherapy. The proportion of residual masses that represent active lymphoma varies between series with relapse rates of ~20% in HL and 10% in NHL (69,70). Radiotherapy has been shown to have significant short- and more worrying long-term toxicity including ischemic heart disease, fibrosis, and radiation induced carcinomas/sarcomas. Refining the criteria for the use of radiotherapy would therefore be a major advance.

A number of studies have confirmed the superiority of [18]FDG PET in determining the activity of residual masses in HL and NHL compared to both CT and [67]gallium scanning. Of the 32 patients studied by de Wit et al. (71), 17 had a negative [18]FDG PET. None of these patients relapsed, although the follow-up period was relatively short, with a median of 62.6 weeks. Bangerter et al. (72) performed [18]FDG PET in 36 patients with residual masses. Twenty five of 27 patients with negative scans remained in clinical remission at 25 months. In those with a positive scan, four of nine patients remained in complete remission. Similar high positive and negative predictive values in the order of 90% have been reported, with a significantly higher specificity than CT, in more recent published series using state of the art dedicated PET (73).

Other Tumors

In seminomatous residual masses,[18]FDG PET has high positive and negative predictive values for the presence of viable tumor. The positive predictive value is equivalent to biochemical markers but with the benefit of localizing areas of active disease (74,75). With teratomas it is generally not possible to differentiate post-treatment necrosis and scar from mature teratoma, unless a more complex kinetic analysis is

(A)   **(B)**

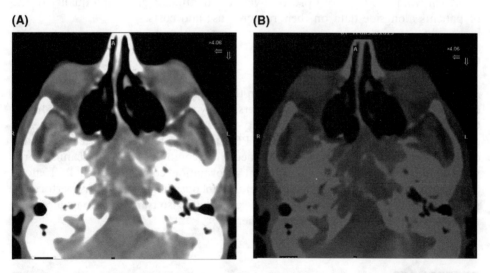

Figure 6 Assessment of residual disease. A patient with NHL involving the skull base. (**A**) Following chemotherapy, residual abnormality was seen on CT. It was not possible to distinguish between active disease and treatment sequelae from the CT appearance. (**B**) FDG PET–CT showed no significant uptake corresponding to the CT abnormalities suggesting inactive disease. (*See color insert for Fig. 6B.*)

made of FDG uptake (76). This latter method is probably not practical in a routine clinical setting. However it is also recommended that PET is performed at least 2 weeks following after completion of therapy for greatest accuracy (77).

COST EFFECTIVENESS OF [18]FDG PET

The ability of [18]FDG PET to consistently change patient management enabling the avoidance of attempted curative invasive treatments in patients with advanced malignancy makes it cost-effective in a number of clinical situations (64,78). In colorectal cancer patients who are potential candidates for hepatic resection, the use of [18]FDG PET in combination with CT has been shown to spare some patients unnecessary surgery by demonstrating unexpected extra-hepatic disease (79). The cost effectiveness of [18]FDG PET in the management of NSCLC patients has been assessed by researchers in the United States and Germany with favorable results. A German study concluded that [18]FDG PET was cost effective in the preoperative staging of patients with NSCLC and normal sized nodes on CT (25). In an U.S.A. setting such a strategy would result in a potential saving of $25,286 per life-year saved (80). However these results were contradicted by a Japanese study where a combination of chest CT plus [18]FDG PET was unlikely to be cost effective (81). This conflicting data illustrate the importance of being cautious about transposing the results of economic studies from one healthcare setting to another. The construction of equivalent sets of decision trees reflecting local practice is required. Variations in clinical practice are known to occur between countries, and it would be unwise to assume that clinical practices in one country would apply universally. Furthermore direct costs in managing patients with NSCLC differ from country to country. To date studies exploring the cost effectiveness of [18]FDG PET have assessed the outcomes solely in terms of life expectancy. A more informative approach would be to record prospectively the treatments given and quality of life of patients alongside data on their resource use and costs.

CONCLUSIONS

Almost all the [18]FDG PET data quoted in this chapter and other literature are based on scans obtained from PET only scanners. Early results show that combined PET CT scanning, improves diagnostic certainty with regard to [18]FDG PET and increases overall accuracy compared with [18]FDG PET and CT alone. Our own preliminary experience also suggests that scans obtained from combined PET-CT scanners provide significantly more clinically relevant information compared with PET alone even when visual correlation with contemporaneous diagnostic CT is performed. Increased ease of combined PET-CT data sets should also translate into its increased utilization in patients undergoing radiotherapy.

REFERENCES

1. Warburg O. On the origin of cancer cells. Science 1954; 123:306–314.
2. Sokoloff L. The deoxyglucose method: theory and practice. Eur Neurol 1981; 20: 137–145.

3. Brown RS, Wahl RL. Over expression of Glut-1 glucose transporter in human breast cancer: an immunohistochemical study. Cancer 1993; 72:2979–2985.

4. Hautzel H, Muller-Gartner HW. Early changes in fluorine-18-FDG uptake during radio-therapy. J Nucl Med 1997; 38:1384–1386.

5. Cook GJ, Fogelman I, Maisey MN. Normal physiological and benign pathological variants of 18-fluoro-2-deoxyglucose positron-emission tomography scanning: potential for error in interpretation. Sem Nucl Med 1996; 26:308–314.

6. Keyes JW. SUV: Standard uptake or silly useless value? J Nucl Med 1995; 36:1836–1839.

7. Hoekstra CJ, Paglianiti I, Hoekstra OS, Smit EF, Postmus PE, Teule GJJ, Lammertsma AA. Monitoring response to therapy in cancer using 18F-2-fluoro-2-deoxy-D-glucose and positron emission tomography: an overview of different analytical methods. Eur J Nucl Med 2000; 27:731–743.

8. Pieterman RM, van Putten JWG, Meuzelaar JJ, et al. Preoperative staging of non-small cell lung cancer with positron emission tomography. N Engl J Med 2000; 343: 254–261.

9. Wong WL, Hussain K, Chevretton E, et al. Validation and clinical application of computer-combined computed tomography and positron emission tomography with 2-[18F]fluoro-2-deoxy-D-glucose head and neck images. Am J Surg 1966; 172(6):628–632.

10. Gould MK, MacLean CC, Kuschner WG, Rydzak CE, Owens DK. Accuracy of positron emission tomography for diagnosis of pulmonary nodules and mass lesions: a meta-analysis. JAMA 2001; 258:914–924.

11. Wong WL, Campbell H, Saunders M. Positron emission tomography (PET)—evaluation of 'indeterminate pulmonary lesions'. Clin Oncol 2002; 14:123–128.

12. Yun M, Kim W, Alnafisi N, Lacorte L, Jang S, Alavi A. 18F-FDG PET in characterizing adrenal lesions detected on CT or MRI. J Nucl Med 2001; 42:1795–1799.

13. Boland GW, Goldberg MA, Lee MJ, et al. Indeterminate adrenal mass in patients with cancer: evaluation of PET with 2-[F-18]-fluoro-2-deoxy-D-glucose. Radiology 1995; 194:131–134.

14. Maurea S, Klain M, Mainolfi C, Ziviello M, Salvatore M. The diagnostic role of radio-nuclide imaging in evaluation of patients with nonhypersecreting adrenal masses. J Nucl Med 2001; 42:893–894.

15. Erasmus JJ, Patz EF, Page McAdams H, et al. Evaluation of adrenal masses in patients with bronchogenic carcinoma using 18F-fluorodeoxyglucose positron emission tomography. AJR 1997; 168:1357–1360.

16. Bury T, Paulus P, Dowlati A, Corhay JL, Rigo P, Radmecker MF. Evaluation of pleural diseases with FDG PET imaging: preliminary report. Thorax 1997; 52:187–189.

17. Erasmus JJ, Page McAdams H, Rossi SE, Goodman PC, Coleman RE, Patz EF. FDG-PET of pleural effusions in patients with non-small cell lung cancer. AJR 2000; 175:245–249.

18. Kinkaid PK, El Saden SM, Park SH, Goy BW. Cerebral gangliogliomas: preoperative grading using FDG PET and 201Tl-SPECT. Am J Neuroradiol 1998; 19:801–806.

19. Massager N, David P, Goldman S. Combined MR and PET guided stereotactic biopsy in brain stem lesions: diagnostic yield in a series of 30 patients. J Neurosurg 2000; 93: 951–957.

20. Gambhir SS, Czernin J, Schwimmer J, Silverman J, Coleman RE, Phelps ME. A tabulated summary of the FDG-PET literature. J Nucl Med 2001; 42:S1–S93.

21. Shreve PD, Anzai Y, Wahl RL. Pitfalls in oncological diagnosis with FDG PET imaging: physiologic and benign variants. Radiographics 1999; 19:61–77.

22. Horiucgi M, Yasuda S, Shohtsu A, Ide M. Four cases of Warthin's tumour of the parotid gland detected with FDG PET. Ann Nucl Med 1998; 12:47–50.

23. Shah N, Townsend E, Saunders M, Wong WL. High FDG uptake in a schwannomma—a PET study. J Comput Assist Tomogr 2000; 24:55–56.

24. Bury T, Barreto A, Daenen F, Barthelemy N, Ghaye B, Rigo P. Fluorine-18 deoxyglucose positron emission tomography for the detection of bone metastases in patients with non-small cell lung cancer. Eur J Nucl Med 1998; 25:1244–1247.

25. Dietlein M, Weber K, Gandjour A, Moka D, Theissen P, Lauterbach KW, Schicha H. Cost-effectiveness of FDG-PET for the management of potentially operable non-small cell lung cancer: priority for a PET-based strategy after nodal-negative CT results. Eur J Nucl Med 2000; 27:1598–1609.

26. Webb WR, Gatsonis C, Zerhouni EA, Heelan RT, Glazer GM, Francis IR, McNeil BJ. CT and MRI imaging in staging non-small cell bronchogenic carcinoma: report of the radiologic diagnostic oncology group. Radiology 1991; 178:705–713.

27. Dwamena BA, Sonnad SS, Angobaldo JO, Wahl RL. Metastases from non-small cell lung cancer: mediastinal staging in the 1990s-meta-analytic comparison of PET and CT. Radiology 1999; 213:530–536.

28. Patz EF, Lowe VJ, Goodman PC, Herndon J. Thoracic nodal staging with PET imaging with 18 FDG in patients with bronchogenic carcinoma. Clin Invest 1995; 108:1617–1621.

29. Malenka DJ, Colice GL, Beck JR. Does the mediastinum of the patient with NSCLC require histological staging/future standards for CT. Am Rev Resp Dis 1991; 144: 1134–1139.

30. Kernstine KH, McLaughlin KA, Menda Y, Rossi NP, Kahn DJ, Bushnell DL, Graham MM, Brown CK, Madsen MT. Can FDG-PET reduce the need for mediastinoscopy in potentially resectable nonsmall cell lung cancer? Ann Thoracic Surg 2002; 73:394–402.

31. Marom EM, Page McAdams H, Erasmus JJ, Goodman PC, Culhane DK, Coleman RE, Herndon JE, Patz EF. Staging non-small cell lung cancer with whole body PET. Radiology 1999; 212:803–809.

32. Graeber GM, Gupta NC, Murray GF. PET imaging with FDG is efficacious in evaluating malignant pulmonary disease. J Thoracic Cardiovasc Surg 1999; 117:719–727.

33. Valk PE, Pounds TR, Hopkins DM, et al. Staging non-small cell lung cancer by whole-body positron emission tomographic imaging. Ann Thoracic Surg 1995; 60:1573–1582.

34. MacManus MP, Hicks RJ, Matthews JP, et al. High rate of detection of unsuspected distant metastases by PET in apparent stage III non-small-cell lung cancer: implications for radical radiation therapy. Int J Rad Oncol Biol Phys 2001; 50:287–293.

35. MacManus MP, Wong K, Hicks RJ, Matthews JP, Wirth A, Ball DL. Early mortality after radical radiotherapy for non-small-cell lung cancer: comparison of PET-staged and conventionally staged cohorts treated at a large tertiary referral centre. Int J Rad Oncol Biol Phys 2002; 52:351–361.

36. Nestle U, Walter K, Schmidt S, Licht N, Nieder C, Motaref B, Hellwig D, Niewald M, Ukena D, Kirsch CM, Sybrecht GW, Schnabel K. 18- F-deoxyglucose positron emission tomography (FDG-PET) for the planning of radiotherapy in lung cancer: high impact in patients with atelectasis. Int J Rad Oncol Biol Phys 1999; 44:593–597.

37. Mah K, Caldwell CB, Ung YC, Danjoux CE, Balogh JM, Ganguli SN, Ehrlich LE, Tirona R. The impact of 18-FDG-PET on target and critical organs in CT-based treatment planning of patients with poorly defined non-small-cell lung carcinoma: a prospective study. Int J Oncol Biol Phys 2002; 52:339–350.

38. Seltzer MA, Yap CS, Silverman DH, et al. The impact of PET on the management of lung cancer: the referring physician's perspective. J Nucl Med 2002; 43:752–756.

39. Kalff V, Hicks RJ, MacManus MP, et al. Clinical impact of 18F fluorodeoxyglucose positron emission tomography in patients with non-small-cell lung cancer: a prospective study. J Clin Oncol 2001; 19:111–118.

40. Laking G, Price P. 18-Fluorodeoxyglucose positron emission tomography (FDG-PET) and the staging of early lung cancer. Thorax 2001; 56:S38–S44.

41. Flamen P, Lerut A, Van Cutsen E, De Wever W, Peeters M, Stroobants S, Dupont P, Bormans G, Hiele M, De Leyn P, Van Raemdonck D, Coosemans W, Ectors N, Haustermans K, Mortelmans L. Utility of positron emission tomography for the staging of patients with potentially operable esophageal carcinoma. J Clin Oncol 2000; 18:3202–3210.

42. Wagner JD, Schauwecker D, Davidson D. Prospective study of FDG PET of lymph node basins in melanoma patients undergoing sentinel node biopsy. J Clin Oncol 1999; 17:1508–1515.

43. Kalff V, Hicks RJ, Ware RE, Greer B, Binns DS, Hogg A. Evaluation of high risk melanoma: comparison of FDG PET with high dose 67-Ga SPECT. Eur J Nucl Med 2002; 29:506–515.

44. Lucas JD, O' Doherty MJ, Cronin BF, et al. Prospective evaluation of soft tissue masses and sarcomas using PET. Br J Surg 1998; 86:550–556.

45. Schwarzbach M, Willeke F, Dimitrakopoulou-Strauss A. Clinical value of FDG PET imaging in soft tissue sarcomas. Ann Surg 2000; 231:380–386.

46. Hain SF, O'Doherty MJ, Timothy AR. FDG PET in the initial staging of germ cell tumours. Eur J Nucl Med 2000; 27:590–594.

47. Larson U, Daugaard G, Rorth M, Eigtved A, Hojgaard L. PET with FDG in clinical stage I germ cell tumours. Proc ASCO 2000; 19:1337.

48. Walsh RM, Wong WL, Chevretton EB, Beaney RP. The use of PET-18FDG imaging in the clinical evaluation of head and neck lymphoma. Clin Oncol 1996; 8(1):51–54.

49. Smith G, Hubner K, McDonald T, Thie J. Avoiding second look surgery and reducing costs in the managing patients with ovarian cancer by applying FDG PET. Clin Positron Imaging 1998; 1:263.

50. Delbeke D, Chapman WC, Pinson CW. FDG imaging with PET has a significant impact on diagnosis and management of pancreatic ductal adenocarcinoma. J Nucl Med 1999; 40:1784–1792.

51. Cook GJ, Houston S, Rubens R, Maisey MN, Fogelman I. Detection of bone metastases in breast cancer by 18 FDG PET: differing metabolic activity in osteoblastic and osteolytic lesions. J Clin Oncol 1998; 16:3375–3379.

52. Moog F, Bangerter M, Diederichs CG, et al. Lymphoma: role of whole-body 2-deoxy-2 [F-18] fluoro-D-glucose (FDG) PET in nodal staging. Radiology 1997; 203:795–800.

53. Hoh CK, Glaspy J, Rosen P, et al. Whole-body FDG-PET imaging for staging of Hodgkin's disease and lymphoma. J Nucl Med 1997; 38:343–348.

54. Stumpe KDM, Urbinelli M, Steinert HC, Glanzmann CH, Buck A, von Schulthess GK. Whole-body positron emission tomography using fluorodeoxyglucose for staging of lymphoma: effectiveness and comparison with computed tomography. Eur J Nucl Med 1998; 25:721–728.

55. Carr R, Barrington SF, Madan B, et al. Detection of lymphoma in bone marrow by whole-body positron emission tomography. Blood 1998; 9:3340–3346.

56. Moog F, Bangerter M, Kotzerke J, Guhlmann A, Frickhofen N, Reske SN. 18-F-fluoro-deoxyglucose-positron emission tomography as a new approach to detect lymphomatous bone marrow. J Clin Oncol 1998; 16:603–609.

57. Ahuja V, Coleman RE, Herndon J, Patz EF. The prognostic significance of fluorodeoxyglucose positron emission tomography imaging for patients with nonsmall cell lung carcinoma. Cancer 1998; 83:918–924.

58. Vansteenkiste JF, Stroobants SG, Dupont PJ, De Leyn PR, Verbeken EK, Deneffe GJ, Mortelmans LA, Demedts MG and the Leuven Lung Cancer Group. Prognostic importance of the standardized uptake value on 18F-fluoro-2-deoxyglucose positron emission tomography scan in non-small–cell lung cancer: an analysis of 125 cases. J Clin Oncol 1999; 17:3201–3206.

59. van Tinteren H, Hoekstra OS, Smit EF, van den Bergh J, Schreurs JM, Stallaert R, van Velthoven P, Gomans E, Diepenhorst FW, Verboom F, van Mourik JC, Postmus PE, Boers M, Tuele G, and the PLUS study group. Effectiveness of positron emission tomography in the preoperative assessment of patients with suspected non-small-cell lung cancer: the PLUS multicentre randomised trial. Lancet 2002; 359:1388–1392.

60. Prabhudesai AG, Kumar D. Adjuvant therapy for colorectal cancer: the next step forward. Current Med Res Opinion 2002; 18:249–257.

61. Cook GJR, Ott RJ. Combining anatomy and function. Eur Radiol 2001; 11:1857–1858.

62. Huebner RH, Park KC, Shepherd JE, Schwimmer J, Czernin J, Phelps ME, Gambhir SS. A meta-analysis of the literature for whole-body FDG PET detection of recurrent colorectal cancer. J Nucl Med 2000; 41:1177–1189.

63. Vitola JV, Delbeke D, Sandler MP. Positron emission tomography to stage metastatic colorectal carcinoma to the liver. Am J Surg 1996; 171:21–26.

64. Valk PE, Abella-Columna E, Haseman MK. Whole body PET imaging with 18FDG in the management of recurrent colorectal cancer. Arch Surg 1999; 134:503–511.

65. Flanagan FL, Dehdashti F, Ogunbiyi OA. Utility of FDG PET for investigating unexplained plasma CEA elevation in patients with colorectal cancer. Ann Surg 1998; 227:319–323.

66. Delbeke D, Vitola J, Sandler MP. Staging recurrent metastatic colorectal cancer with PET. J Nucl Med 1997; 38:1196–1201.

67. Anzai Y, Carroll WR, Quint DJ. Recurrence of head and neck cancer after surgery or irradiation: prospective comparison of FDG PET and MR imaging diagnoses. Radiology 1996; 200:135–141.

68. Ogawa T, Inugami A, Hatazawa J, Kanno I, Murakami M, Yasui N. Clinical PET for brain tumours: comparison of 18FDG and 11C-methionine. Am J Neuroradiol 1996; 17:345–353.

69. Jochelson M, Mauch P, Balikian J, Rosenthal D, Canellos G. The significance of residual mass in treated Hodgkin's disease. J Clin Oncol 1985; 3:637–640.

70. Surbonne A, Longo DL, DeVita VT, et al. Residual abdominal masses in aggressive non-Hodgkin's lymphoma after chemotherapy: significance and management. J Clin Oncol 1988; 6:1832–1837.

71. de Wit M, Bumann D, Beyer W, Herbst K, Clausen M, Hossfield DK. Whole body FDG PET for diagnosis of residual mass in patients with lymphoma. Ann Oncol 1998; 8(suppl 1):57–60.

72. Bangerter M, Moog F, Griesshammer M, Reske SN, Bergman L. Role of whole body FDG PET in predicting relapse in residual masses after treatment of lymphoma. Br J Haematol 1998; 102:148.

73. Mikhaeel NG, Timothy AR, Hain SF, O'Doherty MJ. 18-FDG-PET for the assessment of residual masses on CT following treatment of lymphomas. Ann Oncol 2002; 11(suppl 1): 147–150.

74. Hain SF, O'Doherty MJ, Timothy AR, Leslie MD, Harper PG, Huddart RA. Fluoro-deoxyglucose positron emission tomography in the evaluation of germ cell tumours at relapse. Br J Cancer 2000; 83:863–869.

75. De Santis M, Bokemeyer C, Becherer A, et al. Predictive impact of 2-18fluoro-2-deoxy-D-glucose positron emission tomography for residual postchemotherapy masses in patients with bulky seminoma. J Clin Oncol 2001; 19:3740–3744.

76. Sugawara Y, Zasadny KR, Grossman HB, et al. Germ cell tumour: differentiation of viable tumour, mature teratoma and necrotic tissue with FDG PET and kinetic modelling. Radiology 1999; 211:249–256.

77. Cremerius U, Effert PJ, Adam G. FDG PET for detection and therapy control of metastatic germ cell tumour. J Nucl Med 1998; 39:815–822.

78. Gambhir SS, Valk P, Shepherd J. Cost effective analysis modeling of the role of PET in the management of patients with recurrent colorectal cancer. J Nucl Med 1997; 38:90P.

79. Park KC, Schwimmer J, Shepherd JE, et al. Decision analysis for the cost-effective management of recurrent colorectal cancer. Ann Surg 2000; 233:310–319.

80. Scott WJ, Shepherd J, Gambhir SS. Cost-effectiveness of FDG-PET for staging non-small cell lung cancer: a decision analysis. Ann Thoracic Surg 1998; 66:1876–1885.

81. Kosuda S, Ichihara K, Watanabe M, Kobayashi H, Kusano S. Decision-tree sensitivity analysis for cost-effectiveness of chest 2-fluoro-2-D [18F] fluorodeoxyglucose positron emission tomography in patients with pulmonary nodules (non-small cell lung carcinoma) in Japan. Clin Invest 2000; 117:346–353.

8

Clinical Advances in PET and Tracer Development

Ludwig G. Strauss and Antonia Dimitrakopoulou-Strauss
Medical PET Group—Biological Imaging, Clinical Cooperation Unit Nuclear Medicine, German Cancer Research Center, Heidelberg, Germany

---

A Note from the Editors

*T*he authors of this exciting chapter are well known and respected with an international PET imaging reputation. This chapter begins with general fundamentals of PET technology and focuses on advances made in clinical image reconstruction. Different quantification approaches are discussed and dynamic scanning techniques are explained. There is a brief mention of PET/CT and the advantages associated with this recently introduced imaging modality. In the second section to this chapter the authors have excelled at describing a host of imaging applications utilizing FDG and other newer tracers. These include investigating tumor proliferation (FLT), chemotherapeutic treatment (F-18-FU), amino acid transport (C-11-AIB), melanin synthesis (F-18-DOPA), tumor volume delineation (Ga-68-DOTATOC), and associated therapy (Y-90-DOTATOC). The two main sections to this chapter complement each other well and afford the reader an insight into general PET technology and new imaging applications.*

In contrast to other imaging methods, both instrumentation and radiochemistry are equally important for nuclear medicine procedures. Since the beginning of positron emission tomography (PET) in the 1980s, constant progress had been made regarding instrumentation and radiochemistry. While the first PET systems could only be used for brain studies and provided one to three slices simultaneously, current systems acquire approximately 15 cm or more at each bed position. New PET/CT systems now allow morphology and function to be easily combined. Due to the complex nature of PET, it is important to optimize all steps required for PET studies. Data acquisition and image reconstruction are important topics that must be optimized to achieve best results. Furthermore, for visual and quantitative assessment of PET studies, appropriate software is required to perform more sophisticated quantification procedures.

DATA ACQUISITION, IMAGE RECONSTRUCTION, AND EVALUATION

PET with F-18-deoxyglucose (FDG) is frequently used for oncological and non-oncological applications to assess tissue viability. While visual evaluation is most common for routine PET studies, there is increasing interest in quantitative approaches. Generally, PET provides more accurate radioconcentration measurements than conventional nuclear medicine procedures. The big advantage of PET is the ability to simultaneously detect 511 keV using the electronic coincidence principle. Other factors such as improved attenuation correction based on transmission measurements are important to achieve accurate radionuclide measurements.

One key factor influencing image quantification is the image reconstruction technique. While filtered back-projection (FBP) is frequently used for image reconstruction in single photon emission computer tomography (SPECT), iterative reconstruction algorithms are gaining increasing importance for PET. FBP is a well-known technique for reconstruction applied in computed tomography (CT) and generally provides acceptable quality images due to the high photon flux observed. In contrast to radiological procedures such as CT, nuclear medicine studies have to deal with less useful signal acquired per unit time. Therefore, the application of FBP for reconstruction usually results in images with limited quality (Fig. 1). While the FBP algorithm is fast and images are obtained immediately due to short reconstruction times, limitations exist with respect to image quality and accuracy, especially when high regional activity concentrations are present or in studies with low count rates.

Besides the FBP technique, other approaches can be applied for PET image reconstruction. Iterative image reconstruction techniques were introduced in PET more than 10 years ago and have been found to be useful for quantitative PET (1,2). However, limitations exist for the routine application of this technique due to the higher computational demand and the slow convergence of the algorithm. On the basis of the performance of current computer systems, most manufacturers are providing iterative reconstruction techniques for PET studies. However, it is important to consider additional factors that are important to achieve optimized quantitative PET studies.

A major progression in iterative image reconstruction was shortening of reconstruction times. Introduction of ordered subset method provides a major step forward to speed up the reconstruction process. On the other hand, the method uses

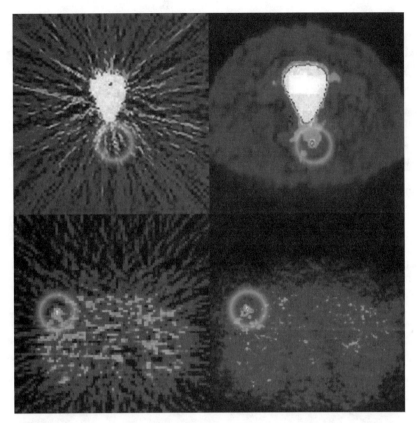

Figure 1   Comparison of FBP (*left images*) and iterative image reconstruction (*right images*). (*Upper row*): Small recurrent colorectal carcinoma, which is not easily detectable with FBP due to severe artifacts caused by excreted FDG accumulating in the bladder. (*Lower row*): Small liver metastasis, which is relatively difficult to detect in the filtered back-projected image (*lower left*) because of the low total number of counts in the image. Superior detection of the lesion is noted when the iterative image reconstruction was used (*lower right*). (*See color insert.*)

only part of the information to reconstruct an image, and this may increase noise significantly. Therefore, it is important to limit the number of subsets, especially with the total number of counts is low, in order to avoid an increase in the noise level (Fig. 2). The example in Figure 2 demonstrates a significant increase of the noise level from 12% (32 iterations, no subsets) to 21% (single iteration, 32 subsets). Furthermore, the structure of the liver parenchyma as well as the tracer distribution in the circular liver metastasis changes according to the reconstruction parameters used.

Another critical aspect of the iterative reconstruction algorithm is the dependency of image quality on the number of iterations. Furthermore, the uptake values used for the semi-quantitative evaluation are dependent on the reconstruction parameters used. Usually the signal increases nonlinearly with the number of iterations, therefore limiting the comparison of PET studies reconstructed with different number of iterations. One solution is the use of the so-called median root prior correction, which limits the increase in the signal (Fig. 3) (3,4). An optimized image quality is important for both the visual and quantitative evaluation of PET studies.

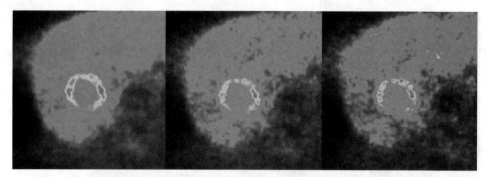

Figure 2 Rim-like FDG uptake in a liver metastasis. The product of the number of iterations and number of subsets was kept constant for the image reconstruction. (*Left*): Thirty-two iterations, no subsets. (*Middle*): Four iterations, eight subsets. (*Right*): One iteration, 32 subsets. Significant increase of the noise level are noted from 12% (*left image*) to 21% (*right image*) when the number of subsets was increased. Furthermore, the distribution of the maxima within the metastasis and the homogeneity of the tracer distribution in the normal liver parenchyma are dependent on the reconstruction parameters. (*See color insert.*)

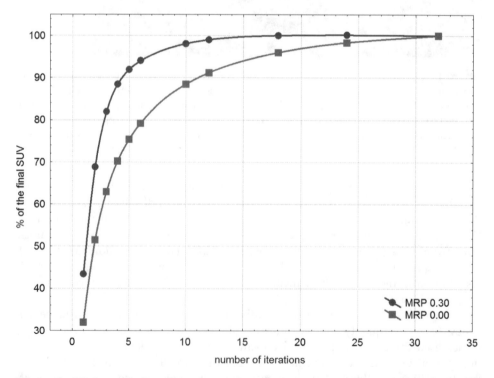

Figure 3 FDG uptake in a liver metastasis, quantified according to the SUV procedure. Slow increase of the uptake value with time without reaching a plateau phase is observed when the median root prior correction is not used. A constant SUV level is not achieved even with 32 iterations (*squares*). Fast convergence of the uptake values when the median root prior correction is applied (*circles*).

Generally, quantitative PET studies can be performed if attenuation corrected PET images are reconstructed from the emission data. To increase the information obtained from a PET examination, the use of a modified whole body protocol is helpful for the data acquisition. One approach is to select a primary target area on the basis of the information provided by the referring physician and to perform a dynamic study for one hour. This protocol is helpful if a full compartment model is used for data evaluation. If the evaluation is confined to a few kinetic data, the acquisition protocol can be shortened to a 10-minute dynamic acquisition beginning with the tracer injection, followed by repositioning of the patient, and acquiring a five-minute image at the same level 55 minutes after tracer injection.

One parameter for the semi-quantitative evaluation is based on normalization of tracer concentrationsnormalization of for the injected dose and body weight, for which the term "standardized uptake value" (SUV) was introduced more than 13 years ago (5). While static measurements one hour after tracer injection reflect the global FDG accumulation at one time point, more information is provided with dynamic data acquisitions. Because FDG uptake one hour after tracer injection is the result of complex dynamic processes, dynamic measurements are the most accurate approach to quantify FDG kinetics.

Several attempts had been made to reduce the complexity of dynamic data acquisitions, which are more time consuming in the patient examination stage and also require sophisticated software for the data evaluation compared to simple static measurements. Matthies et al. (6) performed dual point measurements in patients with pulmonary nodules and found high sensitivity (100%) for detection of malignant tumors, while the specificity was 89%. Hubner et al. (7) compared visual evaluation, SUV, and Patlak analysis in patients with malignant lung lesions and reported that accuracy was improved when both SUV and Patlak values were used for the evaluation. The basic two-compartment model that describes the metabolic fate of FDG was found to be useful for the analysis of FDG kinetics.

One major limitation is the availability of appropriate software for fast evaluation of dynamic data. We are routinely performing dynamic studies in patients undergoing PET for research purposes as well as for clinical tumor diagnostics. Our studies are evaluated using the routines for compartment and noncompartment modeling of a software package available from PMod Technologies Ltd. Burger et al. (8) have developed the software package "PMod," which is extremely useful for the quantitative analysis of dynamic studies. Generally the quantitative evaluation should include most of the target volume to improve statistics for the quantitative assessment. This requirement is supported by PMod via the use of Volumes-of-Interest (VOI) instead of Regions-of-Interest (ROI). The quantitative evaluation is generally based on the calculation of standardized uptake values (SUV). The SUV is calculated according to the formula (5):

SUV (Standardized uptake value) =
Tissue concentration (Bq/g)/[Injected dose (Bq)/Body weight(g)]

One advantage of SUV is the fast calculation and the application to dynamic as well as to static images. In contrast, the calculation of the global FDG influx based on the Patlak approach requires a dynamic data acquisition. The global influx of FDG can be calculated using tracer concentrations for the target area and the plasma (9). The tracer concentration can be obtained via blood sampling, but it is more applicable to retrieve the input function from dynamic images. Ohtake et al. (10) showed that the image-based data obtained from a VOI of a large vessel correlated well with those obtained by arterial blood sampling. Similar results are reported by Keiding et al. (11). However, a VOI consisting of at least seven ROIs should be used to minimize the statistical error. Partial volume correction should be applied if required. The recovery coefficient of the PET system used at our center is 0.85 for lesions exceeding a diameter of 8 mm. Therefore, data from the abdominal aorta can be used usually even without correction in most of the patients.

The most detailed information is obtained by the classical two-compartment analysis of the FDG kinetics. It should be emphasized that the full compartment model should be applied to the data for the analysis of FDG kinetics in tumors. The transport constants $K1$ to $k4$ as well as the distribution volume for FDG can be estimated from the compartment fit procedure (Fig. 4). Especially the estimation of the so-called vessel density, a parameter correlated to the exchange surface of FDG, is important for an accurate quantitative approach, because the kinetics is modulated by this parameter. Furthermore, $k4$ must be considered because some

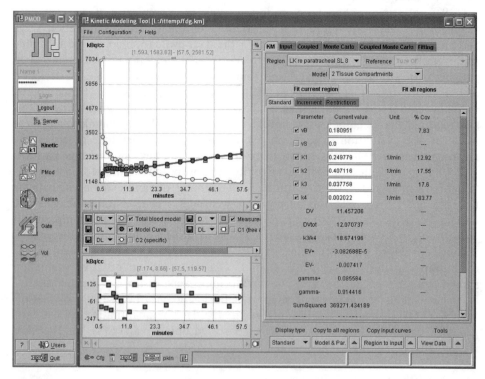

Figure 4 Standard output for a two-compartment fit according to the FDG model. The data are obtained from a metastatic paratracheal lymph node metastasis. The input data (*grey curve*) are used to calculate the compartment parameters for the target area (*dark grey curve*). Twenty-eight measurements are calculated with increasing time intervals for a total of one hour. The iterative compartment fit provides the following parameters (*see right part of the figure*); vB: vessel density, a parameter related to the exchange surface for FDG in the target volume; $K1$: transport of FDG from blood to tissue; $k2$: transport of FDG from tissue to blood; $k3$: phosphorylation of FDG; $k4$: dephosphorylation of FDG.

tumors can show a dephosphorylation of FDG. Using compartment parameters, FDG influx can also be calculated using the formula influx $= (K1^* k3)/(k2 + k3)$.

Compartment modeling can be helpful in the differential diagnosis of malignant tumors, as shown by Dimitrakopoulou-Strauss et al. (12,13). The authors used dynamic PET studies in patients with soft-tissue sarcomas and evaluated the impact on diagnosis as well as the correlation to grading (13). Some overlap existed when SUVs were used to differentiate benign and malignant lesions. Furthermore, SUV was helpful to identify grade III tumors, but the use of full kinetic information permitted the differentiation of further classes. The authors concluded that the evaluation of full FDG kinetics is necessary in these tumors and is superior to a single static data acquisition (13). Similar results were reported by Nieweg et al. (14), who showed a correlation of the metabolic rate and the tumor grade in soft-tissue sarcomas. Sugawara et al. (15) used FDG kinetic modeling in 21 patients with untreated and treated germ cell tumors. The major aim of the study was the evaluation of kinetic analysis for the classification of mature teratoma. The authors were able to differentiate viable tumors using the semi-quantitative SUV approach, but they did not find significant differences between mature teratomas and necrosis when SUV or visual analysis was used. In contrast, statistical significant differences were found for the rate constants $K1$ as well as for the global FDG influx (15). These results demonstrate that a detailed quantitative analysis of the FDG kinetics can help to achieve more accurate diagnoses.

One important improvement in PET technology is the development of combined PET/CT systems. These systems are especially helpful as detailed morphological information is provided by high resolution CT scans. Furthermore, it has been shown that close correlation of PET and CT images is required to achieve optimal diagnoses. It has been repeatedly stated that the use of PET/CT systems decreases the number of equivocal findings, even for experienced readers. According to our own experience, "soft fusion" of CT and PET images using dedicated fusion software is helpful in many cases (Fig. 5). "Hard fusion" using a dedicated PET/CT scanner is generally easier, but demands an additional CT study and therefore adds radiation exposure for patients. Currently PET/CT systems are being used for radiation treatment planning and in the future, the combination of PET and MRI may be even more helpful for functional/morphological correlations.

PET CORRELATES WITH MOLECULAR BIOLOGY

Many studies have been performed to correlate gene expression and prognosis in cancer patients. Lee et al. (16) evaluated the tumor suppressor gene expression in 329 patients with gastric carcinomas and found that the overexpression of p53 and MUC1 as well as the loss of several tumor suppressor genes was associated with patient survival. Grabsch et al. (17) noted that the overexpression of the mitotic checkpoint genes BUB1, BUBR1, and BUB3 are associated with tumor cell proliferation and are therefore important for prognosis in gastric cancer. Due to the dependency of PET radiotracer kinetics on molecular mechanisms, it is important to evaluate possible coexpression of GLUT's and HK's with genes related to malignant lesions.

Several studies have shown that the expression of glucose transporter genes is linked to prognostic parameters. Overexpression of the GLUT-1 transporter is reported to be associated with poor prognosis in patients with oral squamous cell

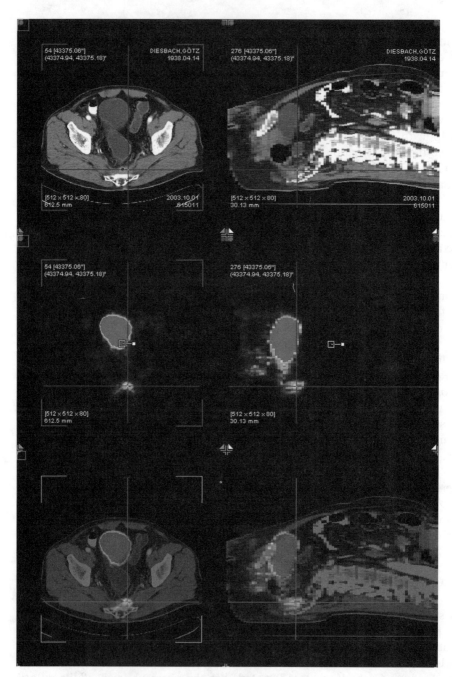

Figure 5 Image fusion of PET and CT in a patient with a recurrent colorectal carcinoma. This patient has a soft-tissue mass in CT in front of the sacrum (*upper images at the intersection of the blue lines*). The corresponding PET image demonstrates a circumscribed hypermetabolic lesion following FDG injection (*images middle row*). Image fusion was done using PMod software using the mutual information technique and demonstrates that the recurrent tumor is only in the left paramedian part of the soft-tissue mass noted in CT, whereas the right lateral area does not contain active tumor tissue. (*See color insert.*)

carcinoma (18). The authors were able to compare GLUT-1 expression as measured by immunohistochemistry and FDG PET in 31 patients with squamous cell carcinoma of the oropharynx and found that GLUT-1 expression was an independent marker of prognosis. Furthermore, an SUV exceeding 5.6 was associated with shorter survival. Comparable results are reported for other tumors. High GLUT-1 expression was associated with a higher risk of death (2.3 times) compared to low GLUT-1 expression in colorectal carcinomas (19). GLUT-1 was compared with the prognostic significance of p53, Ki-67, and VEGF in adenocarcinoma of the lung (20). The authors found that GLUT-1 expression was the most important prognostic factor for survival.

Younes et al. evaluated both GLUT-1 and GLUT-3 in patients with non-small cell lung cancer and found that GLUT-1 was enhanced in 83% of the tumors, while the GLUT-3 expression was increased in 21% of the cases (21). The enhanced expression of both the genes was correlated with poorer survival. The authors conclude that GLUT-1 enhancement reflects aggressive biologic behavior, which is further enhanced by increased GLUT-3 expression. Haberkorn et al. (22) performed experimental studies using a rat Morris hepatoma (MH3924A) model and evaluated glucose transport and apoptosis after gene therapy with HSV thymidine kinase. They found that glucose transport might even be enhanced following treatment with ganciclovir due to a stress reaction of the tumor cells to prevent cell death.

FDG, the most frequently used radiopharmaceutical for PET examinations in the world, is transported like glucose into tumor cells, but then trapped after phosphorylation. However, the knowledge about the correlation of gene expression and FDG kinetics is limited. Experimental studies in several cell lines demonstrated that the deoxyglucose uptake is mainly determined by GLUT-1 expression and not primarily dependent on hexokinase activity (23). Miyakita et al. (24) performed FDG PET in 19 patients with renal cell carcinoma and assessed the GLUT-1 expression in these patients using tumor specimens. The authors report no significant correlation of GLUT-1 expression with FDG uptake. Interestingly, an increased FDG uptake was only observed in 6 of 19 patients with renal cell carcinoma. GLUT-1 expression may be very different according to the tumor type. Higashi et al. (25) evaluated 32 patients with non-small cell lung cancer and found that six of seven bronchoalveolar carcinomas were negative for the expression of GLUT-1 as measured with immunohistochemistry, while only 1 of 23 nonbronchoalveolar adenocarcinomas was negative.

Besides histology, the heterogeneity of the tumor tissue may result in local variations of FDG uptake. Brown et al. (26) examined the intratumoral distribution of tritiated FDG in breast carcinoma and compared the distribution of the tracer with GLUT-1 expression. The authors found comparable distributions of both FDG and GLUT-1 in tumor cells; overall, a positive correlation existed with $r = 0.3$ to 0.6 for FDG uptake and GLUT-1 expression. Comparable data are reported by Higashi et al. (27), who compared both one-hour SUV and a retention index based on dual point measurements at one and two hours after FDG injection with GLUT-1 and hexokinase-II expression. The authors found a low correlation for the one-hour SUV and the GLUT-1 expression, but no correlation with hexokinase-II expression. In contrast, a significant correlation was observed for the retention index and hexokinase-II, indicating that late measurements following FDG application are mainly related to the tracer trapping based on hexokinase activity, but not the images within one hour following FDG application.

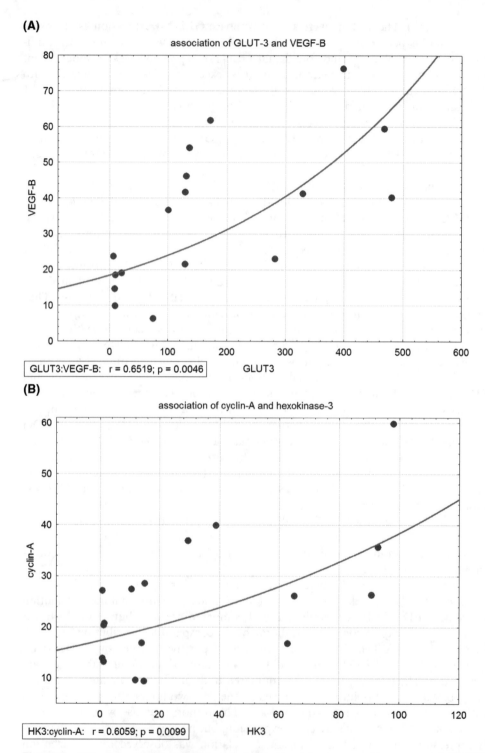

Figure 6 Gene chip analysis of tumor samples (colorectal tumors and bone tumors). VEGF-B and cyclin-A are correlated with glucose transporter GLUT-3 (*upper diagram*) and hexokinase (*lower diagram*). The data gave evidence for a link between angiogenesis, proliferation, and glucose metabolism.

Other genes may also have an impact on FDG kinetics. We are evaluating the correlation of FDG kinetics with gene expression using gene chip technology in colorectal tumors and sarcomas (28). Interestingly, several genes show a coexpression with glucose transporters and hexokinases. One interesting group of genes is the vascular endothelial growth factors (VEGF), which are directly involved in angiogenesis and lymphatic spread of tumors. Another group is cell cycle related genes, which are important for the proliferation of tumors. Our preliminary results obtained from colorectal tumors and sarcomas show that VEGF-B was associated with GLUT-3 and cyclin-A with HK3 (Fig. 6) (29). Therefore, there is evidence that enhanced angiogenesis and proliferation are associated with increased glucose metabolism in these tumors.

OTHER TRACERS

^{18}F-3′-Deoxy-3′-Fluorothymidine

The thymidine analog ^{18}F-3′-deoxy-3′-fluorothymidinethymidine analog (F-18-FLT) is a promising tracer, now finding limited use as a proliferation marker. Originally, FLT was used as a chemotherapeutic agent, but abandoned due to severe side effects. FLT is currently used in its F-18 labeled form for both experimental and patient studies. Rasey et al. (30) evaluated F-18-FLT in cell culture studies using human lung carcinoma cells and noted that the tracer uptake correlates with the thymidine kinase-1 activity with $r^2 = 0.63$. The authors report an excellent correlation of $r^2 = 0.91$ for the F-18-FLT uptake and the percentage of cells in S-phase. The comparison of F-18-FLT and C-14-DG (deoxyglucose) showed that an increase of the percent S-phase cells from 4% to 32% enhanced the F-18-FLT uptake by a factor of 6.4, while the C-14-DG uptake was only increased by 1.8 (30). The data show that DG is dependent on proliferation, but the uptake change varies according to the S-phase fraction and is generally lower. F-18-FLT is likely to be more accurate with regard to tumor proliferation (Fig. 7).

The accurate, noninvasive quantification of tumor proliferation requires a tracer which is incorporated into DNA. However, F-18-FLT is an indirect marker for proliferation, because the majority of the signal is obtained by the thymidine kinase-1 activity. Lu et al. (31) evaluated several radiotracers regarding their use as proliferation markers. The comparison of tracer kinetics demonstrates only for 1-(2′-deoxy-2′-fluoro-β-D-arabinofuranosyl)-5-[^{76}Br]bromouracil (^{76}Br-BFU), a continuous increase of tracer uptake with time. The DNA incorporation was highest for ^{76}Br-BFU with 97%, 80% for 1-(2′-deoxy-2′-fluoro-β-D-arabinofuranosyl)-[methyl-^{11}C]thymine (^{11}C-FMAU), and only 2% for F-18-FLT. Cimetidine, which has an impact on the elimination of nucleosides, altered the uptake of ^{76}Br-BFU, but not ^{11}C-FMAU and F-18-FLT. The data show that the tumor proliferation can be measured with different accuracy. While ^{76}Br-BFU is likely to reflect tumor proliferation most accurately, other tracers like F-18-FLT and FDG are also acceptable for patient studies because they are indirectly involved in the proliferation of cells.

F-18-Fluorouracil

One interesting PET application is the evaluation of tracer kinetics of drugs already used for chemotherapeutic treatment. 5-Fluorouracil (F-18-FU) is the standard cytotoxic agent for the treatment of metastatic colorectal cancer. It has been used

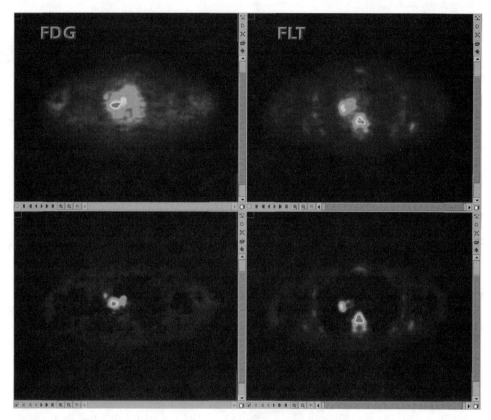

Figure 7 FDG and F-18-FLT in a 66-year-old male patient with a squamous cell carcinoma of the upper lobe of the right lung. (*Upper row*): Uptake images 60 minutes following tracer application. (*Lower row*): Parametric images of the tracer influx. Preferentially enhanced FDG uptake in the malignant tumor (*left images*). F-18-FLT demonstrates the most active, proliferating part of the tumor (*right images*). Enhanced F-18-FLT uptake in the bone marrow is frequently seen in F-18-FLT studies. (*See color insert.*)

in the F-18 labeled form to evaluate the kinetics of the agent using systemic and regional application (32,33). Furthermore, the correlation of tracer retention and therapy result was studied (34). The intravenous application of tracer demonstrated a rapid uptake in normal liver parenchyma, while liver metastases generally showed a low tracer uptake (32). Dimitrakopoulou-Strauss et al. (33) used O-15-water and F-18-FU and compared the systemic and regional application of the tracers in patients with liver metastases from colorectal carcinoma. The authors found that the access to lesions, as measured with O-15-water, was enhanced in 87% of metastatic lesions, which resulted in an improved F-18-FU transport into tumor cells in 83% of the metastases. However, only 33% of the lesions showed an enhanced trapping of F-18-FU two hours after tracer application (Fig. 8). On the basis of data, it can be expected that the retention of 5-FU, which is mandatory for a sufficient treatment result, is limited because of the tracer efflux out of the tumor cells in patients receiving intra-arterial chemotherapy. Enhancement of the treatment effects, therefore, requires a modification of the efflux mechanism.

It is still in discussion as to what resistance mechanisms exist in colorectal tumors. Tseng et al. (35) evaluated the role of Ha-ras overexpression and fluorouracil

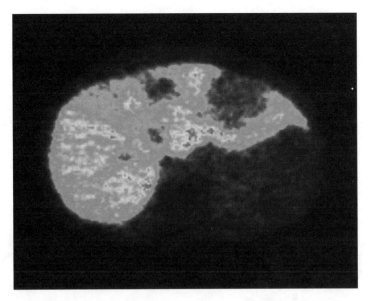

Figure 8 PET image in a patient with multiple metastases from a colorectal carcinoma. Image of the F-18-FU uptake two hours after tracer application. Low retention of the tracer is seen in the metastases, which are visible as defects. Therefore the therapeutic success with FU treatment is limited. (*See color insert.*)

effects. The authors were able to show a close relation between Ha-ras expression and FU sensitivity of the cells. Yoshinare et al. (36) assessed the chemosensitivity to fluorouracil in colorectal cancer specimens and found that a high thymidine phosphorylase mRNA expression correlated well with low sensitivity to FU. Furthermore, the authors emphasize that the levels of dihydropyrimidine dehydrogenase (DHPDH), the key enzyme of FU catabolism, and es-nucleoside transporter, an important transmembrane transporter of nucleosides, are possible predictors of sensitivity to FU. Interestingly, we noted a close correlation for HK3 and DHPDH, which may direct to an association of glucose metabolism and FU catabolism (Fig. 9).

It was shown that for other genes such as the multidrug resistance gene (mdr1) one important resistance mechanism is the fast efflux of cytostatic drugs out of the tumor cells, mediated by membrane located, ATP dependent efflux pumps. Guo et al. (37) performed studies in MRP8 overexpressing cells and found that MRP8 reduces the cAMP and CGMP levels and enhances the elimination of cyclic nucleotides from the cells. As a consequence, the MRP8 overexpressing cells were resistant to a range of clinically used nucleotide analogs, including fluorouracil. Interestingly, studies of fluorouracil transport were performed noninvasively with F-18-fluorouracil in patients with liver metastases from colorectal carcinomas to obtain information about the FU transport mechanisms (32). The perfusion of lesions with O-15-water was evaluated, the FU transport was assessed using SUV measurements following a short infusion of F-18-FU together with nonlabeled FU, and the retention was quantified on the basis of the two-hour F-18-FU uptake. Cluster analysis revealed two groups: 43/53 lesions, the majority of the metastases evaluated with O-15-water and F-18-FU, demonstrated a dependency on blood flow, but the retention of F-18-FU two hours after tracer application was low and less than 2.0 SUV. In contrast, 10 metastases had a nonperfusion dependent F-18-FU transport and 7/10

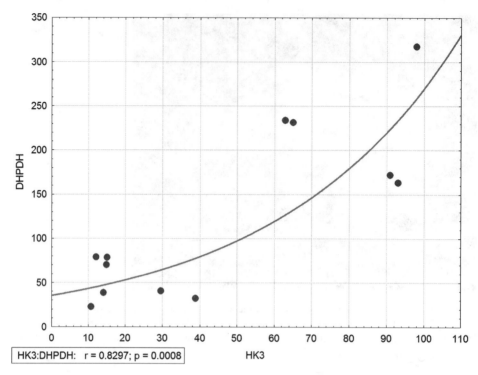

Figure 9 Gene chip analysis revealed a correlation of HK3 and DHPDH, the key enzyme of the FU catabolism.

showed uptake values exceeding 2.0 SUV. The authors conclude that PET with F-18-FU can be used to select those patients showing a higher retention of the tracer in metastatic lesions. With respect to the studies of Tseng et al. (35), the fast efflux of F-18-FU, out of the majority of the metastases, is likely to be due to the enhanced MRP8 expression. Alternatively, different transport pathways for FU must be discussed. F-18-FU is a promising tracer to be used in patients with metastatic color-ectal cancer for the individualization of therapy management.

C-11-AIB

While PET with FDG generally provides a high sensitivity, specificity is limited due to the preferential uptake of FDG in a large number of tumors, and nondesirable uptake in some benign diseases (38). Therefore, the use of other tracers as a multitracer examination can help to gain additional information. Besides glucose metabolism, the transport of amino acids can be important in oncology, because tumors frequently show an increased protein synthesis. Amino acids are transported via several transport mechanisms, from which about 20 different systems are known. One of the main systems which mediate the transport of neutral amino acids is called the A-type transport. This sodium dependent transport mechanism is typically represented by alanine and transports neutral amino acids with a short side chain. Conti et al. (39) were one of the first authors reporting about the use of C-11 labeled alpha-aminoisobutyric acid (AIB) in tumors. The authors evaluated the uptake of C-11-AIB in nude mice bearing human malignant melanoma heterotransplants and found a mean tumor-to-blood ratio of

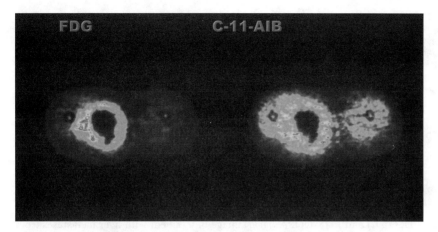

Figure 10 FDG (*left*) and C-11-AIB image of a patient with a liposarcoma on the right leg. Enhanced FDG metabolism and increased amino acid A-type transport. The distribution of the FDG uptake is different from the amino acid uptake. (*See color insert.*)

5.42, 45 minutes following the tracer application. Sordillo et al. (40) used C-11-AIB in 10 patients with metastatic or unresectable malignant melanoma and noted an increased tracer uptake in the primary tumor in six patients. However, no comparison was made with FDG. Uehara et al. (41) evaluated four different tracers in experimental brain tumors in rats and found that viable and necrotic appearing tumor regions could be better distinguished with AIB than with FDG. We noted in most soft-tissue sarcomas a higher uptake for FDG, because it is not only transported but also trapped by phosphorylation, whereas C-11-AIB provides additional information, which is frequently different from FDG regarding the spatial distribution in the tumor (Fig. 10). It was shown that AIB might be helpful for the differentiation of tumor and inflammation (42). In contrast to FDG, it is likely that C-11-AIB is not taken up in granulocytes, therefore inflammatory structures are negative on the AIB scan.

6-[^{18}F] Fluoro-L-Dopa

Several authors have investigated 6-[^{18}F]fluoro-L-dopa (F-18-DOPA) in oncological patients to increase the specificity of PET. Dihydroxyphenylalanine (DOPA) has the potential to be used as a precursor of melanin synthesis. Ishiwata et al. (43) assessed F-18-DOPA uptake in mice bearing B16 melanomas and found that tracer uptake was correlated with melanogenesis. However, it is likely that F-18-DOPA primarily provides information about the transport of the tracer, because the F-18 label is removed after the first metabolic step when DOPA is labeled in the sixth-position (44). Perfusion, FDG, and F-18-DOPA kinetics were compared in 11 patients with metastatic melanoma by Dimitrakopoulou-Strauss et al. (44). Generally FDG uptake was 1.5-fold higher than the F-18-DOPA uptake in 18 of 22 metastases. The authors report that the F-18-DOPA uptake was not perfusion dependent and provided different information as compared with FDG. Jacob et al. (44) used F-18-DOPA and FDG in four patients with small cell carcinoma and noted a lower uptake of F-18-DOPA as compared to FDG. Besides malignant melanoma, F-18-DOPA does accumulate in endocrine tumors (Fig. 11). On the basis of the current literature data, F-18-DOPA seems to be a promising tracer for PET imaging in patients

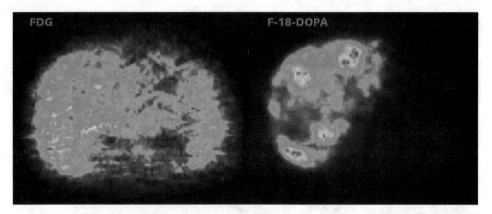

Figure 11 FDG (*left*) and F-18-DOPA (*right*) image of a patient with liver metastases from an endocrine tumor following chemotherapeutic treatment. The metastases show a low FDG uptake and preferentially accumulate F-18-DOPA. (*See color insert.*)

with malignant melanoma and endocrine tumors, additional to FDG. Especially in patients following chemotherapeutic treatment, F-18-DOPA can provide additional information as compared to FDG, because FDG uptake can be low in these patients.

Ga-68-DOTATOC

Somatostatin is a peptide that inhibits the release of growth hormone and proved to be a cyclic peptide consisting of 14 amino acids. Five subtypes of human somatostatin receptors have been cloned and characterized in humans. Somatostatin receptors have been demonstrated in various regions of the brain and leptomeninges, the anterior pituitary, the endocrine and exocrine pancreas, and the mucosa of the gastrointestinal tract, as well as in the immune system. The first somatostatin analog introduced for clinical use is octreotide, which inhibits the release of growth hormone, glucagon, and insulin more powerfully than somatostatin itself. Octreotide binds with a high affinity to somatostatin-receptor (SSTR) subtype 2 and to a lower extent with subtype 5. Somatostatin receptor scintigraphy with In-111-octreotide has been found useful in the diagnostics of endocrine tumors. Belhocine et al. (46) compared PET with FDG and In-11-octreotide scintigraphy in patients with endocrine tumors and noted a higher sensitivity of In-11-octreotide. PET provides higher spatial resolution and better quantification capabilities compared with SPECT. Furthermore, the affinity of DOTATOC for SSTR2 is superior to octeotide. Therefore, it is not surprising that Hofmann et al. (47) report a higher sensitivity for Ga-68 labeled DOTATOC in contrast to In-111-octreotide. Ga-68-DOTATOC is preferentially bound to the SSTR2 receptor and primarily provides information about the expression of this receptor. The radiopharmaceutical is helpful in meningiomas and endocrine tumors to delineate the tumor volume accurately. Furthermore, other tumors such as lung tumors may show a GA-68-DOTATOC tracer accumulation (Fig. 12).

The high, specific uptake of DOTATOC due to enhanced expression of SSTR2 can be used not only for diagnostic purpose but also for treatment. Walherr et al. (48) used Y-90-DOTATOC in 39 patients with progressive neuroendocrine tumors and noted subsequent progressive disease in only 8% of the patients; in most patients, stable disease was achieved. Schumacher et al. (49) used local injections

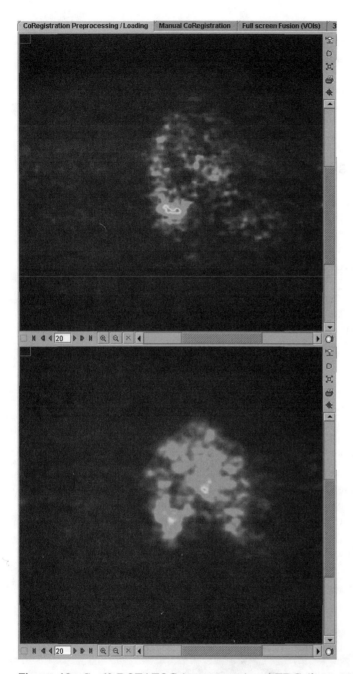

Figure 12 Ga-68-DOTATOC (*upper image*) and FDG (*lower image*) in a patient with non-small cell lung cancer. The patient has a malignant tumor located dorsal above above the right hilar region. The tumor shows a moderate FDG uptake (3.7 SUV) and a circumscribed accumulation of Ga-68-DOTATOC (4.8 SUV). The image contrast is higher for Ga-68-DOTATOC due to the lower background activity. (*See color insert.*)

of Y-90-DOTATOC in five patients with progressive gliomas grades II and III. However, the number of patients is limited, but the local treatment seems to be helpful in these patients. The authors observed that one patient had a slow transformation of a primary inoperable anaplastic astrocytoma into a subsequently resectable multicystic lesion. The data show that Y-90-DOTATOC is an alternative therapeutic approach especially in patients with endocrine tumors, provided that lesions demonstrate an increased uptake of Ga-68-DOTATOC.

OTHER NEW TRACERS

Continuous progress made in the field of molecular biology has led to the development of new radiopharmaceuticals for imaging. One aim is to image gene expression noninvasively using radiotracers. This may be achieved by the use of antisense imaging. Antisense imaging methods are being investigated to modulate the gene expression. Base pairing of messenger RNA with oligonucleotide ultimately results in a downregulation of specific genes. This technique, based on suppression of DNA transcription or RNA translation, can be used for therapeutic and diagnostic purposes. Due to the unique selectivity, oligonucleotides are promising tools for the development of new radiotracers for molecular imaging. Automated synthesis procedures have been developed, which are a pre-requisite for the application of these new radiopharmaceuticals (50).

One currently investigated application of molecular biological techniques is the use of gene therapeutic approaches, e.g., the modification of iodine uptake in malignant tumors to provide a possibility for radioisotope treatment. The therapeutic outcome of differentiated thyroid cancer is dependent on the ability to accumulate iodine for radioisotope therapy. The transport of iodine is mediated by the sodium/iodide transporter (NIS). NIS is regulated by TSH, but also by several other factors. It has been reported that thyroid cancers may show a down-regulation of the NIS, which limits radioisotope therapy. Besides thyroid tissue, NIS expression was found in several other tissues, including pancreas, breast tissue, prostate gland, ovary, and lung (51). Dohán et al. (52) report about an expression rate of 80% in breast cancer samples. The upregulation of NIS in these structures can be used to target radioiodine therapy in thyroid carcinoma as well as in other tumors (Fig. 13). Chung

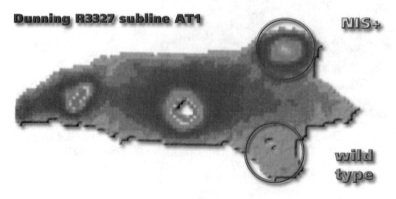

Figure 13 Modification of NIS expression in a prostate carcinoma (Dunning R3327). Significant increase of the iodine uptake in the genetically modified tumor (*yellow circle*) as compared to the wild type (*green circle*). (*See color insert.*)

reviewed the role of the sodium iodide transporter in nuclear medicine and emphasized the role of NIS as an alternative imaging reporter gene (53). However, one major problem for the clinical application is the efflux of iodine out of tumor cells following upregulation of NIS (54). Haberkorn et al. used a Dunning prostate adenocarcinoma model and reported an initially 200-fold enhanced tracer uptake in the genetically modified tumor. However, up to 81% of the radioactivity was released within 20 minutes. Dosimetry calculations revealed that an injected activity resulting in a dose of $1200\,MBq/m^2$ resulted in 3 ± 0.5 Gy dose in the tumor, which is by far too low for any therapeutic effect (54). To extend the retention time for iodine, different modifications were proposed, including the simultaneous transfer of the thyroperoxidase gene, use of lithium, and the application of other more effective radioisotopes such as Re-188. These problems need to be solved prior to the application of the method in patients; however, this approach represents a new and promising procedure to treat malignant tumors.

REFERENCES

1. Schmidlin P, Kübler WK, Doll J, Strauss LG, Ostertag H. Image processing in whole body positron emission tomography. In: Schmidt HAE, Csernay L, eds. Nuklearmedizin. Stuttgart, Germany: Schattauer, 1987:84–87.
2. Strauss LG, Clorius JH, Schlag P, et al. Recurrence of colorectal tumors: PET evaluation. Radiology 1989; 170:329–332.
3. Alenius S, Ruotsalainen U. Bayesian image reconstruction for emission tomography based on median root prior. Eur J Nucl Med 1997; 24:258–265.
4. Alenius S. On noise reduction in iterative image reconstruction algorithms for emission tomography: median root prior. Thesis for the degree of Doctor of Technology, Tampere, Finland, 1999.
5. Strauss LG, Conti PS. The applications of PET in clinical oncology. J Nucl Med 1991; 32:623–648.
6. Matthies A, Hickeson M, Cuchiara A, Alavi A. Dual time point 18F-FDG PET for the evaluation of pulmonary nodules. J Nucl Med 2002; 43:871–875.
7. Hubner KF, Buonocore E, Gould HR, Thie J, Smith GT, Stephens Dickey J. Differentiating benign from malignant lung lesions using "quantitative" parameters of FDG PET images. Clin Nucl Med 1996; 21:941–949.
8. Burger C, Buck A. Requirements and implementation of a flexible kinetic modeling tool. J Nucl Med 1997; 38:1818–1823.
9. Patlak CS, Blasberg RG, Fenstermacher JD. Graphical evaluation of blood-to-brain transfer constants from multiple-time uptake data. J Cereb Blood Flow Metab 1983; 3(1):1–7.
10. Ohtake T, Kosaka N, et al. Noninvasive method to obtain input function for measuring tissue glucose utilization of thoracic and abdominal organs. J Nucl Med 1991; 32:1432–1438.
11. Keiding S, Munk OL, Schiott KM, Hansen SB. Dynamic 2-[18F]fluoro-2-deoxy-D-glucose positron emission tomography of liver tumours without blood sampling. Eur J Nucl Med 2000; 27:407–412.
12. Dimitrakopoulou-Strauss A, Strauss LG, Heichel T, Wu H, Burger C, Bernd L, Ewerbeck V. The role of quantitative (18)F-FDG PET studies for the differentiation of malignant and benign bone lesions. J Nucl Med 2002; 43:510–518.
13. Dimitrakopoulou-Strauss A, Strauss LG, Schwarzbach M, Burger C, Heichel T, Willeke F, Mechtersheimer G, Lehnert T. Dynamic PET 18F-FDG studies in patients with

primary and recurrent soft-tissue sarcomas: impact on diagnosis and correlation with grading. J Nucl Med 2001; 42:713–720.

14. Nieweg OE, Pruim J, van Ginkel RJ, et al. Fluorine-18-fluorodeoxy-glucose PET imaging of soft-tissue sarcoma. J Nucl Med 1996; 37:257–261.

15. Sugawara Y, Zasadny KR, Grossman HB, Francis IR, Clarke MF, Wahl RL. Germ cell tumor: differentiation of viable tumor, mature teratoma, and necrotic tissue with FDG PET and kinetic modeling. Radiology 1999; 211(1):249–256.

16. Lee HS, Lee HK, Kim HS, Yang HK, Kim WH. Tumour suppressor gene expression correlates with gastric cancer prognosis. J Pathol 2003; 200:39–46.

17. Grabsch H, Takeno S, Parsons WJ, et al. Overexpression of the mitotic checkpoint genes BUB1, BUBR1, and BUB3 in gastric cancer-association with tumour cell proliferation. J Pathol 2003; 200:16–22.

18. Kunkel M, Reichert TE, Benz P, Lehr HA, Jeong JH, Wieand S, Bartenstein P, Wagner W, Whiteside TL. Overexpression of Glut-1 and increased glucose metabolism in tumors are associated with a poor prognosis in patients with oral squamous cell carcinoma. Cancer 2003; 97:1015–1024.

19. Haber RS, Rathan A, Weiser KR, Pritsker A, Itzkowitz SH, Bo-dian C, Slater G, Weiss A, Burstein DE. GLUT1 glucose transporter expression in colorectal carcinoma: a marker for poor prognosis. Cancer 1998; 83(1):34–40.

20. Minami K, Saito Y, Imamura H, Okamura A. Prognostic significance of p53, Ki-67, VEGF and Glut-1 in resected stage I adenocarcinoma of the lung. Lung Cancer 2002; 38:51–57.

21. Younes M, Brown RW, Stephenson M, Gondo M, Cagle PT. Overexpression of Glut1 and Glut3 in stage I normal cell lung carcinoma is associated with poor survival. Cancer 1997; 15:1046–1051.

22. Haberkorn U, Altmann A, Kamencic H, et al. Glucose transport and apoptosis after gene therapy with HSV thymidine kinase. Eur J Nucl Med 2001; 28:1690–1696.

23. Waki A, Kato H, Yano R, et al. The importance of glucose transport activity as the rate-limiting step of 2-deoxyglucose uptake in tumor cells in vitro. Nucl Med Biol 1998; 25:593–597.

24. Miyakita H, Tokunaga M, Onda H, Usui Y, Kinoshita H, Kawamura N, Yasuda S. Significance of 18F-fluorodeoxyglucose positron emission tomography (FDG-PET) for detection of renal cell carcinoma and immunohistochemical glucose transporter 1 (GLUT-1) expression in the cancer. Int J Urol 2002; 9:15–18.

25. Higashi K, Ueda Y, Sakurai A, et al. Correlation of Glut-1 glucose transporter expression with [18][F]FDG uptake in non-small cell lung cancer. Eur J Nucl Med 2000; 27:1778–1785.

26. Brown RS, Leung JY, Fisher SJ, Frey KA, Ethier SP, Wahl RL. Intratumoral distribution of tritiated-FDG in breast carcinoma: correlation between Glut-1 expression and FDG uptake. J Nucl Med 1996; 37(6):1042–1047.

27. Higashi T, Saga T, Nakamoto Y, et al. Relationship between retention index in dual-phase (18)F-FDG PET, and hexokinase-II and glucose transporter-1 expression in pancreatic cancer. J Nucl Med 2002; 43:173–180.

28. Strauss LG, Dimitrakopoulou-Strauss A, Koczan D, et al. Glucose transporters and hexokinases: correlation with FDG kinetics and coexpression with other genes. J Nucl Med 2003; 44(suppl):80P.

29. Dimitrakopoulou-Strauss A, Strauss LG, Koczan D, Thiesen HJ, Bernd L, Haberkorn U. FDG kinetics and association with cyclin-A and VEGF. J Nucl Med 2003; 44(suppl):80P.

30. Rasey S, Grierson JR, Wiens LW, Kolb PD, Schwartz JL. Validation of FLT uptake as a measure of thymidine kinase-1 activity in A549 carcinoma cells. J Nucl Med 2002; 43:1210–1217.

31. Lu L, Samuelsson L, Bergström M, Sato K, Fasth KJ, Langström B. Rat studies comparing ^{11}C-FMAU, ^{18}F-FLT, and [76]BR-BFU as proliferation markers. J Nucl Med 2002; 43:1688–1698.

32. Dimitrakopoulou A, Strauss LG, Clorius JH, et al. Studies with positron emission tomography after systemic administration of Fluorine-18-Uracil in patients with liver metastases from colorectal carcinoma. J Nucl Med 1993; 34:1075–1081.

33. Dimitrakopoulou-Strauss A, Strauss LG, Schlag P, et al. Intravenous and intra-arterial Oxygen-15 labeled water and Fluorine-18-labeled Fluorouracil in patients with liver metastases from colorectal carcinoma. J Nucl Med 1998; 39:465–473.

34. Dimitrakopoulou-Strauss A, Strauss LG, Schlag P, et al. Fluorine-18-Fluorouracil to predict therapy response in liver metastases from colorectal carcinoma. J Nucl Med 1998; 39:1197–1202.

35. Tseng YS, Tzeng CC, Chiu AWH, et al. Ha-ras overexpression mediated cell apoptosis in the presence of 5-fluorouracil. Exp Cell Res 2003; 288:403–414.

36. Yoshinare K, Kubota T, Watanabe M, et al. Gene expression in colorectal cancer and in vitro chemosensitivity to 5-fluorouracil: a study of 88 surgical specimens. Cancer Sci 2003; 94:633–638.

37. Guo Y, Kotova E, Chem ZS, et al. MRP8, ATP-binding Cassette C11 (ABCC11), is a cyclic nucleotide efflux pump and a resistance factor for fluoropyrimidines 2′,3′-dideoxycytidine and 9′-(2′-phosphonylmethoxyethyl)adenine. J Biol Chem 2003; 278: 29,509–29,514.

38. Strauss LG. Fluorine-18 deoxyglucose and false-positive results: a major problem in the diagnostics of oncological patients. Eur J Nucl Med 1996; 23:1409–1415.

39. Conti PS, Sordillo EM, Sordillo PP, Schmall B. Tumor localization of alpha-aminoisobutyric acid (ABI) in human melanoma heterotransplants. Eur J Nucl Med 1985; 10:45–47.

40. Sordillo PP, DiResta GR, Fissekis J, et al. Tumor imaging with carbon-11 labeled alphaaminoisobutyric acid (AIB) in patients with malignant melanoma. Am J Physiol Imaging 1991; 6:172–175.

41. Uehara H, Miyagawa T, Tjuvajev J, et al. Imaging experimental brain tumors with laminocyclopentane carboxylic acid and alpha-aminoisobutyric acid: comparison to fluorodeoxyglucose and diethylenetriaminepentaacetic acid in morphologically defined tumor regions. J Cereb Blood Flow Metab 1997; 17:1239–1253.

42. Dimitrakopoulou-Strauss A, Strauss LG, Goldschmidt H, Oberdorfer F, Kriesten J, van Kaick G. PET with C-11-aminoisobutyric acid (AIB) for diagnostics and therapy management of oncological patients. Radiology 1997; 205:P221.

43. Ishiwata K, Kubota K, Kubota R, Iwata R, Takahashi T, Ido T. Selective 2-[18F]fluorodopa uptake for melanogenesis in murine metastatic melanomas. J Nucl Med 1991; 32:95–101.

44. Dimitrakopoulou-Strauss A, Strauss LG, Burger C. Quantitative PET studies in pretreated melanoma patients: a comparison of 6[^{18}F]Fluoro-L-Dopa with ^{18}F-FDG and ^{15}O-Water using compartment and noncompartment analysis. J Nucl Med 2001; 42:248–256.

45. Jacob T, Grahek D, Younsi N, et al. Positron emission tomography with [^{18}F]FDOPA and [^{18}F]FDG in the imaging of small cell lung carcinoma: preliminary results. Eur J Nucl Med Mol Imaging 2003; 30:1266–1269.

46. Belhocine T, Foidart J, Rigo P, et al. Fluorodeoxyglucose positron emission tomography and somatostatin receptor scintigraphy for diagnosing and staging carcinoid tumours: correlations with the pathological indexes p53 and Ki-67. Nucl Med Commun 2002; 23:727–734.

47. Hofmann M, Maecke H, Borner R, et al. Biokinetics and imaging with the somatostatin receptor PET radioligand (68)Ga-DOTATOC: preliminary data. Eur J Nucl Med 2001; 28(12):1751–1757.

48. Waldherr C, Pless M, Maecke HR, et al. Tumor response and clinical benefit in neuroendocrine tumors after 7.4 GBq [90]YDOTATOC. J Nucl Med 2002; 43:610–616.

49. Schumacher T, Hofer S, Eichhorn K, et al. Local injection of the ^{90}Y-labelled peptidic vector DOTATOC to control gliomas of WHO grades II and III: an extended pilot study. Eur J Nucl Med 2002; 29:486–493.

50. Wagner S, Eritja R, Zuhayra M, et al. Synthesis and properties of radiolabeled CPTA-oligonucleotides. J Label Compd Radiopharm 2003; 46:175–186.

51. Filetti S, Bidart JM, Arturi F, Caillou B, Russo D, Schlumberger M. Sodium/iodine symporter: a key transport system in thyroid cancer cell metabolism. Eur J Endocrinol 1999; 141:443–457.

52. Dohán O, de la Vieja A, Paroder V, et al. The sodium/iodide symporter (NIS): characterization, regulation, and medical significance. Endocrine Rev 2003; 24:48–77.

53. Chung JK. Sodium iodide symporter: its role in nuclear medicine. J Nucl Med 2002; 43:1188–1200.

54. Haberkorn U, Kinscherf R, Kissel M, et al. Enhanced iodide transport after transfer of the human sodium iodide symporter gene is associated with lack of retention and low absorbed dose. Gene Therapy 2003; 10:774–780.

9

Molecular Targeted Imaging in Oncology with Radioscintigraphy

David J. Yang and E. Edmund Kim
Division of Diagnostic Imaging, The University of Texas M.D. Anderson Cancer Center, Houston, Texas, U.S.A.

A Note from the Editors

*W*hile PET imaging has garnered much of the attention in oncologic imaging, there have been parallel and exciting developments in more conventional gamma radioscintigraphy. Conventional radioscintigraphy with 99m-technetium offers a substantially lower cost alternative to PET both in terms of synthesis and in instrumentation. This chapter describes a "platform technology" in which a surprising variety of ligands can be chelated to technetium. Examples of oncologic agents already in preclinical testing are provided. The authors, who are leaders in the field of radioligand synthesis, demonstrate how this "plug and play" construct lends itself to automation and portends a future in which versatile radioligands, tailored to the individual needs of the patient, can be created on demand.

INTRODUCTION

While the use of ^{18}F-fluorodeoxyglucose (FDG)-PET in oncology has generated intense interest, conventional gamma-emitting radionuclides remain important and are possibly a cost-effective alternative in molecular imaging techniques for clinic use. New advances in chelate chemistry include the development of "plug and play" platform technology in which the imaging beacon and chelate remain the same, while a host of small molecule ligands can be substituted as needed. Combining this chemistry with automated synthesis devices creates the opportunity to generate, perhaps, hundreds of radioligands for imaging, allowing customization of patient workup in the future.

This chapter reviews developments in the synthesis of Technetium99m (^{99m}Tc) chelates for radiolabeling of ligands to assess tumor targets in man. A family of new ligands bound to ^{99m}Tc ethyelendicysteine (EC) has been developed for single photon emission computed tomography (SPECT) imaging of neoplasms. Several of these new agents are discussed in detail including ^{99m}Tc-EC–deoxyglucose (EC–DG) for glycolysis imaging, ^{99m}Tc-EC C225 antibody, endostatin, and celebrex for angiogenesis imaging, ^{99m}Tc-EC–metronidazole (EC–MN) for hypoxia imaging, ^{99m}Tc-EC–annexin V for apoptosis imaging, ^{99m}Tc-EC–doxorubicin for multidrug resistance (MDR) imaging, ^{99m}Tc-EC–LHRH for imaging of hormone sensitive tumors such as prostate cancer, and ^{99m}Tc-C–guanosine for nucleic acid synthesis or proliferation imaging. The sheer breadth of possibilities for expanding imaging and the ease with which these agents can be developed and substituted for each other argues well for a future in which individual patients could undergo serial imaging studies to characterize the nature of their tumor without the need for biopsy. On the basis of these results the treatment regimen could be designed with the maximal likelihood of success. Herein, the details of the chemical synthesis are discussed and early preclinical results with these new molecular imaging methods.

Several imaging modalities including computed tomography (CT), magnetic resonance imaging (MRI), ultrasound, optical imaging, and gamma scintigraphy have been used to assess cancer. Although CT and MRI provide detailed anatomic information about the location and the extent of tumors, they are inherently non-specific. For instance, in the case of brain tumors they cannot reliably differentiate residual or recurrent tumors from edema, radiation necrosis, or gliosis. Doppler ultrasound images are of lower resolution but enable regional blood flow measurements to be made. Despite this advantage, ultrasound suffers from relatively poor specificity and poor penetration of air-containing body cavities thus limiting its applications; and is also highly operator dependent. Although optical imaging shows promise, its inability to penetrate deeply into tissue will limit its human imaging applications. Optical imaging may prove useful for surface imaging such as during endoscopy or surgery. Radionuclide imaging modalities (positron emission tomography, PET; SPECT) are diagnostic cross-sectional imaging techniques that map the location and concentration of radionuclide-labeled compounds (1–3). In addition to localizing tumors, PET and SPECT are making it possible to "see" the molecular makeup of the tumor and its metabolic activity. PET and SPECT can provide a very accurate picture of metabolically active areas, whereas their ability to show anatomic features is limited by constraints on resolution. As a result, PET and SPECT images are commonly fused with CT scans (obtained at either the same time or later) and these "fused" images can subsequently be used for treatment planning. Thus, PET-CT or SPECT-CT scanners combine the advantages of anatomic and functional imaging into a single study, leading to better image registration and improved convenience for the patient.

To improve the diagnosis, prognosis, planning, and monitoring of cancer treatment, pretherapy characterization of tumor tissue may be improved by the development of more tumor specific imaging agents. Radiolabeled ligands as well as radiolabeled antibodies have opened a new era in the scintigraphy detection of tumors and some of these have already undergone extensive preclinical development and evaluation. The most well-known agent is FDG-PET. ^{18}F-FDG–PET has been used to diagnose and stage tumors myocardial infarction and neurological disease (4–17). Although tumor metabolic imaging using ^{18}F-FDG has been successfully integrated into oncology practice, its expansion is limited by factors such as availability of PET emitting isotopes and equipment cost (18). In addition, ^{18}F chemistry is complex and requires more time for synthesis (e.g., ^{18}F-FDG, 40–75 minutes). In addition to ^{18}F-FDG–PET, several gamma ray emitting radionuclide imaging agents are employed to image and characterize tumors. Researchers have used radiotracers such as; I-123, In-111, Ga-67, and others when developing novel imaging agents. While these other tracers may provide diagnostic quality imaging, they are higher in cost, lower in availability, and in some cases lead to increased radiation exposures. Thus, it would be desirable to develop simple chelation techniques for labeling agents with a gamma ray emitter suitable for SPECT imaging using less costly radioisotopes for tissue specific imaging.

SPECT imaging with ^{99m}Tc radiolabeling is much less expensive than PET, owing to the lower cost of ^{99m}Tc and the imaging equipment. This is because the detector costs associated with higher energy gamma rays (511 keV for ^{18}F vs. 140 keV for ^{99m}Tc) are much higher. Moreover, ^{99m}Tc can be obtained from a desktop generator and has a longer half-life than the radioisotopes typically used with high-energy imaging cameras such as PET (^{99m}Tc six hours compared with [18]F—110 minutes), so additional images can be taken without readministering the radiopharmaceutical.

Several ^{99m}Tc-labeling techniques have been reported, and they include N_4 (e.g., DOTA), N_3S (e.g., MAG-3), N_2S_2 (e.g., ECD), NS_3, S_4 (e.g., sulfur colloid), diethylenetriamine pentaacetic acid (DTPA), tricarbonyl, and hydrazinenicotinamide (HYNIC) [19–24]. Among these chelators, the DTPA moiety does not chelate with ^{99m}Tc with the same stability as with 111In. The HYNIC technique requires two additional chemicals (tricine and triphenylphosphine) to form a ^{99m}Tc complex, thus making it inconvenient and higher in cost. The tricarbonyl technique requires the use of carbon monoxide as a reducing agent, which is toxic and inconvenient. The nitrogen and sulfur combination has been shown to be a stable chelator for [99m]Tc. Bis-aminoethanethiol tetradentate ligands, also called diaminodithiol compounds, are known to form very stable Tc(V)O-complexes on the basis of efficient binding of the oxotechnetium group to two thiolsulfur and two amine nitrogen atoms. ^{99m}Tc–L,L-ethylenedicysteine (^{99m}Tc-EC) is the most recent and successful example of N_2S_2 chelates [25,26]. EC can be labeled with ^{99m}Tc easily and efficiently with high radiochemical purity and stability. A series of ^{99m}Tc-EC–agent conjugates for functional imaging in oncology have been reported (27–30).

In addition to assessing molecular targets, ^{99m}Tc might be useful in planning internal targeted radionuclide therapy with [188]Re-labeled agents using the same chelate–ligand combination. [188]Re has good characteristics for imaging and therapeutic use, because of its β energy (2.1 MeV), its relatively short physical half-life (16.9 hours), and its 155 keV γ-ray emission for dosimetry and imaging purposes. The shorter physical half-life of [188]Re compared with other therapeutic radioisotopes allows for higher doses of radionuclides having longer half-life. Furthermore, the shorter half-life reduces the problems of radioactive waste handing and storage. In particular, [188]Re is available from an in-house generator system similar to a ^{99m}Tc generator. [188]Re can be obtained from a [188]W/[188]Re generator, which makes it very convenient for clinical use. Both ^{99m}Tc and [188]Re emit gamma rays, so the dosimetry generated based on ^{99m}Tc images is expected to be more accurate than that produced using the current standard treatment radioisotope, Y-90. Herein, various ^{99m}Tc-EC–conjugates bound to functional ligands to measure relevant tumor processes such as angiogenesis, hypoxia, signaling, and apoptosis are discussed. In addition to characterizing tumors, these agents also provide the opportunity to monitor therapeutic response of tumors to treatment.

PRODUCTION OF ^{99m}Tc-EC–AGENT CONJUGATE

The EC conjugate is prepared in a two-step synthesis according to methods described by Blondeau et al. (25) and Ratner and Clarke (26). Briefly, cysteine–HCl is dissolved in water; to this, formaldehyde is added and the reaction mixture is stirred overnight at room temperature. Pyridine is then added and the precipitate formed. The crystals are separated, washed with ethanol at room temperature, and filtered. The crystals are triturated with petroleum ether and filtered. The precursor, L-thiazolidine-4-carboxylic acid (m.p. 195°C, reported 196–197°C), is used for synthesis of EC. The precursor is dissolved in liquid ammonia and refluxed. Sodium metal was added until a persistent blue color appears. Ammonium chloride is added to the blue solution, and the solvents are evaporated to dryness. The residue is dissolved in water and the pH is adjusted to two. A precipitate is formed and is filtered and washed with water. The solid phase is dried in a calcium chloride dessicator. EC is then prepared (m.p. 237°C, reported 251–253°C).

Sodium bicarbonate solution is added to a stirred solution of EC in water (5 mL). To this colorless solution, sulfo-N-hydroxysuccinimide (NHS) and ethyl carbodiimide (EDC) are added. The desired agent is then added. The mixture is stirred at room temperature for 24 hours. The mixture is dialyzed for 48 hours using Spectra/POR molecular porous membrane with specific molecular cut-off. After dialysis, the product is frozen and dried using lyophilizer. Radiosynthesis of ^{99m}Tc-EC–agent is achieved by adding the required amount of EC-agent, tin (II) chloride ($SnCl_2$, 100 µg), and pertechnetate ($Na^{99m}TcO_4$). Radiochemical purity is assessed by radio-TLC scanner.

In Vitro Cellular Uptake Assay

In vitro cellular uptake assays of the newly formed conjugates are conducted by using various cancer cell lines chosen for binding of the ligand. Each well contains 80,000 cells and 2 µCi of ^{99m}Tc-EC–agent is added. After incubation at 0.5 to 4 hours, the cells are washed with phosphate buffered saline three times and this is followed by trypsin to loosen the cells. The cells are then counted by a gamma counter to determine the amount of cellular binding. It should be emphasized that successful in vitro results do not always correlate with successful in vivo activity.

In Vitro [³H] Thymidine Incorporation Assay

[³H] Thymidine incorporation assays are conducted to demonstrate that the agents are incorporated into the DNA. Tumor cells are plated at 50,000 cells/well in

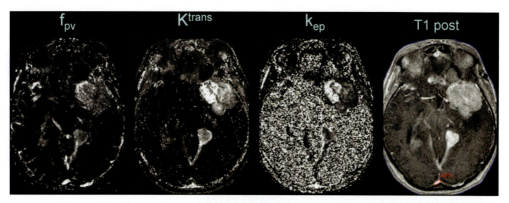

Figure 2-7 See text p. 31.

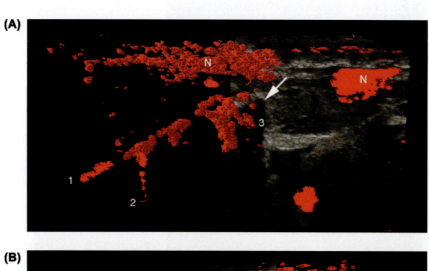

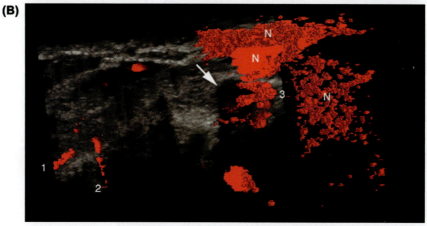

Figure 3-4 See text p. 43.

(A)

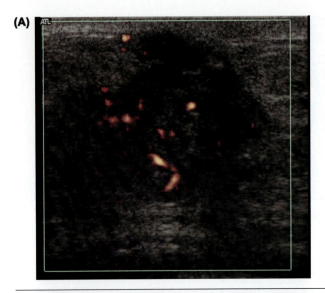

Figure 3-5A See text p. 48.

(B)

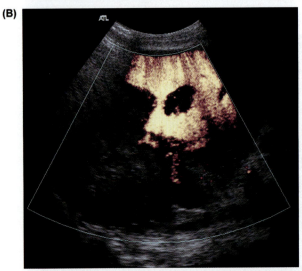

Figure 3-7B See text p. 51.

(B)

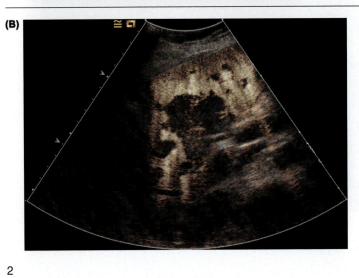

Figure 3-8B See text p. 52.

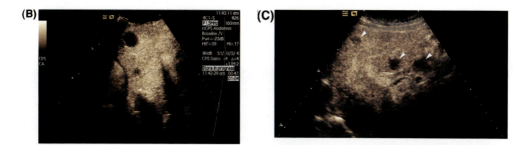

Figure 3-9B,C See text pp. 54 and 55.

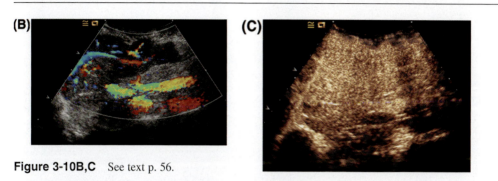

Figure 3-10B,C See text p. 56.

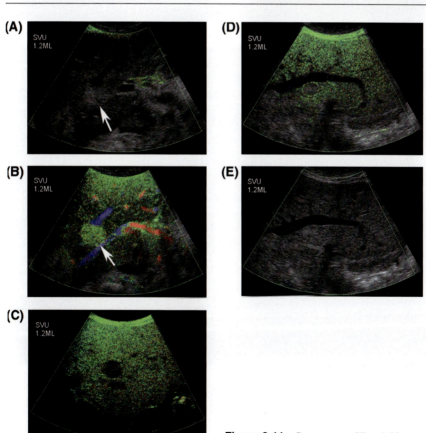

Figure 3-11 See text pp. 57 and 58.

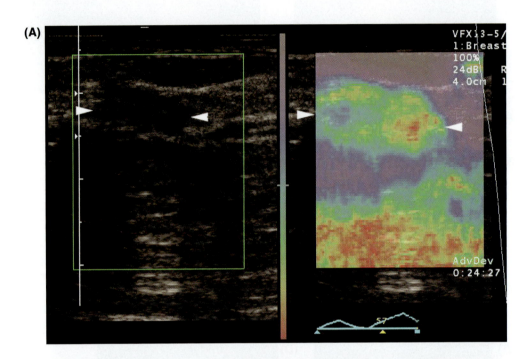

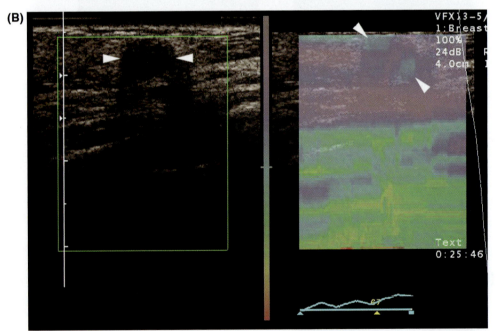

Figure 3-12 See text p. 61.

(B)

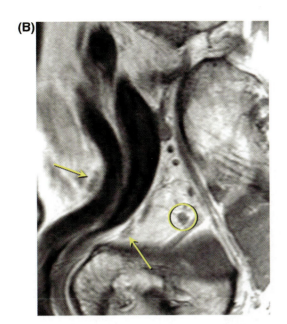

Figure 4-3B See text p. 69.

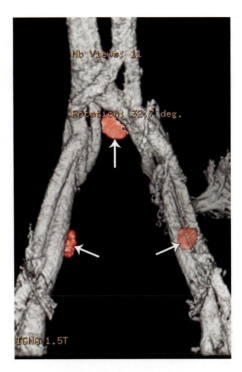

Figure 4-7 See text p. 73.

(A)

(B)

(C)

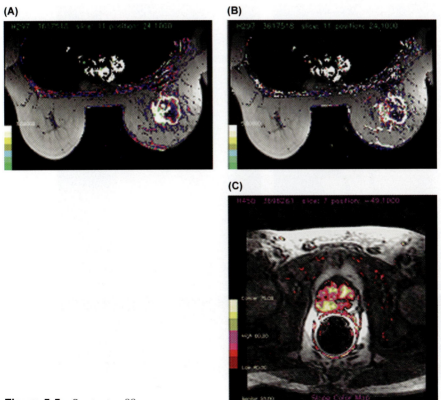

Figure 5-5 See text p. 88.

5

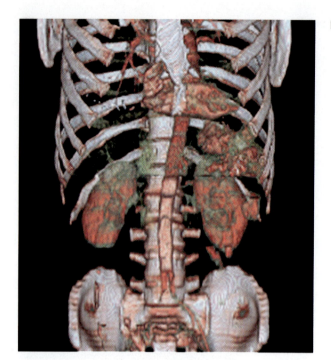

Figure 5-9 See text p. 92.

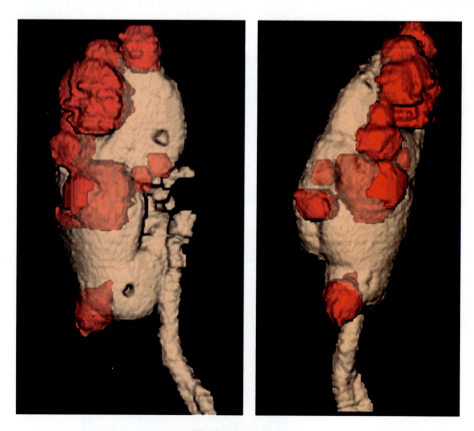

Figure 5-11 See text p. 94.

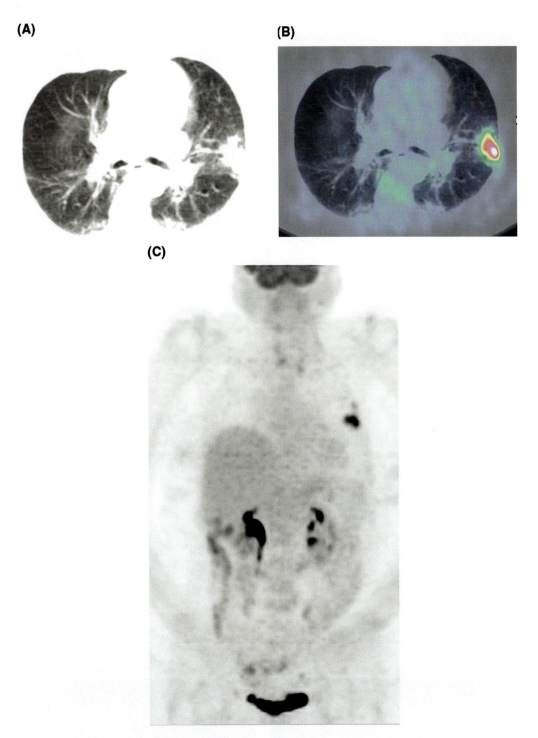

Figure 7-2 See text p. 129.

(A)

(B)

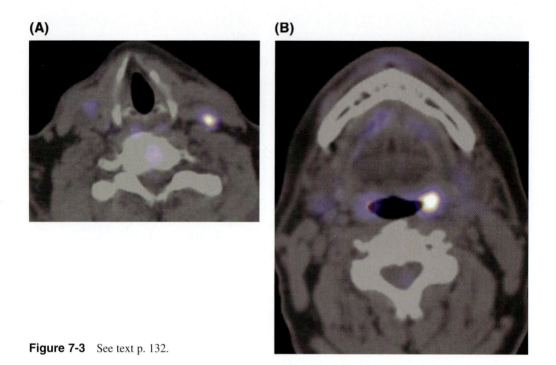

Figure 7-3 See text p. 132.

(A)

(B)

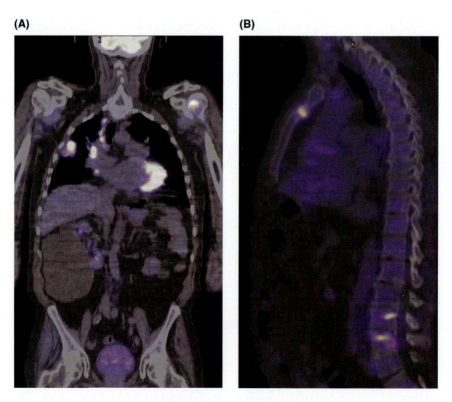

Figure 7-4 See text p. 134.

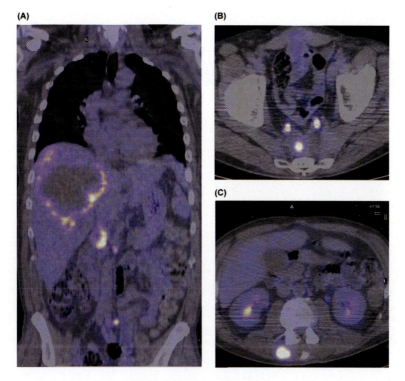

Figure 7-5   See text p. 138.

(B)

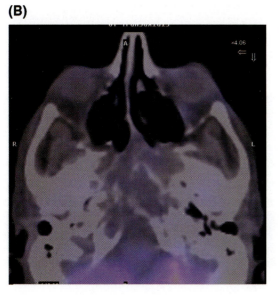

Figure 7-6B   See text p. 139.

9

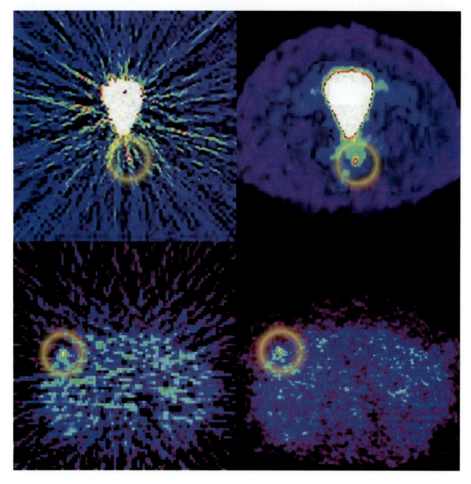

Figure 8-1 See text p. 147.

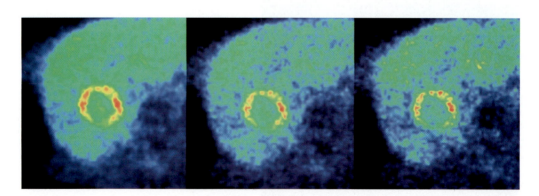

Figure 8-2 See text p. 148.

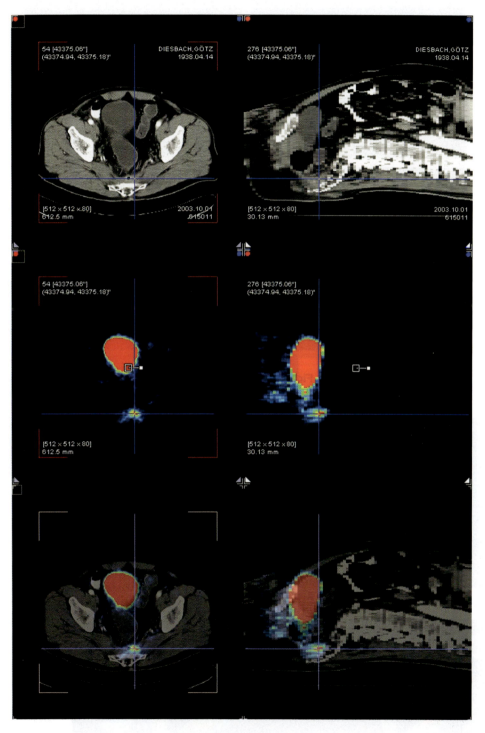

Figure 8-5 See text p. 152.

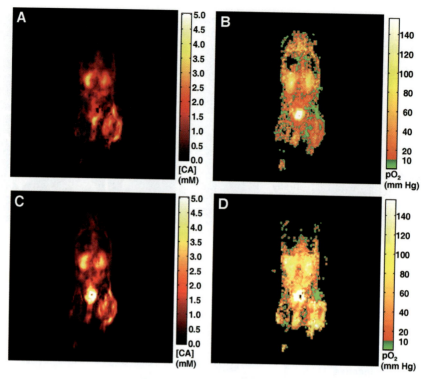

Figure 17-5 See text p. 348.

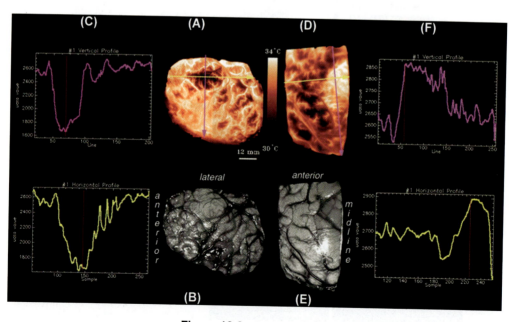

Figure 18-2 See text p. 355.

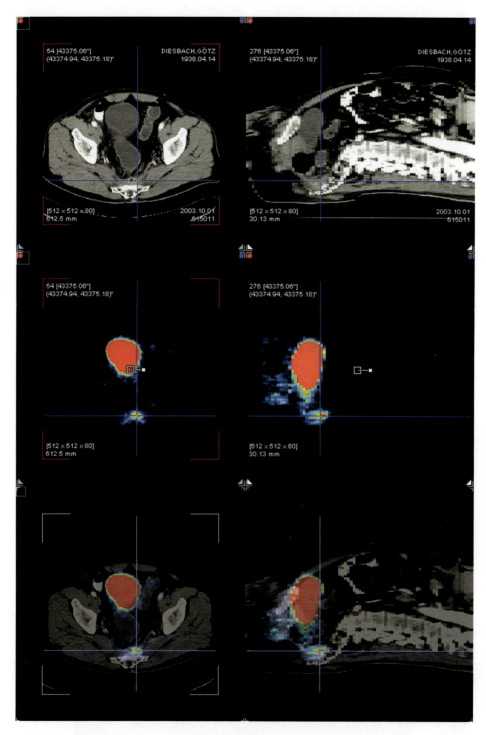

Figure 8-5 See text p. 152.

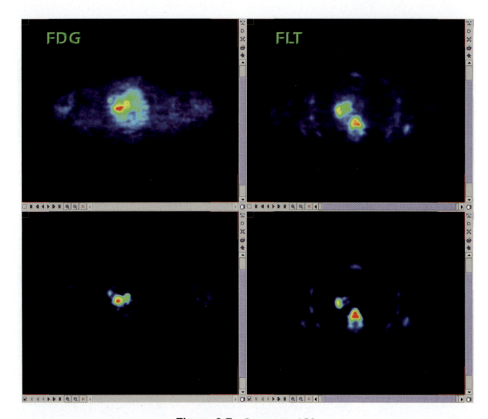

Figure 8-7 See text p. 156.

Figure 8-8 See text p. 157.

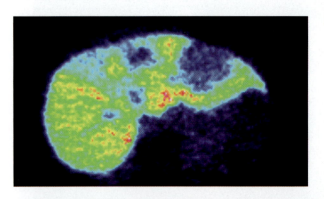

Figure 8-10
See text p. 159.

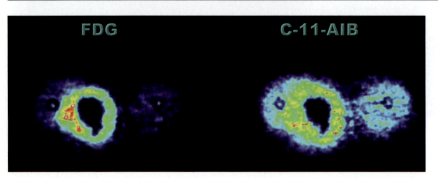

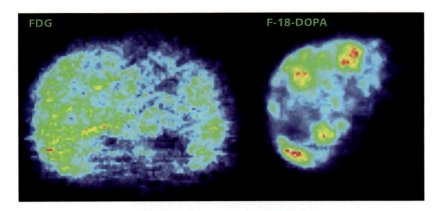

Figure 8-11 See text p. 160.

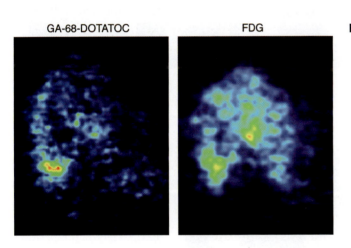

Figure 8-12 See text p. 161.

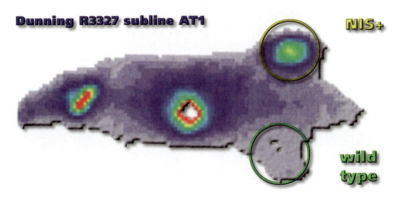

Figure 8-13 See text p. 162.

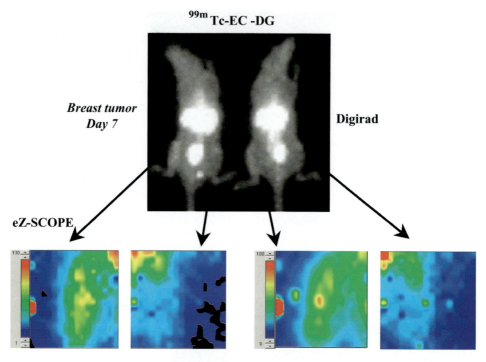

Figure 9-3 See text p. 173.

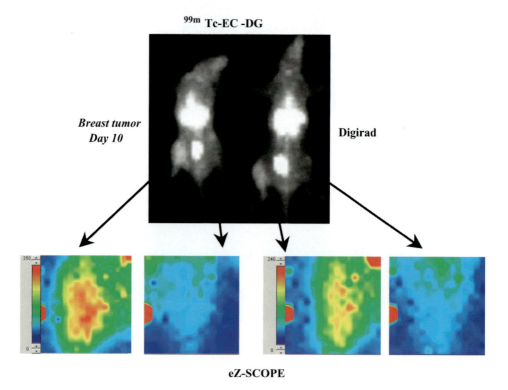

Figure 9-4 See text p. 174.

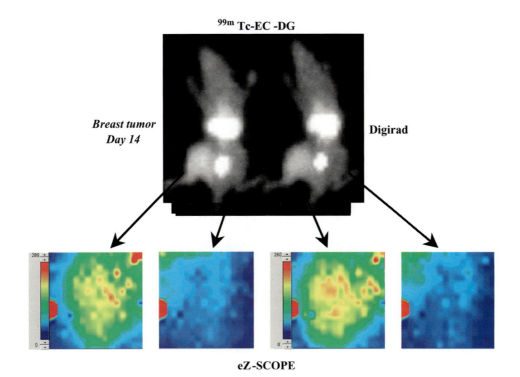

^{99m} Tc-EC -DG

*Breast tumor
Day 14*

Digirad

eZ-SCOPE

Figure 9-5   See text p. 175.

Nuclear Medicine Imaging

eZ-SCOPE   Digirad   Autoradiogram

T

T

Figure 9-7   See text p. 176.

**Autoradiography of
^{99m}Tc-EC-DG & [¹⁸F]FDG**

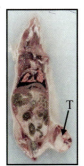
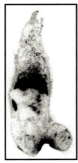
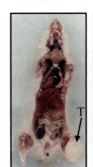
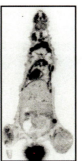

T

T

Figure 9-8   See text p. 176.

Scintigraphic Images of ^{99m}Tc-EC-COXi

$-^{99m}$Tc EC$^-$-COXi ^{99m}Tc-EC

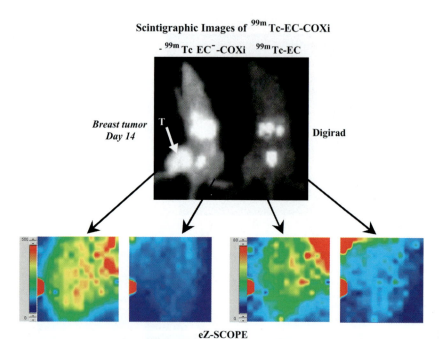

Breast tumor Day 14   T   Digirad

eZ-SCOPE

Figure 9-11
See text p. 179.

Breast cancer (right leg, rat)

^{99m}Tc-COXi
(at 1h after injection)

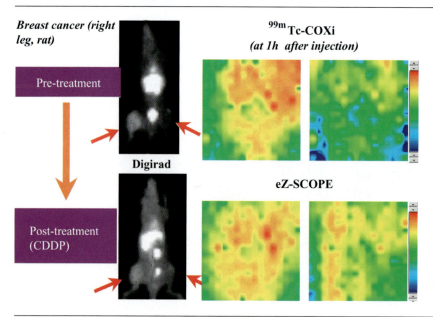

Pre-treatment

Digirad

eZ-SCOPE

Post-treatment (CDDP)

Figure 9-12
See text p. 180.

(B)

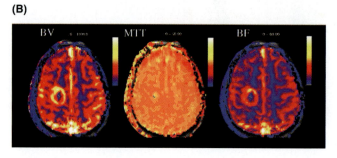

BV   MTT   BF

Figure 11-4   See text p. 219.

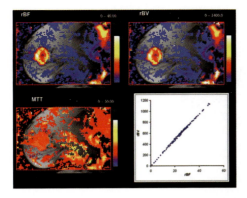

Figure 11-5 See text p. 220.

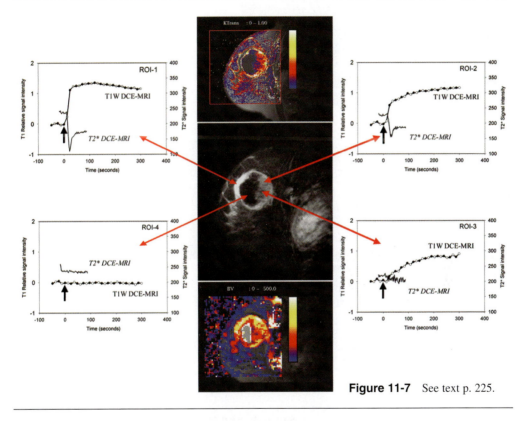

Figure 11-7 See text p. 225.

(B)

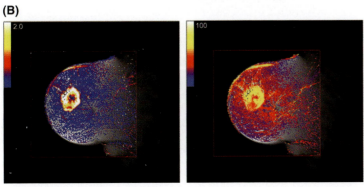

Figure 11-8B See text p. 226.

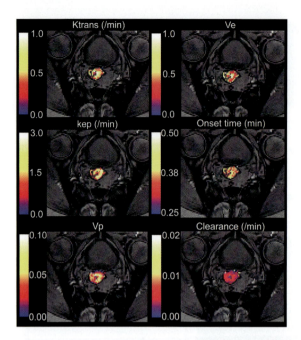

Figure 11-9 See text p. 229.

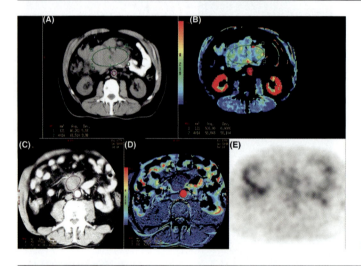

Figure 12-1 See text p. 251.

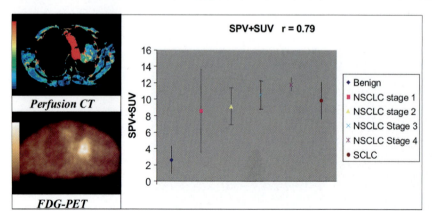

Figure 12-2
See text p 253.

(B)

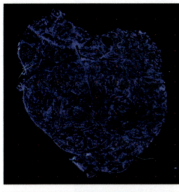

Figure 13-3B See text p. 265.

H216
10/26/01

H287
01/22/02

Figure 14-7 See text p. 285.

	K^{trans}	k$_{\text{ep}}$	f$_{\text{pv}}$	v$_{\text{e}}$
10/26/01 ROI	0.029	0.242	0.023	0.121
01/22/02 ROI	0.011	0.111	0.019	0.099

H430
08/28/02

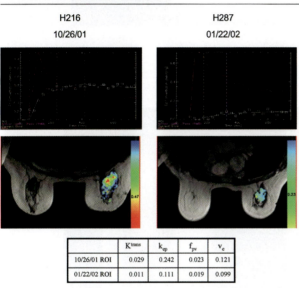

ROIs	K^{trans}	k$_{\text{ep}}$	f$_{\text{pv}}$	v$_{\text{e}}$
ROI 2 (core)	0.025	0.082	0.030	0.310
ROI 3 (rim)	0.118	0.331	0.252	0.356

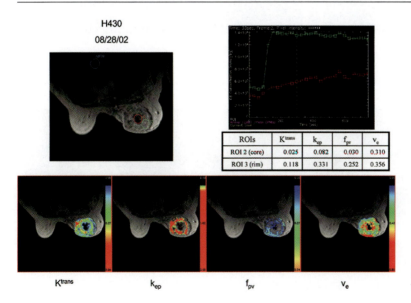

K^{trans} k$_{\text{ep}}$ f$_{\text{pv}}$ v$_{\text{e}}$

Figure 14-8 See text p. 286.

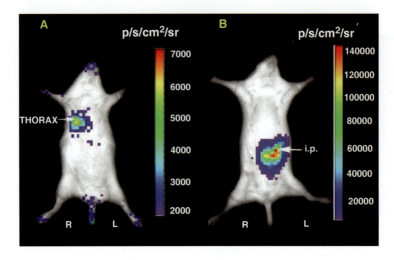

Figure 15-3 See text p. 303.

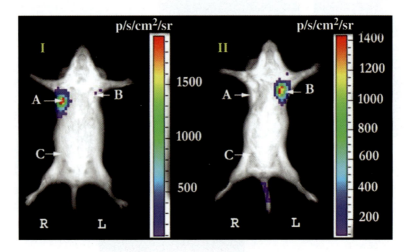

Figure 15-4 See text p. 303.

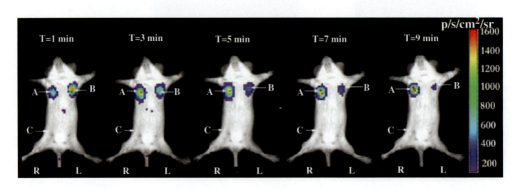

Figure 15-5 See text p. 304.

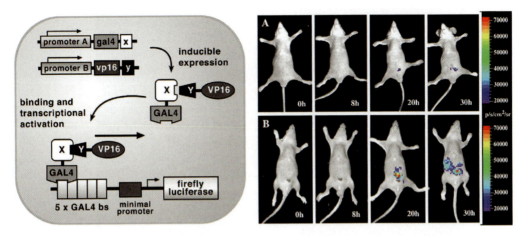

Figure 15-6 See text p. 308.

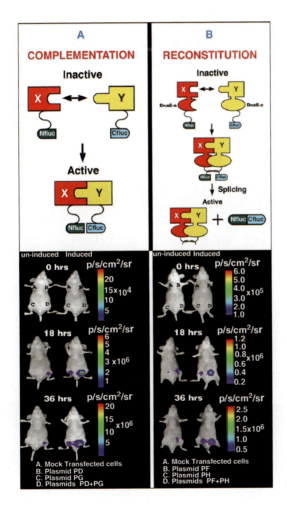

Figure 15-7 See text p. 310.

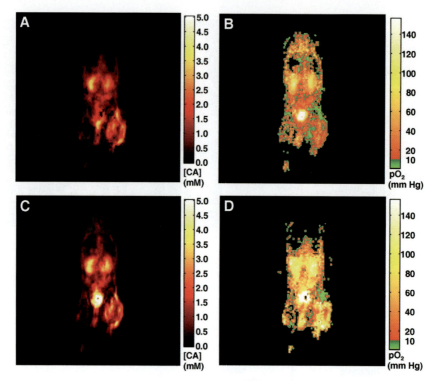

Figure 17-5 See text p. 348.

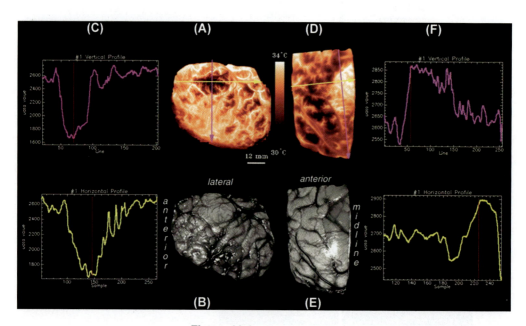

Figure 18-2 See text p. 355.

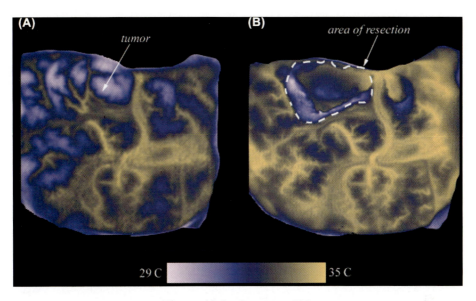

Figure 18-3 See text p. 356.

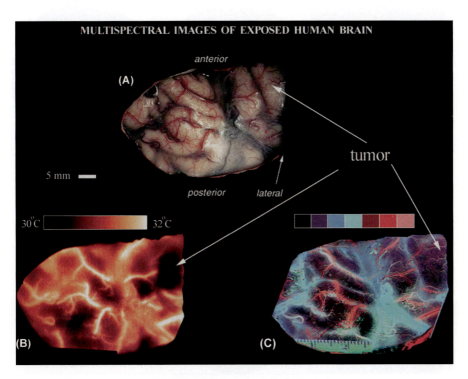

Figure 18-4 See text p. 358.

(A)

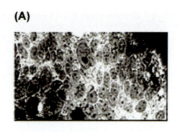

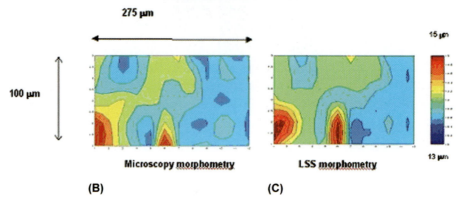

275 µm

100 µm

15 µm

Microscopy morphometry

LSS morphometry

13 µm

(B)   **(C)**

Figure 18-9   See text p. 363.

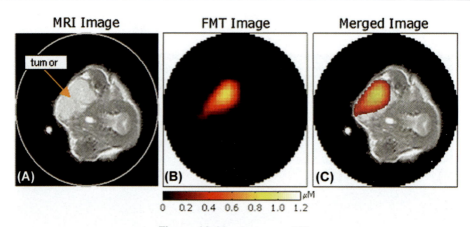

MRI Image   FMT Image   Merged Image

tumor

(A)   **(B)**   **(C)**

0   0.2   0.4   0.6   0.8   1.0   1.2   µM

Figure 18-10   See text p. 365.

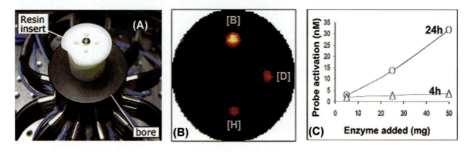

Figure 18-11   See text p. 366.

200 µL RPMI, 10% FCS. Concentration of the EC-agents (0.1–1 mg/well) and saline (control) are added to this 96-well culture plate and incubated in 5% CO_2/air at 37°C. After 24 hours, each well is pulsed with 0.5 µCi/10 µL [^{3}H] thymidine and incubated for 24 hours. Cells are then harvested, typsinized with 100 µL of typsin, and incubated for 10 minutes in the incubator. The cells are counted with a liquid scintillation counter. Cellular uptake of [^{3}H] thymidine in the control group is normalized to be 100 (baseline).

Tissue Biodistribution Studies of ^{99m}Tc-EC–agent

To ascertain the in vivo biodistribution of the conjugates, rodents are inoculated subcutaneously with cancer cells from various tumor cell lines as appropriate for the ligand. After the tumor reaches 8 to 10 mm, biodistribution studies using ^{99m}Tc-EC–agent (1–3 µCi/mouse, 10–20 µCi/rat, IV) is performed. The mice are divided into three groups, each group representing a time interval (0.5, 2, and 4 hours) and each containing three rodents. Following the administration of the radio-tracers, the rodents are sacrificed and the selected tissues are excised, weighed, and counted for radioactivity. The biodistribution of tracer in each sample is calculated as percentage of the injected dose per gram of tissue wet weight (%ID/g). Tumor/nontarget tissue count density ratios are calculated from the corresponding %ID/g values.

Preclinical Gamma Scintigraphy Imaging Studies

Prior to the introduction in man, in vivo imaging studies are conducted in animals. To perform these studies, rodents are inoculated subcutaneously with cancer cells from various tumor cell lines. Scintigraphic imaging is serially performed at 0.5 to 4 hours after injection of 100 to 300 µCi (mouse and rat) of ^{99m}Tc-EC–agents via tail vein. Imaging is performed with a planar gamma camera (Digirad, San Diego, California, U.S.) equipped with a low-energy parallel-hole collimator. The intrinsic spatial resolution is 3 mm and the matrix is 64 × 64.

Autoradiography

Another method of assessing in vivo distribution of the agent is to utilize whole-body autoradiographs with a quantitative image analyzer (Cyclone Storage Phosphor System, Packard, Meridian, Connecticut, U.S.). Following IV injection of 100 to 300 µCi of ^{99m}Tc-EC–agent, tumor-bearing rodents are killed at one hour and the body is fixed in carboxymethyl cellulose (3%). The frozen body is mounted onto a cryostat (LKB 2250 cryomicrotome, Ijamsville, Maryland, U.S.) and cut into 100 µm coronal sections. Each section is thawed and mounted on a slide. The slide is then placed in contact with phosphor storage screen (MP, 7001480) and exposed for 15 hours.

Tc-EC Targeted Imaging Agents

Glycolysis Targets

Owing to the structural similarity between glucosamine (2-amino deoxyglucose) and FDG (2-fluoro deoxyglucose), it was predicted that ^{99m}Tc-EC–glucosamine (EC–DG) could act as the SPECT analog of FDG-PET. The chemical structure of

^{99m}Tc-C–DG is shown in Figure 1. The labeling efficiency of this adduct is 95% to 100%. However,^{99m}Tc-EC–DG is also predicted to be taken up by the nucleic acid synthesis. To demonstrate whether ^{99m}Tc-EC–DG was involved in DNA/RNA incorporation, thymidine incorporation assays were conducted with EC–DG, FDG, and glucose. Tissue distribution, dosimetry, autoradiographic, and gamma scintigraphic imaging studies of ^{99m}Tc-EC–DG and ^{18}F-FDG were conducted in tumor bearing animal models. Tumor/nontarget tissue count density ratios were calculated from the corresponding %ID/g values.

Biodistribution studies with ^{99m}Tc-EC–DG revealed that tumor/brain and tumor/muscle ratios of ^{99m}Tc-EC–DG in rodents were higher than ^{18}F-FDG (57). Data obtained from thymidine incorporation assays indicated that EC–DG and glucose was involved in cell nuclei activity whereas FDG was not (Fig. 2). In vivo imaging studies showed that changes in tumor volume could be monitored with ^{99m}Tc-EC–DG (Figs. 3–5). Compared to the images of nontargeted ^{99m}Tc-EC (control), the tumor was visualized quite clearly only with ^{99m}Tc-EC–DG (Fig. 6). A xenograft human uterine sarcoma implanted in nude mice could be visualized by autoradiography with ^{99m}Tc-EC–DG but not controls (Figs. 7 and 8). Compared to ^{18}F-FDG, less brain or myocardial radioactivity was observed with ^{99m}Tc-EC–DG groups. These findings support the potential use of ^{99m}Tc-EC–DG as a functional imaging agent.

Synthesis of ^{99m}Tc-EC-DG

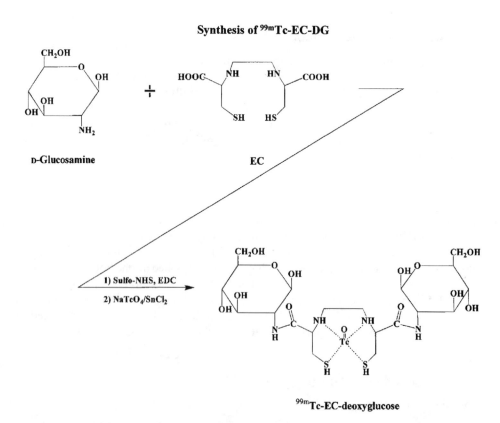

D-Glucosamine   EC

1) Sulfo-NHS, EDC

2) NaTcO$_4$/SnCl$_2$

^{99m}Tc-EC-deoxyglucose

Figure 1 Synthetic procedure for conjugation of D-glucosamine to ethlenedicysteine (EC). Stablizing/activating agents (**1**) and (**2**) radioisotope/reducing agent are then added to form radiolabeled EC–DG.

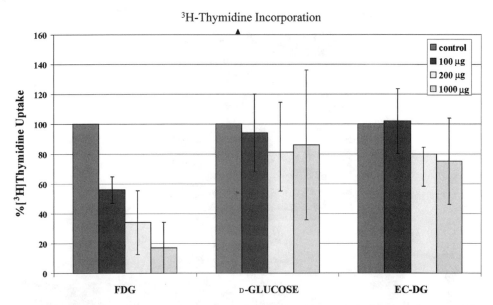

Figure 2 Thymidine incorporation assay indicated that both EC–DG and D-glucose exhibited similar DNA/RNA incorporation values. FDG showed decreased cell nuclei activity in a dose-dependent manner. The findings suggest that EC–DG is a more tumor-specific agent than FDG.

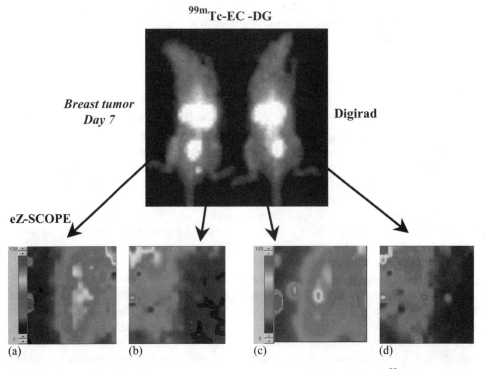

Figure 3 On day 7 postinoculation of tumor cells, planar scintigraphy of ^{99m}Tc-EC–DG in breast tumor-bearing rats (100 μCi/rat, IV) was conducted at 90 minutes. Uptake in the tumor (**a** and **c**) is greater than that of muscle tissue (**c** and **d**) by using an eZ-scope. (*See color insert*)

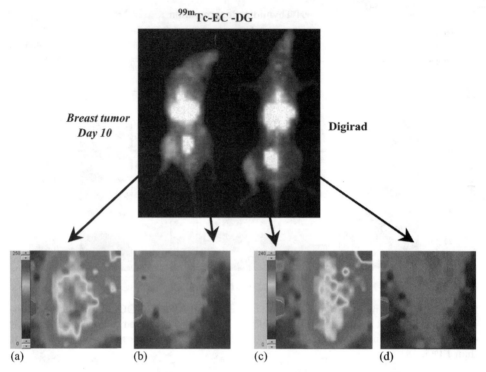

Figure 4 On day 10 postinoculation of tumor cells, planar scintigraphy of ^{99m}Tc-EC–DG in breast tumor-bearing rats (100 μCi/rat, IV) shows the tumors (1 cm) well. The imaging study was conducted at 90 minutes. Uptake in the tumor (**a** and **c**) is greater than that in muscle tissue by using an eZ-scope. (*See color insert.*)

Angiogenesis Targets

The identification of tumor-specific regulators of angiogenesis offers new hope for cancer treatment. Antiangiogenesis is a strategy for starving tumors by interrupting their blood supply. Currently, assays for the effectiveness of antiangiogenic therapy rely on serial tissue biopsies with measurements of microvessel density, interleukin 8, VEGF, bFGF, wound healing, and tumor apoptotic rate. Serial biopsies are far from ideal for monitoring therapies. There are issues of patient selection, patient availability, tumor heterogeneity, and adequate sized sample when using serial biopsies. Importantly, neither patients nor their physicians like serial biopsies. Radioactive ^{15}O water has been used to assess blood perfusion and diffusion within tumors however, this is a nonspecific agent and provides only bulk properties of the tumor (32).

Antiangiogenic therapeutic agents can be divided into two groups: angiotoxic and angioregulatory agents. Angiotoxic agents are focused on specific molecular targets of tumor cells, but not necessarily to endothelial cells. Many anticancer agents (e.g., paclitaxel, doxorubicin, bleomycin, 5-FU, thalidomide, herceptin, camptothecin, and C225 antibody) belong to this category. Angioregulatory agents are targeted to endothelial cells and stromal cells. Endostatin, angiostatin, thromospondin, cytokines, VEGF, bFGF, PDGF, TGFα, and pO$_2$ modulators belong to this category. Angio-regulatory agents are relatively nontoxic, although some side effects such as poor wound healing and hypertension are reported (33). Radiolabeled angioregulatory

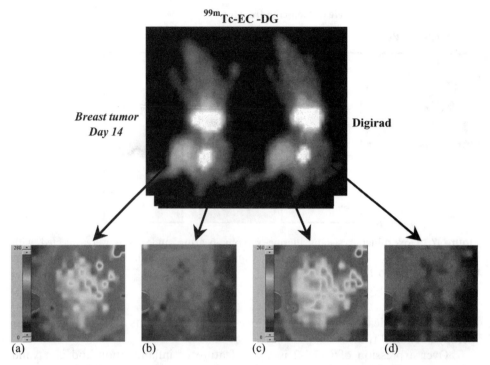

Figure 5 On day 14 postinoculation of tumor cells, planar scintigraphy of ^{99m}Tc-EC–DG in breast tumor-bearing rats (100 μCi/rat, IV) shows tumors (2 cm). The imaging study was conducted at 90 minutes. Uptake in the tumor (**a** and **c**) is greater than that in muscle tissue by using an eZ-SCOPE®. (*See color insert.*)

Rabbit Imaging

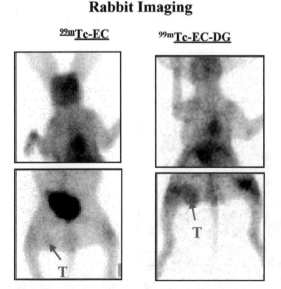

Figure 6 Planar scintigraphic images of VX-2 tumor-bearing male rabbits after administration of ^{99m}Tc-EC and ^{99m}Tc-EC–DG (1 mCi, IV) show that the tumor can be well visualized one hour post injection. Arrow designates tumor (T).

Nuclear Medicine Imaging

eZ-SCOPE   Digirad   Autoradiogram

Figure 7 Doxorubicin-resistant uterine sarcome-bearing nude mice were injected with 100 μCi of ^{99m}Tc-EC–DG kit and sacrificed 70 minutes post injection. Arrow designates tumor (T). (*See color insert.*)

agents would be ideal candidates for the assessment of endpoints of targeted molecular therapy in clinical trials.

Over expression of COX-2 is a key feature of inflammation and is a valid angiogenic target for the treatment colorectal cancer since COX-2 inhibitors can down-regulate a number of important angiogenic factors including VEGF, FGF, and PDGF and reduce capillary tube formation in vitro (34–37). Two distinct COX isoenzymes referred to as COX-1 and COX-2 have been identified. COX-1 is constitutively expressed in most of the tissues with highest levels found in stomach, platelet, renal tubules, and liver. COX-1 produces prostaglandins necessary for maintaining the integrity of the gastrointestinal tract and platelet function (35). In contrast, COX-2 is not expressed in normal tissues, however, it is greatly induced

Autoradiography of
^{99m}**Tc-EC-DG & [**^{18}**F]FDG**

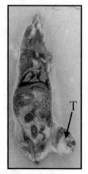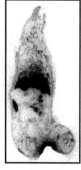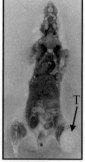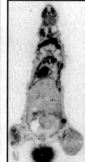

Figure 8 Doxorubicin-sensitive uterine sarcoma-bearing nude mice were injected with 100 μCi of ^{99m}Tc-EC–DG kit (*left*) and (^{18}F) FDG (*right*) and sacrificed 60 minutes post injection. Sections were cut at 100 μm and exposed for 16 hours. Arrow designates tumor (T). (*See color insert.*)

during inflammation or tumorigenesis (38–40). Celebrex, a specific COX-2 inhibitor is a treatment for osteoarthritis or rheumatoid arthritis based on its potent anti-inflammatory activity and favorable toxicity profile with reduced incidence of peptic ulcer (39). Noninvasive molecular imaging of celebrex expression in vivo would be of paramount clinical value in validating the COX-2 response in future anti–COX-2 based clinical studies. Thus, ^{99m}Tc-EC–C225, ^{99m}Tc-EC–endostatin, and ^{99m}Tc-EC–celebrex were developed as markers of angiogenesis.

In vivo biodistribution of ^{99m}Tc-EC–C225 in tumor-bearing rodents showed increased tumor versus tissue ratios as a function of time. SPECT images confirmed that the tumors could be visualized with ^{99m}Tc-EC–C225 from 0.5 to 4 hours. In vitro and biodistribution studies demonstrated the possibility of using ^{99m}Tc-EC–C225 to assess EGFR expression (58). Biodistribution of ^{99m}Tc-EC–endostatin in tumor-bearing rats also showed increased tumor versus tissue count density ratios as a function of time. Tumor uptake (%ID/g) of ^{99m}Tc-EC–endostatin was 0.2 to 0.5. Planar images confirmed that the tumors could be visualized clearly with ^{99m}Tc-EC–endostatin. The optimal time for imaging using radiolabeled endostatin was two hours. Tumor response to endostatin therapy in tumor-bearing animal models was assessed by correlating tumor uptake dose with microvessel density, VEGF, bFGF, and IL-8 expression during endostatin therapy. The results indicated that ^{99m}Tc-EC–endostatin could assess treatment response. There was a correlation between tumor uptake and cellular targets expression (33).

To assess COX-2 activity, N-4-(5-p-tolyl-3-trifluoromethyl-pyrazol-1-yl) benzenesulfonylamide (Celebrex, COXi) has been used as a starting material. COXi was converted to ester form and reacted with ethylenediamine. The amino analog of COXi was then conjugated to EC (Fig. 9). In vitro cell culture using tumor cells (RBA CRL-1747) was incubated with ^{99m}Tc-EC–COXi at 0.5 to 2 hours in. There was a significant increase in uptake compared to ^{99m}Tc-EC (Fig. 10). Scintigraphic imaging studies were performed in mammary tumor-bearing rats and squamous tumor-bearing rabbits at 0.5 to 4 hours (0.3 mCi/rat; 1 mCi/rabbit, $n = 3$, IV). Planar images confirmed that the tumors could be visualized clearly with ^{99m}Tc-EC–COXi (Figs. 11–13). Acute toxicity studies indicated that at the dosage of 20 to 40 mg/kg, all mice tolerated the doses well and no marked decrease in body weight was observed.

Tumor Hypoxia Targets

[^{18}F] Fluoromisonidazole (FMISO) has been used to assess the hypoxia in brain ischemia, myocardial infarction, and various tumors (41–46). Moreover, the assessment of tumor hypoxia with labeled MISO prior to radiation therapy could provide a rational means of selecting patients for treatment with radiosensitizing or bioreductive drugs. Actual hypoxia measurements within tumors requires intratumoral pO$_2$ measurements using Eppendorf probes and a computerized histographic system. Typically, 20 to 25 pO$_2$ measurements are obtained along with each of the two to three linear tracks at 0.4 mm intervals on each tumor (40–75 measurements total). This invasive procedure produces accurate results but is time consuming and invasive. To measure hypoxia in vivo ^{99m}Tc-EC–MN was synthesized and its potential as a tumor hypoxic imaging agent was evaluated in comparison to nontargeted ^{99m}Tc-EC, (^{18}F) FMISO, and [^{131}I] IMISO (Figs. 14 and 15).

In vivo biodistribution of ^{99m}Tc-EC–MN in breast tumor-bearing rats showed increased tumor versus blood and tumor versus muscle ratios as a function of time. Conversely, tumor-to-blood values showed time-dependent decrease with

Synthesis of EC-COX2

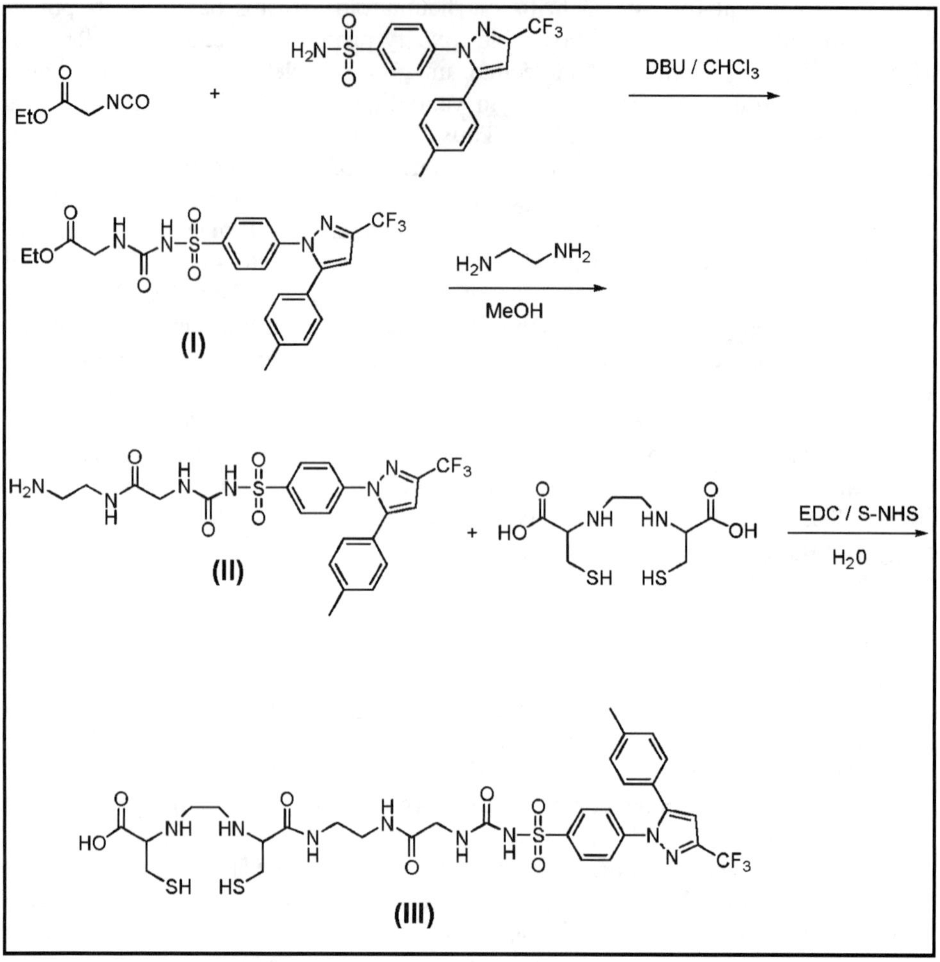

Figure 9 Chemical synthesis of EC-COXi.

nontargeted ^{99m}Tc-EC in the same period. Intratumoral pO_2 measurements of tumors indicated that the tumor oxygen tension was 4.6 ± 1.4 mmHg as compared to normal muscle of 35 ± 10 mmHg indicating that tumors were hypoxic. Planar scintigraphy images and autoradiographs confirmed that the tumors could be visualized clearly with ^{99m}Tc-EC–MN at 0.5 to 4 hours. There was no significant difference of tumor-to-blood values between 99^mTc-EC–MN and [^{131}I] iodomisonidazole (IMISO) at two to four hours postinjection. From 0.5 to 4 hours, both ^{99m}Tc-EC–MN and [^{131}I] IMISO had higher tumor versus muscle ratios compared to [^{18}F] FMISO. These results indicated that it is feasible to use ^{99m}Tc-EC–MN to assess tumor hypoxia (29).

Apoptosis Targets

Apoptosis, or programmed cell death, is a natural, orderly, energy-dependent process that causes cells to die without inducing an inflammatory response (48,49). Apoptosis

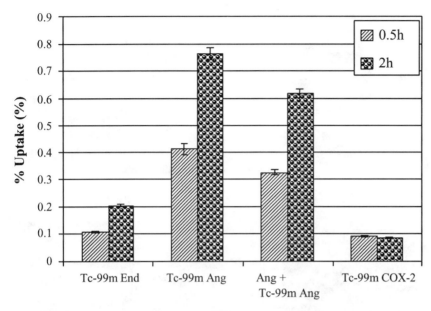

Figure 10 In vitro cellular uptake of ^{99m}Tc-EC-agents in breast cancer cells.

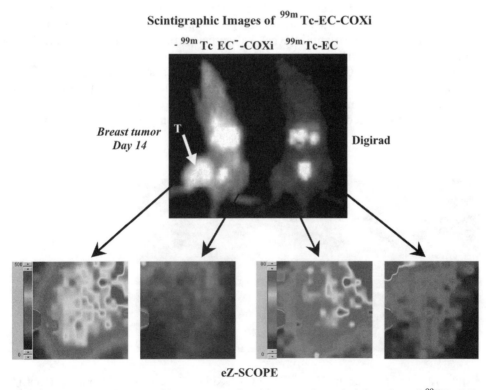

Figure 11 Planar images of breast tumor-bearing rats after administration of ^{99m}Tc-EC–COXi (left rat) and ^{99m}Tc-EC (right rat) show that tumor can be visualized. (*See color insert.*)

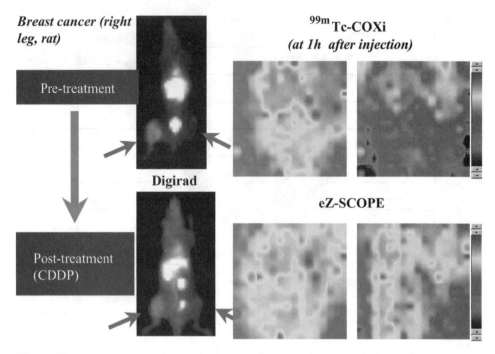

Figure 12 Post treatment changes in tumor volume can be assessed. (*See color insert.*)

is triggered either by a decrease in factors required to maintain the cell in good health or by an increase in factors that cause damage to the cell (50,51). When these factors tilt in the direction of death and the cell has sufficient time to respond, a proteolytic cascade involving cysteine aspartic acid–specific proteases (caspases) is activated to initiate apoptosis (52). Cells that die by apoptosis autodigest their DNA and nuclear proteins, change the phospholipid composition on the outer surface of their cell membrane, and form lipid enclosed vesicles, which contain noxious intracellular contents, organelles, autodigested cytoplasm, and DNA. The compositional cell membrane

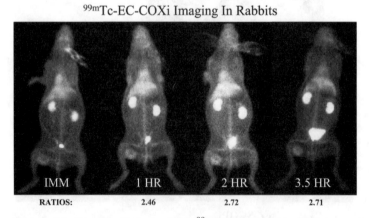

Figure 13 Planar scintigrapy with ^{99m}Tc-EC-COXi in VX2 tumor-bearing rabbits (1 mCi/ rabbit, IV) demonstrated that tumor could be well visualized. Tumor versus nontumor ratios are shown (T, tumor).

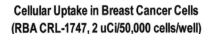

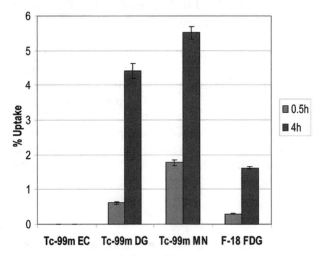

Figure 14   Cellular uptake of ^{99m}Tc-EC-agents shows that EC-MN makes the highest uptake compared to that with other agents.

phospholipid change that occurs with the onset of apoptosis is marked by the expression of phosphatidylserine (PS). PS, a phospholipid that constitutes 10% to 15% of phospholipid content and appears on the inner leaflet of the cell membrane is redistributed onto the external leaflet of the membrane during apoptosis (53). Annexin V binds to phosphatidylserine during apoptosis and radiolabeled annexin V may be useful in evaluating the efficacy of therapy and disease progression or regression (54–56).^{99m}Tc-EC–annexin V was synthesized to determine if this agent could image apoptosis.

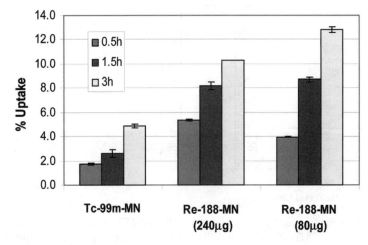

Figure 15   Cellular uptakes of Tc-99m and Re-188 EC-MN show a similarity.

In vitro cellular uptake showed that there was significantly increased uptake of ^{99m}Tc-EC–annexin V in apoptotic cells induced by irradiation (10–30 Gy) and paclitaxel treatment (Figs. 16 and 17). In vivo biodistribution of ^{99m}Tc-EC–annexin in breast tumor-bearing rats showed increased tumor versus blood, tumor versus lung, and tumor versus muscle count density ratios as a function of time. Planar images confirmed that the tumors could be visualized clearly with ^{99m}Tc-EC–annexin (Fig. 18). To demonstrate in vivo cellular apoptosis induced by chemotherapy, a group of rats was treated with paclitaxel and planar imaging studies were conducted at 0.5 to 4 hours. Computer outlined region of interest (ROI) measurements were used to quantify tumor uptake on day three and day five post-treatment. There was a significant difference of ROI ratios between pre- and post-paclitaxel treatment groups at two and four hours postinjection. The results indicate that apoptosis can be quantified using ^{99m}Tc-EC–annexin and that it is feasible to use ^{99m}Tc-EC–annexin to image tumor apoptosis (30).

MDR Targets

Adriamycin (Doxorubicin, Rubex), a potent topoisomerase II inhibitor as well as a MDR substrate, has been widely used to treat breast and ovarian cancers, leukemia, lymphoma, as well as other forms of cancer. Noninvasive imaging using ^{99m}Tc-EC–adriamycin may predict the response of adriamycin therapy for breast cancer. Additionally, such a radiotracer may provide an early indicator of MDR.

Two breast cancer cell lines (sensitive and resistant to doxorubicin) were used to evaluate the specificity of ^{99m}Tc-EC–doxorubicin. In vitro cell culture indicated that there was more ^{99m}Tc-EC–doxorubicin uptake in doxorubicin-sensitive cells (MDA 231, low HER2) than doxorubicin-resistant cells (MDA 453, high HER2)

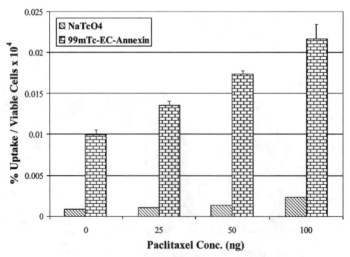

Figure 16 Viable cells were determined by methylene tetrazolium (MTT) assay. There was a markedly increased uptake of ^{99m}Tc-EC–annexin V in paclitaxel treated groups (50 and 100 ng) compared to nontreated groups at four hours incubation.

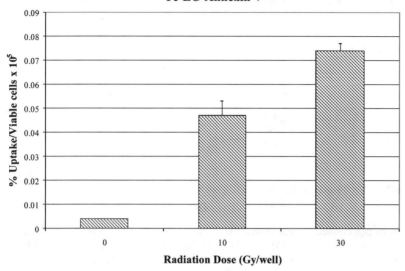

Figure 17 Breast tumor cells (2.5×10^5 cell/5 mL buffer/well) were irradiated with a Cs-137 external beam source. After three-day incubation, cell viability was determined by MTT assay. Significantly increased uptake of ^{99m}Tc-EC–annexin V was observed in radiation-treated groups (10 and 30 Gy) compared to nontreated groups at two hours incubation.

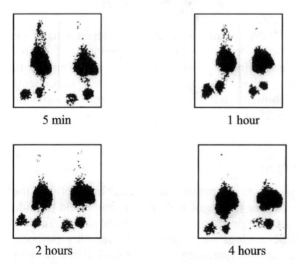

Figure 18 Planar images of tumor-bearing rats following administration of ^{99m}Tc-EC–annexin V (100 μCi/rat, IV) showed that tumor uptake could be visualized from five minutes to four hours on day 14 after inoculation of tumor cells.

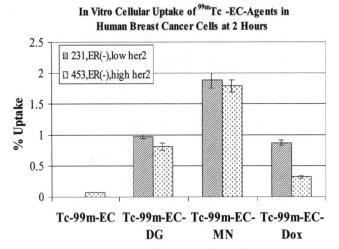

Figure 19 In vitro cell culture indicated that there was more ^{99m}Tc-EC-doxorubicin uptake in doxorubicin-sensitive cells (MDA 231, low HER2) than dozorubicin-resitant cells (MDA 453, high HER2).

(Fig. 19). The findings suggest that ^{99m}Tc-EC–doxorubicin might be a useful in vivo marker for MDR.

Markers of LHRH Receptor Targets

Gonadotrophin-releasing hormone receptors (GnRH and LHRH) are found in cancers of reproductive tissues, including those of the prostate, ovarian, and breast, and gonadotrophin-releasing hormone can inhibit growth of cell lines derived from such cancers. A radiolabeled LHRH ligand could be useful in diagnosing diseases that produce high levels of LHRH-receptors, such as ovarian cancer, endometriosis, uterine carcinoma, and prostate cancer.

Two prostate cancer cell lines (LNCap: androgen and PSA dependent; PC-3: androgen and PSA independent) were used to evaluate the specificity of ^{99m}Tc-EC–LHRH. In vitro cell culture assays indicated that there was more uptake in PC-3 cells (androgen independent) than LNCap cells (androgen dependent) (Fig. 20). Planar imaging studies showed that tumor (LHRH positive) could be imaged with ^{99m}Tc-EC–LHRH (Fig. 21).

Markers of Tumor Cell Proliferation

Noninvasive imaging assessment of tumor cell proliferation could be helpful in the evaluation of tumor growth potential, the degree of malignancy, and could provide an early assessment of treatment response prior to changes in tumor size. ^{99m}Tc-EC–adenosine and ^{99m}Tc-EC–guanosine analogs were synthesized for this purpose. These radioligands could improve the understanding of the biological behavior of malignant tumors, and lead to better prognostic evaluation, treatment follow-up, and patient management. To assess tumor proliferative activity and cellular uptake, autoradiographs and radionuclide imaging of these ligands were performed.

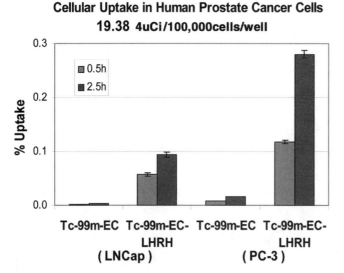

Figure 20   In vitro cell culture assays indicate more uptake in PC-3 cells (androgen independent) than LNCap cells (androgen dependent).

    The synthesis of EC-guanosine analog (EC-Guan) is shown in Fig. 22. In vitro thymidine incorporation assays indicated that ^{99m}Tc-EC–Guan was involved in DNA/RNA cell nuclei activities (Fig. 23). Cellular uptake of ^{99m}Tc-EC–Guan was time dependent and proportional to cellular uptake (Fig. 24). Such an agent has also been used as a reporter molecule for HSV-tk expression in reporter–gene constructs. In this setting, the herpes simplex thymidine kinase phosphorylates ^{99m}Tc-EC–Guan leading to accumulation within the cell. Thus,[99m]Tc-EC–Guan acts as a "reporter" for the presence of HSV-tk and other genes cotransfected with the same viral transcript. There was no marked difference in cellular uptake of ^{99m}Tc-EC– Guan pre- and post-viral transfection of prostate cancer cells (Fig. 25). Planar imaging in tumor-bearing rabbits showed that tumors could be visualized with

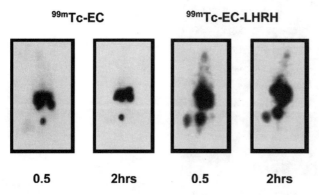

Figure 21   Planar images of breast tumor-bearing rats after administration of ^{99m}Tc-EC and ^{99m}Tc-EC-LHRH (100 µCi/rat, IV) show that the tumor could be well visualized from 0.5 to 2 hours post injection.

Synthesis of EC-Guan

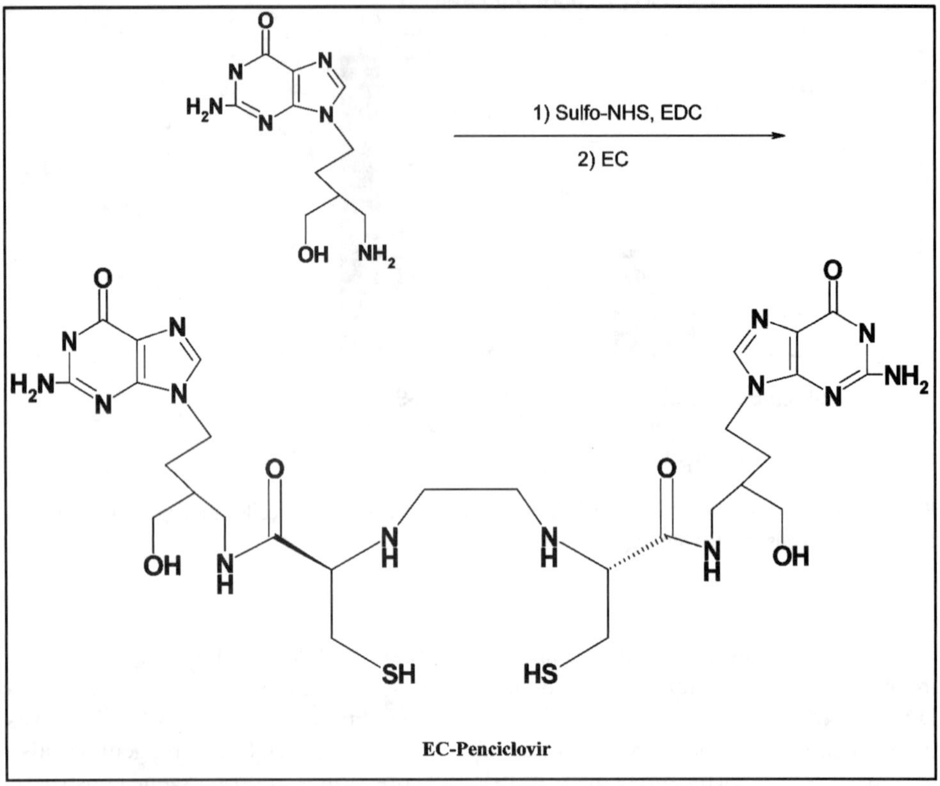

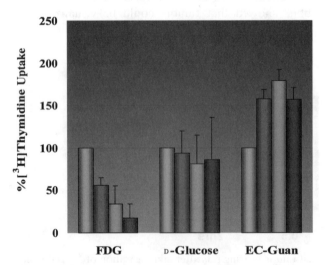

Figure 22 Chemical synthesis of EC–Guan.

[H-3]Thymidine Incorporation Assay

Figure 23 In vitro thymidine incorporation assays indicated that ^{99m}Tc-EC–Guan was involved in cell nuclei DNA/RNA activity.

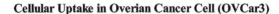

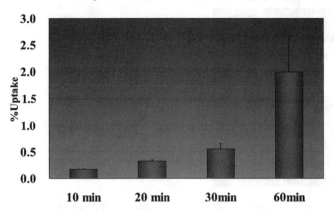

Figure 24 Cellular uptake of ^{99m}Tc-EC–Guan is time dependent.

^{99m}Tc-EC–Guan. The uptake was higher than the nontargeted ^{99m}Tc-EC (control group) (Figs. 26 and 27).

CONCLUSION

The ^{99m}Tc-EC platform enables many different ligands to be radiolabeled without resorting to new, highly complex radiochemistry each time a new ligand is introduced. Such a "reductionist" approach presupposes the development of automated synthesis chambers, which could allow the onsite radiolabeling of a wide range of ligands in a single radiopharmacy. The use of a ubiquitous isotope, a uniform chelation method along with imaging with conventional planar or SPECT imaging can dramatically lower study costs associated with molecular imaging. In this chapter,

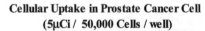

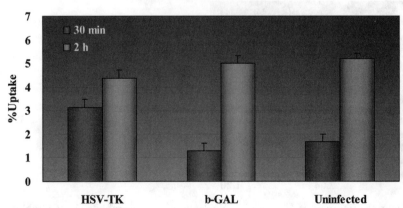

Figure 25 No marked differences of cellular uptake of ^{99m}Tc-EC–Guan between viral tansfection of HSV tk expression and without HSV tk expression.

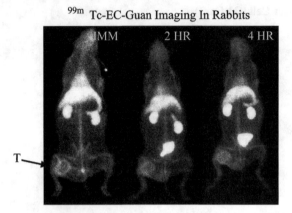

Figure 26 Planar scintigraphy of ^{99m}Tc-EC–Guan in VX2 tumor-bearing rabbits (1mCi/ rabbit, IV) demonstrates that the tumor could be well visualized.

only a few of the many radioligands that can be produced by the ^{99m}Tc-EC– construct is discussed.

The ^{99m}Tc-EC–DG, for instance, could serve as a substitute for FDG-PET and thus, provide metabolic information about glycolysis and cell turnover. Angiogenesis imaging is another potentially important target for this technology. Imaging with radiolabeled antiangiogenic agents has the following potential advantages over biopsy: (i) noninvasive assessment, (ii) easily quantifiable, (iii) can be used to access anatomical regions that are difficult to biopsy, and (iv) whole body evaluations. Though histological assessments of angiogenesis (blood vessel density) and/or its main regulators such as IL-8, VEGF, and bFGF in solid tumors may provide sensitive markers for tumor progression, metastasis, and prognosis, the therapeutic response of tumors may not be adequately reflected by these histologic measurements. The role of ^{99m}Tc-EC–endostatin in imaging tumors that over-express endothelial markers associated with angiogenesis needs to be evaluated. The findings

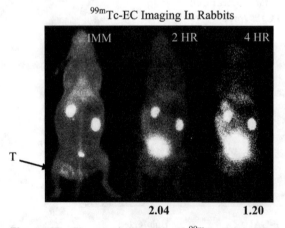

Figure 27 Planar scintigraphy of ^{99m}Tc-EC in VX2 tumor-bearing rabbits (1 mCi/rabbit, IV) demonstrate that the tumor could be well visualized. Tumor versus nontumor ratios were 2.04 and 1.20.

suggest that the combination use of endostatin with cytotoxic chemotherapeutic agents or radiation therapy may enhance the efficiency of endostatin therapy. &132#However, radiolabeled endostatin was found to be useful as a biological response marker in assessing endostatin therapy. Scintigraphic images showed good visualization of the tumor, as well as a correlation between tumor uptake and treatment effects. Decreased tumor versus nontumor uptake of radiolabeled endostatin following endostatin or paclitaxel treatment correlated with decreased tumor volume at the end of treatment as well as decreased expression of angiogenic factors. In other words, the decrease in tumor uptake of ^{99m}Tc-EC–endostatin signified effective anti-tumor activity. For anti-EGFR antibody and COX-2 antagonist, in vitro and in vivo biodistribution studies demonstrated the feasibility of using ^{99m}Tc-EC–C225 and ^{99m}Tc-EC–celebrex to assess EGFR and cox-2 expression. EGFR is over expressed in a significant percentage of human A431 cells, which correlates well with ^{99m}Tc-EC–C225 uptake. Animal studies and preliminary clinical imaging studies suggest that ^{99m}Tc-EC–C225, a specific marker for EGFR, may be useful in selecting patients most likely to benefit from C225 therapy.

Tissue hypoxia is another important predictor of therapeutic response. There was a significantly increased tumor versus tissue uptake ratio as a function of time in the ^{99m}Tc-EC–MN group. When compared with [^{18}F]FMISO and [^{131}I]IMISO, the tumor versus tissue uptake ratios for ^{99m}Tc-EC–MN were similar to those of [^{131}I]IMISO. Thyroid tissue uptake was not altered after ^{99m}Tc-EC–MN, whereas thyroid uptake increased with [^{131}I] IMISO. The findings suggest that ^{99m}Tc-EC–MN is more metabolically stable than [^{131}I] IMISO. Tumor oxygen tension was determined to be 3.2 to 6.0 mmHg within the hypoxic regions, whereas normal muscle tissue demonstrated oxygen tension readings of 30 to 40 mmHg. The findings support further studies to determine normal tissue dosimetry, measuring sensitizer enhancement ratio (SER) and identifying whether ^{99m}Tc-EC–MN can provide a rational means of selecting patients for treatment with radiosensitizing (e.g., SR-2508 and Ro-03–8799) or bioreductive agents.

Apoptosis occurs during treatment with chemotherapy and radiation (25,26,59–62). Apoptosis can occur early, before tumor volume changes, and thus, is an early marker of treatment efficacy. Annexin V is known to bind phosphatidylserine, which is overexpressed by apoptotic cells as a signal for clearance by macrophages. Assessment of apoptosis by annexin V could be useful to evaluate the efficacy of therapy and disease progression or regression. Increased uptake of annexin V at earlier time points, and later decreased uptake after treatment would reflect a positive treatment response. Unfortunately, not all apoptotic cells express phosphatidylserine in their outer membrane. Thus, this agent could become a critical pathway common for the assessment of tumor treatment regimens as many of them eventually cause apoptosis.

Other agents such as ^{99m}Tc-EC–doxorubicin, ^{99m}Tc-EC–LHRH, and ^{99m}Tc-EC–guanosine analog could be useful markers of MDR, sensitivity to hormone therapy, and proliferation markers. The diversity of radiolabeled biomarkers could lead to a more complete assessment of the biological characteristics of tumors.

In summary, EC-conjugates to Technetium can be used to synthesize radiolabeled targeted molecular imaging agents. The chemical synthesis of these agents lends itself to automation and the broad range of ligands that are "chelatable" means that this is a highly flexible and versatile system for radiolabeling. The use of technetium, which can be produced by a desktop generator at low cost, with good energy levels for external detection and a six hour half-life makes this radioisotope suitable for molecular imaging in man.

ACKNOWLEDGMENTS

This work was supported by the John S. Dunn Foundation and Cell Point Research Grant. Animal research was supported by the Cancer Center Core Grant, NIH-NCI CA-16672.

REFERENCES

1. Bar-Shalom R, Valdivia AY, Blaufox MD. PET imaging in oncology [review]. Semin Nucl Med 2000; 30(3):150–185.
2. Plowman PN, Saunders CA, Maisey M. On the usefulness of brain PET scanning to the paediatric neuro-oncologist. Br J Neurosurg 1997; 11(6):525–532.
3. Weber WA, Avril N, Schwaiger M. Relevance of positron emission tomography (PET) in oncology. Strahlenther Onkl 1999; 175:356.
4. Lau CL, Harpole DH, Patz E. Staging techniques for lung cancer [review]. Chest Surg Clin N Am 2000; 10(4):781–801.
5. Schulte M, Brecht-Krauss D, Heymer B, et al. Grading of tumors and tumor-like lesions of bone: evaluation by FDG PET. J Nucl Med 2000; 41(10):1695–1701.
6. Yutani K, Shiba E, Kusuoka H, et al. Comparison of FDG-PET with MIBI-SPECT in the detection of breast cancer and axillary lymph node metastasis. J Comput Assist Tomogr 2000; 24(2):274–280.
7. Franzius C, Sciuk J, Daldrup-Link HE, Jurgens H, Schober O. FDG-PET for detection of osseous metastases from malignant primary bone tumours: comparison with bone scintigraphy. Eur J Nucl Med 2000; 27(9):1305–1311.
8. Folpe AL, Lyles RH, Sprouse JT, Conrad EU, Eary JF. (F-18) fluorodeoxyglucose positron emission tomography as a predictor of pathologic grade and other prognostic variables in bone and soft tissue sarcoma. Clin Cancer Res 2000; 6(4):1279–1287.
9. Meyer PT, Spetzger U, Mueller HD, Zeggel T, Sabri O, Schreckenberger M. High F-18 FDG uptake in a low-grade supratentorial ganglioma: a positron emission tomography case report. Clin Nucl Med 2000; 25(9):694–697.
10. Franzius C, Sciuk J, Brinkschmidt C, Jurgens H, Schober O. Evaluation of chemotherapy response in primary bone tumors with F-18 FDG positron emission tomography compared with histologically assessed tumor necrosis. Clin Nucl Med 2000; 25(11):874–881.
11. Carretta A, Landoni C, Melloni G, et al. 18-FDG positron emission tomography in the evaluation of malignant pleural diseases—a pilot study. Eur J Cardiothorac Surg 2000; 17(4):377–383.
12. Torre W, Garcia-Velloso MJ, Galbis J, Fernandez O, Richter J. FDG-PET detection of primary lung cancer in a patient with an isolated cerebral metastasis. J Cardiovasc Surg 2000; 41(3):503–505.
13. Brunelle F. Noninvasive diagnosis of brain tumours in children [review]. Childs Nerv Syst 2000; 16(10–11):731–734.
14. Mankoff DA, Dehdashti F, Shields AF. Characterizing tumors using metabolic imaging: PET imaging of cellular proliferation and steroid receptors. Neoplasia 2002:71.
15. Fitzgerald J, Parker JA, Danias PG. F-18 fluoro deoxyglucose SPECT for assessment of myocardial viability. J Nucl Cardiol 2000; 7(4):382–387.
16. Schwarz A, Kuwert T. Nuclear medicine diagnosis in diseases of the central nervous system (Review). Radiology 2000; 40(10):858–862.
17. Roelcke U, Leenders KL. PET in neuro-oncology [review]. J Cancer Res Clin Oncol 2001; 127(1):2–8.
18. Brock CS, Meikle SR, Price P. Does ^{18}F-fluorodeoxyglucose metabolic imaging of tumors benefit oncology? Eur J Nucl Med 1997; 24:691–705.

19. Ohtsuki K, Akashi K, Aoka Y, et al. Technetium-99m HYNIC-annexin V: a potential radiopharmaceutical for the in-vivo detection of apoptosis. Eur J Nucl Med 1999; 26(10):1251–1258.

20. Vriens PW, Blankenberg FG, Stoot JH, et al. The use of technetium ^{99m}Tc annexin V for in vivo imaging of apoptosis during cardiac allograft rejection. J Thorac Cardiovasc Surg 1998; 116:844–853.

21. Verbruggen AM, Nosco DL, Van Nerom CG, Bormans GM, Adriaens PJ, De Roo MJ. Evaluation of ^{99m}Tc-L,L-ethylenedicysteine as a potential alternate to ^{99m}Tc-MAG3. Eur J Nucl Med 1990; 16:429.

22. Canet EP, Casali C, Desenfant A, et al. Kinetic characterization of CMD-A2-Gd-DOTA as an intravascular contrast agent for myocardial perfusion measurement with MRI. Magn Reson Med 2000; 43(3):403–409.

23. Laissy JP, Faraggi M, Lebtahi R, et al. Functional evaluation of normal and ischemic kidney by means of gadolinium-DOTA enhanced TurboFLASH MR imaging: a preliminary comparison with 99Tc-MAG3 dynamic scintigraphy. Magn Reson Imaging 1994; 12(3):413–419.

24. Kao CH, ChangLai SP, Chieng PU, Yen TC. Technetium-99m methoxyisobutylisonitrile chest imaging of small cell lung carcinoma: relation to patient prognosis and chemotherapy response—a preliminary report. Cancer 1998; 83:64–88.

25. Blondeau P, Berse C, Gravel D. Dimerization of an intermediate during the sodium in liquid ammonia reduction of L-thiazolidine-4-carboxylic acid. Can J Chem 1967; 45:49–52.

26. Ratner S, Clarke HT. The action of formaldehyde upon cysteine. J AM Chem Soc 1937; 59:200–206.

27. Ilgan S, Yang DJ, Higuchi T, et al. ^{99m}Tc-Ethylenedicysteine-Folate: A new tumor imaging agent. Synthesis, labeling and evaluation in animals. Cancer Biotherapy Radiopharm 1998; 13:427–435.

28. Zareneyrizi F, Yang DJ, Oh CS, et al. Synthesis of ^{99m}Tc-ethylenedicysteine-colchicine for evaluation of antiangiogenic effects. Anti-Cancer Drugs 1999; 10:685–692.

29. Yang DJ, Ilgan S, Higuchi T, et al. Noninvasive assessment of tumor hypoxia with ^{99m}Tc-labeled metronidazole. Pharm Res 1999; 16(5)743–750.

30. Yang DJ, Azhdarinia A, Wu P, et al. In vivo and in vitro measurement of apoptosis in breast cancer cells using ^{99m}Tc-EC-annexin V. Cancer Biother Radiopharm 2001; 16(1):73–84.

31. Xie W, van de Werve G, Berteloot A. An integrated view of the kinetics of glucose and phosphate transport, and of glucose 6-phosphate transport and hydrolysis in intact rat liver microsomes. J Membr Biol 2001; 179(2):113–126.

32. Mullani N, Herbst R, Abbruzzese J, et al. Antiangiogenic treatment with endostatin results in uncoupling of blood flow and glucose metabolism in human tumors. Clin Positron Imaging 2000; 3:151.

33. Yang DJ, Kim KD, Schechter NR, et al. Assessment of antiangiogenic effect using ^{99m}Tc-EC-endostatin. Cancer Biother Radiopharm 2002; 17:233–245.

34. Sheehan KM, Sheahan K, O'Donohue DP. The relationship between cyclooxygenase-2 expression and colorectal cancer. JAMA 1999; 282:1254–1257.

35. Cianchi F, Cortesini C, Bechi P, et al. Up-regulation of cyclooxygenase 2 gene expression correlates with tumor angiogenesis in human colorectal cancer. Gastroenterology 2001; 121:1339–1347.

36. Leahy KM, Ornberg RL, Wang Y, Zweifel BS, Koki AT, Masferrer JL. Cyclooxygenase-2 inhibition by Celecoxib reduces proliferation and induces apoptosis in angiogenic endothelial cells in vivo. Cancer Res 2002; 62(3):625–631.

37. Sun WH, Tsuji S, Tsujii M, et al. Cyclooxygenase regulates angiogenesis induced by colon cancer cells. Cell 1998; 93(5)705–716.

38. Gupta RA, DuBois RN. Colorectal cancer prevention and treatment by inhibition of cyclooxygenase. Nat Rev Cancer 2001; 1:11–21.

39. Howe LR, Dannenberg AJ. A role for cyclooxygenase-2 inhibitors in the prevention and treatment of cancer. Semin Oncol 2002; 29(3 suppl 11):111.

40. Alshafie GA, Abou-Issa HM, Seibert K, Harris RE. Chemotherapeutic evaluation of Celecoxib, a cyclooxygenase-2 inhibitor, in a rat mammary tumor model. Oncol Rep 2000; 7(6):1377–1381.

41. Koh W-J, Rasey JS, Evans ML, et al. Imaging of hypoxia in human tumors with ^{18}F fluoromisonidazole. Int J Radiat Oncol Biol Phys 1992; 22:199–212.

42. Valk PET, Mathis CA, Prados MD, Gilbert JC, Budinger TF. Hypoxia in human gliomas: Demonstration by PET with [^{18}F]fluoromisonidazole. J Nucl Med 1992; 33:2133–2137.

43. Martin GV, Caldwell JH, Rasey JS, Grunbaum Z, Cerqueia M, Krohn KA. Enhanced binding of the hypoxic cell marker [^{18}F]fluoromisonidazole in ischemic myocardium. J Nucl Med 1989; 30:194–201.

44. Rasey JS, Koh WJ, Grieson JR, Grunbaum Z, Krohn KA. Radiolabeled fluoromisonidazole as an imaging agent for tumor hypoxia. Int J Radiat Oncol Biol Phys 1989; 17:985–991.

45. Rasey JS, Nelson NJ, Chin L, Evans ML, Grunbaum Z. Characterization of the binding of labeled fluoromisonidazole in cells in vitro. Radiat Res 1990; 122:301–308.

46. Yang DJ, Wallace S, Cherif A, et al. Development of F-18-labeled fluoroerythro-nitroimidazole as a PET agent for imaging tumor hypoxia. Radiology 1995; 194: 795–800.

47. Teicher BA, Sotomayor EA. Chemical radiation sensitizers and protectors. In: Foye WO, ed. Cancer Chemotherapeutic Agents. Washington, D.C.: American Chemical Society, 1995:501–527.

48. Saikumar P, Dong Z, Weinberg JM, Venkatachalam MA. Mechanisms of cell death in hypoxia/reoxygenation injury. Oncogene 1998; 17:3341–3349.

49. Yun JK, McCormick TS, Villabona C, Judware RR, Espinosa MB, Lapetina EG. Inflammatory mediators are perpetuated in macrophages resistant to apoptosis induced by hypoxia. Proc Natl Acad Sci USA 1997; 94:13,903–13,908.

50. Dive C, Gregory CD, Phipps DJ, Evans DL, Milner AE, Wyllie AH. Analysis and discrimination of necrosis and apoptosis (programmed cell death) by multiparameter flow cytometry. Biochem Biophys Acta 1992; 1133:275–285.

51. Narula J, Hajjar RJ, Dec GW. Apoptosis in the failing heart. Cardiol Clin 1998; 16: 691–710.

52. Bossenmeyer-Pourie C, Koziel V, Daval J. CPP32/CASPASE-3-like proteases in hypoxia-induced apoptosis in developing brain neurons. Brain Res Mol Brain Res 1999; 71: 225–237.

53. Banasiak KJ, Cronin T, Haddad GG. bcl-2 prolongs neuronal survival during hypoxia-induced apoptosis. Brain Res Mol Brain Res 1999; 72:214–225.

54. Bronckers AL, Goei SW, Dumont E, et al. In situ detection of apoptosis in dental and periodontal tissues of the adult mouse using annexin-V-biotin. Histochem Cell Biol 2000; 113(4):293–301.

55. Tait JF, Smith C. Site-specific mutagenesis of annexin V: role of residues from Arg-200 to Lys-207 in phospholipid binding. Arch Biochem Biophys 1991; 288:141–144.

56. Blankenberg FG, Katsikis PD, Tait JF, et al. Imaging of apoptosis (programmed cell death) with ^{99m}Tc-annexin. J Nucl Med 1999; 40:184–191.

57. Yang DJ, Kim CG, Schechter NR, et al. Imaging with 99mTc ECDG targeted at the multifunctional glucose transport system: feasibility study with rodents. Radiology 2003; 226(2):465–473.

58. Schechter NR, Yang DJ, Azhdarinia A, et al. Assessment of epidermal growth factor receptor with 99mTc-ethylenedicysteine-C225 monoclonal antibody. Anticancer Drugs 2003; 14(1):49–56.

10

Magnetic Resonance Spectroscopy in Cancer

Jeffry R. Alger
Department of Radiological Sciences, Ahmanson-Lovelace Brain Mapping Center,
Brain Research Institute, Jonsson Comprehensive Cancer Center,
David Geffen School of Medicine at UCLA, University of California,
Los Angeles, California, U.S.A.

A Note from the Editors

*M*agnetic resonance spectroscopy (MRS)
evaluates in situ biochemistry by detecting signals
from chemical compounds other than water.
Proton or hydrogen spectroscopy is most commonly employed
because it produces the strongest MRS signal and requires no
modification of conventional high field MRI units. However,
only a limited number of low molecular weight molecules with
characteristic resonance properties can be detected with
MRS. Among the most important in cancer are choline
(cell membrane turnover), N-acetylaspartate (reduced in
brain tumors), mobile lipids (reduced in breast cancer), and
citrate (reduced in prostate cancer). Studies have shown
MRS can detect cancers by demonstrating elevations of
choline and reductions in normal metabolites. MRS provides
information not attainable with conventional MRI without
exposure to radio-isotopes or ionizing radiation.

INTRODUCTION

Research studies aimed at defining the value of magnetic resonance spectroscopy (MRS) for the evaluation of cancer have been undertaken since the early 1980s (1). Readers can refer to the reviews by Negendank and Barker et al. for summaries of the first studies (2,3). MRS accessories for 1.5 Tesla (T) magnetic resonance imaging (MRI) equipment that were cleared for marketing by the Food and Drug Administration (FDA) became available in the late 1990s and this promoted further growth in the use of MRS for the evaluation of various cancers (4,5). Of all human cancers, brain cancer has been the most thoroughly explored by MRS (6–9). However, the use of MRS in the evaluation of breast and prostate cancers is also currently expanding (10–13).

This chapter will introduce and review the fundamental concepts related to cancer evaluation by MRS in humans. Space limitations prevent an exhaustive review of the entire literature relevant to the clinical oncologic uses of MRS and to the large number of MRS studies of cultured cancer cells and of tumors in animals. However, the chapter strives to provide the reader with a starting point to evaluate and understand this growing literature. MRS studies of brain, breast, and prostate cancers in humans will be discussed to illustrate fundamental concepts.

TECHNICAL BACKGROUND

The development of a detailed understanding of the physics principles that underlie MRS is not achievable in a short chapter such as this. However, the following paragraphs provide a succinct, accurate but somewhat superficial description of important principles and concepts.

MRS is closely related to nuclear magnetic resonance (NMR) spectroscopy, which has been used in chemistry and physics since the late 1940s. The term "MRS" is now commonly used for biomedical applications, in preference to "NMR" or "NMR spectroscopy," when NMR spectroscopy studies of living human or animal subjects or cultured living cells are undertaken. MRS is viewed by the radiology and medical imaging communities as member of a large family of MRI techniques. MRS differs from MRI in that MRS detects signals from chemical compounds other than water to evaluate in situ biochemistry, whereas MRI detects tissue water or lipid signals to form images that depict anatomy. However, even this distinction is somewhat simplistic; MRS techniques that image the spatial distribution of in situ biochemicals have been used for the evaluation of cancers since the early 1990s (14,15). MRS and MRI are each performed with an MRI scanner. There are thousands of MRI scanners installed in academic radiology departments and in some private radiology practices throughout the world that are capable of performing MRS. However some MRI scanners are not suitable for MRS. Typically, MRS requires a static magnetic field strength of greater than 1.0 T. Low-field MRI scanners can not therefore be used. As is the case with MRI, MRS requires only exposure to time invariant (static) and oscillatory magnetic fields. Hence, one of the greatest attributes of MRS is that it can evaluate in situ biochemistry without exposing the subject to ionizing radiation or to radioactive isotopes.

Discussion of the component terms of MRS (i.e. magnetic, resonance, and spectroscopy) provides a slightly more detailed understanding. The term "magnetic" is used because MRS utilizes several special types of magnetic fields. Certain atomic nuclei behave as if they were spinning and this causes such nuclei to appear as if they were minute bar magnets. This "nuclear magnetism" can interact with a number of external magnetic fields including (i) the static magnetic field created by the MRI magnet, (ii) the oscillating magnetic fields produced by the MRI scanner's radiofrequency (RF) coils, and (iii) the pulsed magnetic field distortions produced by the MRI scanner's magnetic field gradient system. These "magnetic interactions" lead to a particular type of energy exchange, referred to as "resonance," between the scanner and the nuclear magnetic fields and it is this exchange that is detected as the "MRS signal." The term "spectroscopy" conveys the idea that the magnetic resonance occurs only at specific frequencies and that the signal-producing nuclei can be identified by the presence of resonance only at specific characteristic frequencies. For clinical MRS studies, the characteristic resonance frequency has a time dependence that is similar to that of the "radio waves" used in radio and television broadcasting (Fig. 1). Hence MRS is sometimes described as using radio waves. The basic MRS result is the "spectrum," which is a two-dimensional plot of frequency on the horizontal axis and intensity of resonance interaction on the vertical axis (Fig. 1).

Only certain atomic nuclei (isotopes) of biological significance (e.g., ^{1}H,^{31}P, ^{13}C,^{7}Li, and ^{19}F) have suitable magnetic properties and are therefore capable of producing MRS signals (Fig. 1). MRS signals produced by these isotopes are easily distinguished from each other by their much different characteristic frequencies. The ability of MRS to detect unique signals from different chemicals results from the fact that the magnetic resonance frequency is directly proportional to the static magnetic field strength at the nucleus. The electrons which surround the atomic nuclei located within molecules circulate in ways that tend to alter the magnetic field at the atomic nucleus to a small but significant extent. This causes a small but detectable alterations in the MRS signal frequency which are dependent on the chemical structure surrounding an atomic nucleus, allowing the identification of specific resonance signals from individual nuclei within individual molecules (Figs. 1 and 2). The differences in frequency resulting from chemical structure are referred to as "chemical shifts," which are frequently rather small. Important MRS signals from a particular isotope, such as ^{1}H, may be separated from each other in frequency by only a few cycles per second [Hertz (Hz)] with each of their signals having a frequency of millions of cycles per second [Megahertz (MHz)]. For this reason, it is a common practice to specify the chemical shift in "parts per million (ppm)."

The different nuclei of biological significance have different attributes and practical limitations with respect to MRS detection. The proton [^{1}H] produces the strongest most easily detected MRS signal and is therefore most frequently used for routine clinical MRS. Moreover,^{1}H-MRS is convenient in that it can be performed using the same hardware as is used for conventional MRI. ^{31}P produces the second most intense MRS signal. Figures 1 and 2 illustrate general features that are seen in ^{1}H- and ^{31}P-MRS of normal and neoplastic brain tissue. ^{31}P-MRS has been the basis for some clinical MRS examinations. Indeed, many of the early MRS studies of cancer were performed with ^{31}P-MRS, but the difficulty associated with detection of ^{31}P signals compared to ^{1}H-MRS signals has led to far more common use of ^{1}H-MRS in recent years. Other atomic nuclei are of research interest, but are not used in routine clinical MRS studies of cancer. For this reason, this chapter will discuss only ^{1}H- and ^{31}P-MRS.

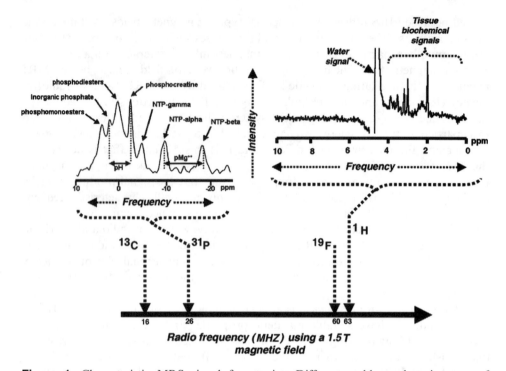

Figure 1 Characteristic MRS signal frequencies. Different stable nuclear isotopes of biological significance produce MRS signals at unique and characteristic frequencies. The characteristic nuclear frequencies differ by a great amount and are easily distinguished. For instance, all ^{1}H nuclei produce signals proximal to 63 MHz in a magnetic field of 1.5 T, whereas all ^{31}P nuclei produce signal proximal to 26 MHz when the same magnetic field strength is used. Within a narrow band of frequencies surrounding the characteristic signal frequency of each nucleus are found distinct signals from chemically unique nuclei. Typical ^{1}H and ^{31}P spectra of normal living brain tissue are shown in the insets. The ^{1}H spectrum shows a large signal produced by tissue water that frequently needs to be suppressed to detect the smaller signals from biochemicals within the tissue. Assignments for chemically unique signals relevant to cancer are given in Figure 2. The ^{31}P spectrum shows signals from NTP and other tissue metabolities associated with energy metabolism. The phosphomonoester signal is the most relevant for cancer studies because many cancers show an elevation of this signal. In addition, the frequency difference between the phosphocreatine and inorganic phosphate signals is sensitive to intracellular pH permitting the noninvasive determination of pH within cancer cells tumors. *Abbreviations*: NTP, nucleotide triphosphate; MHz, megahertz; T, Tesla; ppm, parts per million.

Clinical MRS research studies involving cancer have most frequently sought to evaluate neoplastic mass lesions. In order to evaluate a mass lesion with MRS, there is a need for procedures that can localize the anatomic source of the MRS signals that are detected and studied. Figures 2 and 3 provide illustrations of the two complementary methodologies that are available for attaining volume localization. In localized single volume MRS (Fig. 2), a conventional MR image is used to identify a location of interest within or adjacent to the tumor which is typically defined as a rectilinear "voxel," and MRS signal is acquired from only this location (5,16). If it is desired to obtain MRS from other locations, the localized single volume MRS procedure is repeated. In magnetic resonance spectroscopic imaging (MRSI),

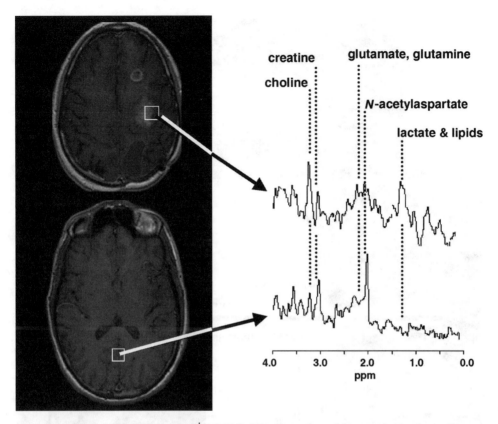

Figure 2 Single volume localized ¹H-MRS data from normal human brain tissue (*bottom panel*) and from a contrast enhancing brain tumor (*top panel*). When using the single volume localized MRS technique, a region of interest is defined using MRI. Without moving the patient, ¹H-MRS data are then collected from the region of interest using a localized spectroscopy pulse sequence. Regions of interest for the two studies on the MRIs are shown (*white rectangles*). The resultant spectra are shown to the right of the MRIs. Key ¹H-MRS signals are labeled. Note that the choline signal is substantially more elevated above baseline in the tumor spectrum compared to the normal spectrum. Furthermore, there is a lactate signal present in the tumor spectrum but not in the normal spectrum and the NAA signal is reduced in the tumor spectrum compared to the normal spectrum. Note that some tumors can also produce strong lipid signals which can often not be distinguished from lactate signals, although this is not the case in this example (44). There is, in fact, a great deal of variability in the spectroscopic patterns exhibited by different tumors at different stages of treatment and response. Moreover there is even variation of spectroscopic patterns displayed by normal brain tissue. *Abbreviations*: NAA, *N*-acetylaspartate; ¹H-MRSI, ¹H-magnetic resonance spectroscopic imaging; ppm, parts per million.

MRS signals are simultaneously acquired from a grid containing a large number of rectilinear voxels that include the tumor and surrounding tissues that is prescribed from a preliminary MRI study (Fig. 3) (8,14,15,17). MRSI is also sometimes referred to as "spectroscopic imaging (SI)" or "chemical shift imaging (CSI)." Figure 3 illustrates that MRSI is capable of providing either localized spectra of individual voxels that can be chosen in a post hoc fashion, or "SI" of the anatomic distribution of the intensity of a particular signal.

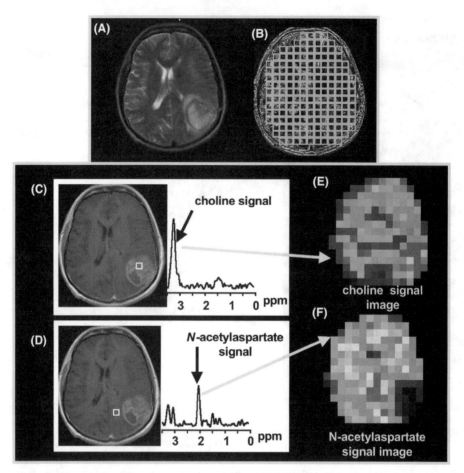

Figure 3 Typical ¹H-MRSI results from a glioblastoma multiforme. (**A**) When using the ¹H-MRSI technique, a slice or volume of tissue of interest is defined from MRI. (**B**) Spectroscopic imaging procedures are then used to obtain a spectrum from each of the locations shown by the grid. Selected spectra sampled from this grid are shown for (**C**) tumor tissue and (**D**) nearby normal tissue. The area under relevant signals is then determined in each of the spectra over the entire grid. These signal measures are then represented with color spectroscopic images [(**E**) the choline signal image and (**F**) the NAA signal image]. Note that the spectra [(**B**) and (**C**)] and spectroscopic images [(**E**) and (**F**)] show NAA signal decrease and choline signal increase in the tumor compared to normal tissue. As with Figure 2, it is important to emphasize that these patterns are characteristic of tumor and normal tissue, but that each type of tissue displays considerable variability. *Abbreviations*: ¹H-MRSI, ¹H-magnetic resonance spectroscopic imaging; NAA, *N*-acetylaspartate; ppm, parts per million.

TECHNICAL LIMITATIONS

MRS signals generated by molecules having molecular weights greater than a few thousand daltons or by smaller molecules that are bound to macromolecular arrays (e.g., proteins, membranes, or nucleic acid polymers) cannot be detected using currently available technology. This effectively means that only small relatively mobile molecules present within tissue can be detected with MRS. Typically, such tissue-associated small molecules are "metabolites" involved in intermediary metabolism.

Accordingly, MRS is often said to detect "tissue metabolites," and from this comes the somewhat inaccurate generalization that MRS "measures" metabolism. In this light, MRS is frequently discussed in association with certain radionuclei imaging procedures, such as fluorodeoxyglucose positron emission tomography (FDG-PET), which are designed to measure metabolic rates through the use of radioactively labeled tracer molecules. In fact, radiotracer imaging technologies and MRS do not sense metabolism in precisely the same manner (18). MRS detects the presence of certain metabolite signals that are inherently present in the tissue. With appropriate calibration, such measures can be used to obtain the tissue concentration of certain metabolites (19). This is inherently different from measuring the rate of a metabolic pathway, which is done in radiotracer imaging. In complex metabolic pathways, metabolite concentrations and metabolite fluxes are not always related in simple ways, and therefore radiotracer imaging and MRS offer distinct and complementary views of metabolism.

MRS has an inherently low sensitivity compared to many destructive techniques for detecting molecules in tissue. Indeed, only a few of the most heavily concentrated tissue molecules are readily detected with MRS. Figures 1 and 2 show the signals that can be readily detected with MRS. For ^{1}H-MRS signal detection, the standard rule of thumb is that there must be at least one micromole of the molecules of interest within the volume of interest. Frequently, the sample or tissue volume that is examined must be upwardly adjusted to meet this requirement. For human cancer, the minimal volume that can be evaluated with MRS has been about $0.2\,cm^3$ under the most favorable circumstances (17). The majority of studies evaluate larger volumes. The normally evaluated volume is $1\text{--}8\,cm^3$ as is illustrated in Figures 2 and 3. In the MRS evaluation of cancers, it is important to consider that tumors usually display a substantial degree of microscopic disorganization. Edema and necrosis are often present and the cells are not as closely packed, as is the case for normal organized tissue. This disorganized cellular ultrastructure further limits the sensitivity with which intracellular tumor metabolites can be detected, because there tend to be fewer cells per unit volume in tumor in comparison to normal tissue (20). Indeed, many studies have pointed out that the inability to assess tumor microstructure is a substantial limitation for MRS evaluation of cancer.

MRS has a strict requirement for a spatially homogeneous static magnetic field. It is the most demanding of all the MRI techniques in this regard. The applied static magnetic field intensity must vary by less than approximately 100 parts per billion over the intended sampling volume. Anatomic features surrounding the tumor can distort the shape and intensity of the applied magnetic field to an unacceptable extent introducing problems with detection of MRS signals from certain regions of the body or in certain tumors. Furthermore, tumors also sometimes have hemorrhages that contain hemoglobin-derived iron particles. Such particles are magnetic, and may also distort the magnetic field homogeneity to an unacceptable extent. In addition to these naturally occurring magnetic field distortions, patients who have had surgeries prior to their MRS examinations sometimes retain magnetic materials as a result of surgery.

Magnetic resonance instruments can provide a highly accurate measure of signal frequency, but are limited in their ability to provide exact measures of signal amplitude (the area under the signal) that are calibrated against a defined universal standard (19). Hence, MRS permits ready conclusions about whether a particular molecule's signal is present above the noise level, but it is somewhat more difficult to determine the exact tissue concentration of the molecule, exactly. Measures of signal intensity must be quoted with reference to some calibration signal that is also present in the spectrum being analyzed or can be acquired from some other MRS or MRI measurement of the same tissue region in the same subject. For this reason, MRS results are often reported as the ratio of two signals although more recent studies have emphasized the utility of more absolute quantification of the concentration of signal-producing compounds (21,22).

MRS has limited resolution for detecting all the molecules that are present in tissue. It is frequently the case, that the MRS signal from one molecule cannot be distinguished from the MRS signal of a different molecule. This introduces uncertainties regarding whether a particular signal is actually detected and may introduce errors in concentration estimation.

In summary, while the ability to detect MRS signals from the molecules within tumors and cancer cells nondestructively and in situ would seem to open the door to exceedingly intricate studies of the biochemistry and metabolism of these entities, the key technical limitations inherent to MRS that are discussed in the this section impair this realization to a great extent.

CANCER BIOCHEMISTRY RELEVANT TO MRS

Cancers have specific and unique biochemical features that are exploited in MRS studies. This section provides a brief introduction to and an overview of these features. It must be emphasized at the outset that a complete and systematic understanding of the metabolic underpinnings of the MRS signal alterations associated with cancer is yet to be attained. Much of the altered biochemistry that is exploited in clinical MRS studies of cancer was "discovered" by doing exploratory in vivo MRS studies. As a result, there is a distinct need for further study, to fully understand the relevant biochemistry within the context of cancer and its treatment. There is very little fundamental understanding of the extent to which the altered biochemical features that are exploited in MRS studies are uniform across all cancer types or all stages of malignancy. Furthermore, it is generally not known how a particular therapeutic regimen will influence the biochemical features that are seen with MRS. Indeed, many research efforts over the past two decades have sought to use MRS studies of patient populations to empirically define how the relevant biochemical alterations may be related to cancer cell type, to degree of malignancy, or to therapeutic successes and failures (see below), but there are only a few examples of fundamental research to characterize and understand the underlying biochemical alterations.

^{1}H-MRS studies of cancer have revealed that many tumors and proliferating cells display an elevation of the "choline signal." Figures 2 and 3 illustrate this finding for brain cancer. The analogous finding in ^{31}P-MRS is elevation of the "phosphomonoester signal." Each of these MRS alterations is related to altered phospholipid metabolism. A simplified rendering of the relevant metabolism based on the studies by Gillies et al. is provided in Figure 4 (23,24). Choline (Cho) is transported from the blood into the cell and then phosphorylated to phosphocholine (PCho) in the Cho kinase reaction. PCho can then be utilized in further anabolic reactions to synthesize phosphatidylcholine (PtdylCho) that can ultimately be incorporated into membranes. Ethanolamine (Ea) follows a similar anabolic pathway to phosphoethanolamine (PEa) and ultimately to membranes. Balancing pathways exist in which the phospholipids PtdylCho and phosphatidylethanolamine (PtdylEa) are catabolized to PCho, PEa, and glycerophosphocholine (GPC). Furthermore, PCho can be formed via catabolism of PtdylCho that arises from methyltransfer

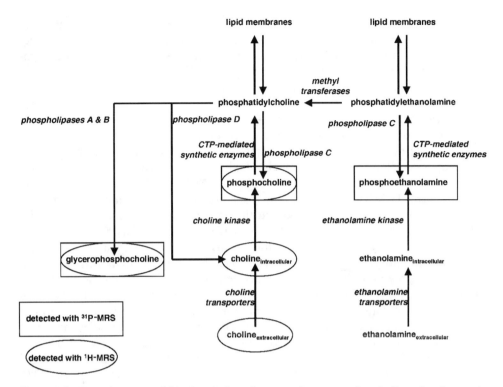

Figure 4 Key elements of biochemical pathways relevant to the choline signal seen in ¹H-MRS and the phosphomonoester signal seen in ³¹P-MRS. Biochemical compounds detectable by ¹H-MRS are surrounded by ellipses and those detectable by ³¹P-MRS are surrounded by rectangles. Anabolic pathways are represented by upward arrows. Catabolic pathways are represented by downward arrows. *Abbreviations:* ¹H-MRS,¹H-magnetic resonance spectroscopy; ³¹P-MRS, ³¹P-magnetic resonance spectroscopy; CTP, cytidine triphosphate. *Source:* From Ref. 23.

of methyl groups from methionine to PtdylEa. In certain glioma (23) and mammary carinoma cells (25), this latter route accounts for very little of the total PCho synthesis, suggesting that the majority of the choline compounds within tumors composed of these cell types is obtained via transport from blood.

In a typical in vivo ¹H-MRS study, the signals produced by Cho, PCho, and GPC cannot be resolved due to the characteristic resonance broadening seen in vivo, although it is possible to resolve the signals arising from these three molecules in MRS studies of cell-free extracts (26). Hence the "choline signal" seen in a typical in vivo ¹H-MRS study is generated by all three molecules and is therefore sometimes referred to as the "total choline signal" or just the "choline signal." It is not likely that PtdylCho phospholipid molecules will make an appreciable contribution to the total choline ¹H-MRS signal because, the majority of these molecules are associated with various membranes which are not sufficiently mobile to permit detection (see previous section). The inability to distinguish the signals produced by the three unique choline-containing metabolites (Cho, PCho, and GPC) leads to uncertainty about the underlying cause for the elevated choline signal seen in cancers and proliferating cells compared to that in normal tissues. The following possibilities exist: (i) Extracellular or blood Cho may be elevated. (ii) Intracellular Cho may be elevated as a result of enhanced transport. (iii) PCho may be elevated as a result of increased choline kinase activity coupled with enhanced Cho transport. (iv) Cho or GPC may be elevated as a result of enhanced catabolic activity of the phospholipases. In other words, elevated total choline MRS signal may be the result of either elevated anabolic activity (possibilities i–iii) or elevated catabolic activity (possibility iv) associated with membrane phospholipid metabolism. Without being able to resolve PCho, Cho, and GPC signals, it is not possible to know whether acceleration of anabolic or catabolic activity is responsible for the choline signal elevation seen in cancers. This uncertainty has led some authors to use terminology like "increased membrane turnover" and "altered membrane or phospholipid metabolism" as means of acknowledging uncertainty about whether enhanced anabolic or catabolic activity is responsible for the increased choline ^{1}H-MRS signal seen in cancers. More recent in vitro ^{1}H-MRS analyses of biopsy material from brain tumor, prostate cancer, and colon cancer have suggested that the predominant cause for the choline signal elevation seen with in vivo ^{1}H-MRS is increased intracellular PCho (12,26–30). Studies of mammary carcinoma and glioma cells have shown enhanced Cho transport and phosphorylation suggesting that acceleration of the anabolic pathway to PCho is probably more important than acceleration of catabolic pathways (23,25). The view that cancers have enhanced synthesis of PCho from Cho is further supported by studies that have shown that inhibitors of choline kinase have antineoplastic activity and may be the basis for chemotherapeutic drugs, and studies that show oncogenic transformation is associated with PCho increase (31,32). However, there is also some evidence to suggest that certain more benign cancer cells have elevated GPC, so the enhancement of catabolic activity cannot be completely ruled out (27).

Elevation of the ^{31}P-MRS phosphomonoester signal has been identified as a feature of neoplasms and proliferating cells for many years (2,10,33). In a typical in vivo ^{31}P-MRS study, the signals produced by PCho and PEa have nearly the same frequency and cannot be distinguished. They are unresolved components of the "phosphomonoester signal" shown in Figure 1. The ^{31}P-MRS signal produced by GPC is however a component of the phosphodiester signal which is readily distinguished from the phosphomonoester signal. The ^{31}P-MRS phosphomonoester signal elevation that is seen in cancer could therefore be the result of PCho or PEa elevation or both. Specialized decoupling techniques sharpen the components of the in vivo ^{31}P-MRS phosphomonoester signal allowing resolution of PCho and PEa (34,35). Studies that have used this technique have demonstrated that both the PCho and PEa signals are elevated in neoplasms (36). A variety of studies reviewed by Podo (33) indicate that the ratio of PEa ^{31}P-MRS signal areas to PCho ^{31}P-MRS signal areas is correlated with the cell proliferation rate and may therefore become useful as an indicator of therapeutic response.

Classical biochemical studies of tumors revealed derangements of glucose metabolism leading to the prediction that tumors should display elevated lactate levels on ^{1}H-MRS and acidic readings on ^{31}P-MRS (15,18,37). Figure 5 illustrates the key concepts that underlie this prediction. Glucose is catabolized in a pathway that includes anaerobic and aerobic steps. It can be metabolized to pyruvate without oxygen, while the further catabolism of pyruvate to carbon dioxide and water requires oxygen. Both the aerobic and anaerobic pathways yield energy in the form of adenosine triphosphate (ATP), however the aerobic portion of the pathway does so much more efficiently than the anaerobic portion. Tumors, frequently, can have defects which lead to inefficient operation of the aerobic portion of the pathway. Tumor microstructure may be such that oxygen cannot be delivered in sufficient amounts to permit optimal utilization of the aerobic pathway. Alternatively, tumors may have

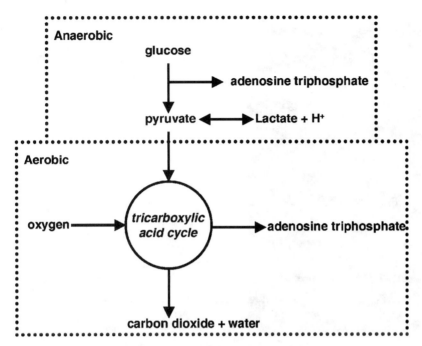

Figure 5 Key elements of the biochemical pathway of glucose metabolism.

deranged mitochondria, which are responsible for integration of the aerobic pathway. Furthermore, there may be loss of feedback regulation between the aerobic and anaerobic pathways that causes the anaerobic pathway to produce pyruvate and lactate at a very high uncontrolled rate despite adequate oxygenation. Lactate, which produces an identifiable signal in ^{1}H-MRS (Fig. 2) may be elevated as a result of any of these possibilities. Furthermore, the anaerobic pathway produces acid suggesting that tumors having such metabolic defects should be somewhat acidic compared to normal tissues. pH can be determined with ^{31}P-MRS by measuring the frequency difference between the inorganic phosphate and the phosphocreatine signals (Fig. 1). Many studies have sought to use ^{1}H-MRS and ^{31}P-MRS as a means of detecting defects in glucose metabolism associated with cancer (37).^{1}H-MRS studies have frequently shown that tumors have abnormally elevated levels of lactate signals, however, there can be considerable variability between tumors and within tumors. Similarly, ^{31}P-MRS studies have shown variable intracellular pH. In some cases somewhat acidic tumors can be identified, while other tumors may be slightly alkaline. These findings are likely a reflection of variable degree of between-tumor vascularization and the heterogeneous vascularization within an individual tumor.

MRS studies also make use of the fact that a neoplastic lesion can cause a decrease or absence of some biochemical signal that would otherwise be present in normal tissue. The most common example is the *N*-acetylaspartate (NAA) signal detected with ^{1}H-MRS. The NAA molecule is produced only within normal neurons (38,39). Astrocytes and other prominent differentiated central nervous system cell types do not contain NAA. Accordingly, brain tumors of glial origin and metastatic deposits do not contain NAA and the NAA signal is not present in ^{1}H-MRS of such tumors. Figures 2 and 3 illustrate the typical NAA signal loss associated with brain tumors. In such circumstances, the NAA signal reduction is attributed to the

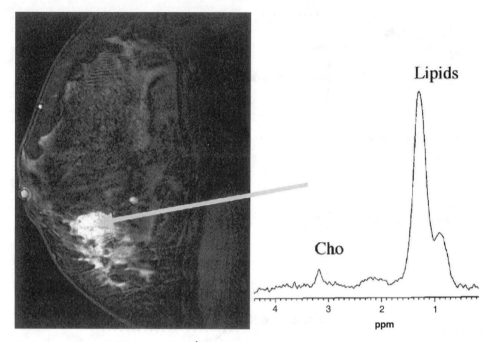

Figure 6 Single volume localized ^{1}H-MRS of an invasive ductal carcinoma. Signals from lipids and Cho are shown. Recent studies suggest that the presence of choline signal above baseline in a breast lesion is an indication of malignancy. *Abbreviations*: ^{1}H-MRSI,^{1}H-magnetic resonance spectroscopic imaging; Cho, choline; ppm, parts per million. *Source*: From Ref. 40.

neuronal death or to loss of neuronal function as the neurons become engulfed by neoplastic cells. Caution must be exercised in asserting the cause of an observed NAA signal loss. Any process that leads to the destruction of functional neurons will lead to NAA signal loss; Cancer may not be the only cause. Certain therapeutic maneuvers may also cause neuron death and therefore, NAA signal loss. Analogous signal losses can be appreciated in ^{1}H-MRS studies of prostate and breast cancers. Normal breast tissue contains a large amount of materials that produce a distinct set of lipid signals on ^{1}H-MRS (Fig. 6) (40,41). These lipid signals can be reduced in breast cancers as neoplastic tissue replaces normal tissue. Normal prostate tissue contains relatively large amounts of citrate and polyamines that produce detectable signals on ^{1}H-MRS, and spectra taken from neoplastic regions show a loss of these citrate and polyamines signals (Fig. 7) (12,42).

CLINICAL USES OF MRS

Numerous studies have been performed to define the clinical utility of MRS for the cancer patient. To a large extent, these have been based on empiricism. Preliminary studies first demonstrated that cancers produced unique features on MRS and this prompted further studies to evaluate whether MRS might be useful for diagnosis, staging treatment, surgical planning, assessing treatment response, and defining when there has been treatment failure, disease progression, or recurrence. There are a growing number of publications that indicate that MRS is a valuable assessment tool for

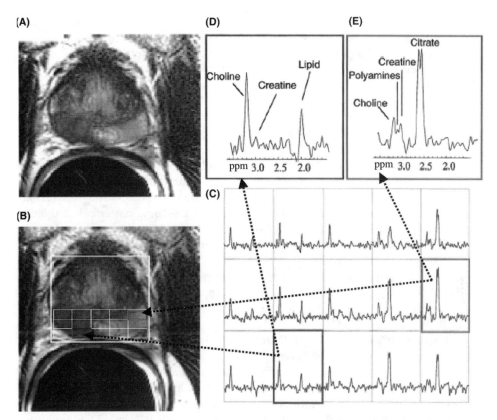

Figure 7 ^{1}H-MRSI of prostate. (**A**) MRI data. (**B**) The voxel grid used for MRSI. (**C**) Spectra from the voxel grid. (**D**) Spectra of tumor tissue. (**E**) Spectra of normal tissue. Note that the cancer displays a pronounced choline signal increase with a reduced citrate signal compared to normal prostatic tissues. *Abbreviations*: ^{1}H-MRSI, ^{1}H-Magnetic resonance spectroscopic imaging; ppm, parts per million. *Source*: From Ref. 12.

each of these cancer management problems. As was discussed above, much of this work has not relied on a detailed fundamental understanding of the biochemistry responsible for the MRS signal alterations associated with cancer.

Although much of the early exploratory work was done with ^{31}P-MRS, there is now a much more substantial interest in using ^{1}H-MRS as a routine clinical tool for mostly technical and logistical reasons. The following paragraphs will therefore summarize current thinking about the use of ^{1}H-MRS in the evaluation of cancers of the brain, breast, and prostate. However some investigators continue to explore the clinical utility of ^{31}P-MRS (34,43).

Brain cancer assessment has been the area of most substantial ^{1}H-MRS application. This is most certainly related to a number of factors, including the absence of severe technical limitations in MRI and MRS studies of the head. However clinical factors have played a role as well. Brain cancer represents a serious health problem with very limited therapeutic alternatives. There are dangers and difficulties associated with neurosurgical procedures and with cranial radiation therapy. Furthermore, chemotherapeutic treatments for brain cancer are frequently not effective. These clinical factors suggest the need for better noninvasive diagnostic procedures that enable more exact definition of regional pathology, that provide a measure of therapeutic response (or failure), and that are capable of detecting tumor regrowth following therapy. ^{1}H-MRS is believed to offer significant opportunities in each of these areas. As result, many brain cancer patients now undergo ^{1}H-MRS studies as part of their routine assessments.

Considerable effort has been expended toward using ^{1}H-MRS technology for defining histological tumor type and grade, prior to biopsy, with the eventual goal being to reduce the need for surgeries that are performed only for diagnostic purposes (21,44–47). Early ^{1}H-MRS studies of cerebral neoplasia suggested that the MRS signal patterns served to identify tumor type and grade (48). Subsequent studies have generally supported this concept, although there are yet to be clearly defined diagnostic standards for typing or grading brain tumors with ^{1}H-MRS with absolute certainty. Different grades and types of intracranial neoplastic mass lesions have statistically significant differences in mean spectroscopic patterns but there is also considerable between subject variability that limits application on a case-by-case basis (44,45). Nevertheless present knowledge permits one to use the ^{1}H-MRS signal patterns to suggest the most likely pathology and, in some cases, it may be possible to rule out certain types of disease. It is clear that pattern analysis systems now being developed will likely provide the most efficient approach by using ^{1}H-MRS for pre-operative diagnosis in preference to the evaluation of a single spectroscopic signal (44,46,49,50).

Other presurgical uses of ^{1}H-MRS have also been promoted (49,51–54). It appears to provide a means of defining the most appropriate locations to perform biopsies and can also be helpful in defining the spatial extent of neoplastic invasion prior to surgery or radiation therapy. Here, the low spatial resolution of ^{1}H-MRS has been a limiting factor, although with the appropriate techniques, assessments can be made with a spatial resolution of approximately $0.2\,cm^3$. The significant MRS pattern differences between normal and neoplastic tissues indicate that MRS can augment conventional MRI in the delineation of lesion extent. There have been exploratory studies in a number of areas that are related to treatment of brain tumors. For instance, studies have demonstrated that progressive or recurrent glioma manifests itself through pronounced change in the choline signal elevation (55–58). Accordingly, many clinicians hope to use ^{1}H-MRS as a means of distinguishing recurrent and progressing tumor from radiation necrosis as a means of better defining when to initiate neoadjuvant therapies. Furthermore, certain ^{1}H-MRS features appear to predict which tumors are most likely to respond to chemotherapeutic treatment (59).

Evaluation of prostate cancer has been an area of substantial ^{1}H-MRS application during the past few years (12,60). This has been the result of technical progress in many areas including design of endorectal RF coils, spectroscopic imaging, and techniques for suppressing the strong lipid signals arising from tissues that surround the prostate gland. From a clinical perspective, the introduction of prostate specific antigen (PSA) blood tests during the past decade has created a need for diagnostic imaging methods that can survey the prostate for disease that is not apparent to conventional imaging techniques in men who have equivocal PSA findings.^{1}H-MRS is clearly capable of identifying the presence and the location of neoplastic disease in the prostate through detection of elevated choline signal and decreased citrate signal (Fig. 7). Accordingly, studies are beginning to demonstrate utility for defining the sites that will provide the most descriptive biopsies. Furthermore, there is evidence to suggest that the choline signal elevation is sensitive to the level of malignancy and provides a means of assessing therapeutic response.

^{1}H-MRS also shows promise of playing a role in the clinical evaluation of breast cancers (11). Currently, the most promising ^{1}H-MRS approach is to determine whether a particular mass produces a detectable choline signal (Fig. 7). Detection of choline signal in such a mass appears to be an indicator of the presence of malignant neoplastic disease. Benign lesions tend to produce no detectable choline signal. Katz-Brull et al. have performed a meta-analysis of five previously published ^{1}H-MRS studies of breast cancer (11). They conclude that ^{1}H-MRS is a useful secondary characterizing tool having reasonable sensitivity and specificity for malignant disease. However, there are several confounds which must be taken into account when using such choline detectability criteria. Lactating breast tissue produces detectable choline signal because there is a strict dietary requirement for choline in developing humans (41). Furthermore, the ability of ^{1}H-MRS to assess small breast lesions is limited. False negative diagnoses of benign disease are sometimes made in small lesions because there is not sufficient tumor tissue within the volume sampled by MRS to produce a detectable choline signal.

FUTURE OF MRS IN ONCOLOGY

Past trends suggest an increased use of MRS for the purpose of addressing clinical management problems in cancer patients, and also to further our understanding of the unique biochemistry and physiology of cancer. Two attributes of MRS provide compelling support for this assertion. First, MRS clearly provides information beyond that provided by other forms of MRI. MRI provides a vivid anatomic depiction as well as some physiological information (e.g., perfusion or oxygenation), while MRS provides complementary biochemical information. The ease with which MRS can be incorporated into an MRI study protocol therefore guarantees it an increased use even though the biochemical information provided by MRS is not fully understood in many cases. Many relevant studies have emphasized that MRS augments MRI and that the two techniques should be used in concert. Second, MRS provides one of the few means of assessing aspects of tissue biochemistry without exposure to radioisotopes or to ionizing radiation. Therefore, MRS can be performed in an individual patient at a frequency that is only limited by finances and logistics. This suggests that MRS may become a diagnostic tool of considerable significance for long-term management of cancer patients, because an individual patient can undergo almost unlimited MRS surveillance during different treatments.

A major factor that limits the increased acceptance of MRS is the problem of interpretation. There simply is not sufficient knowledge of relationships between the relevant metabolism and key clinical features, such as grade of disease or therapeutic response. Future studies will therefore need to address two specific areas. First, there is need for detailed studies of the biochemistry and metabolism of specific cancers. Ultimately, such studies must be related to genetic control of specific metabolic pathways in specific cancers. Most of this work may not even use MRS as an assessment tool, and the techniques of modern molecular biology are likely to significantly augment this discovery process. Second, even if a detailed understanding of relevant biochemisty is lacking, there is a need for large-scale clinical studies that support the role of MRS in addressing specific problems associated with cancer management. Existing studies typically come from a single center and rarely include more than 50 subjects. While such studies are unquestionably useful for defining the appropriate directions for future study, they cannot adequately define the attributes and pitfalls of routine assessment of cancer by MRS.

Finally, it is most important to emphasize that MRS is a "moving technology." There has been sustained technological progress in its implementation during the past ten years. It is clear that this technological progress will continue for at least another decade and will cause a further acceleration in the use of MRS for the clinical assessment of the cancer patient.

REFERENCES

1. Griffiths JR, Cady E, Edwards RH, McCready VR, Wilkie DR, Wiltshaw E. 31P-NMR studies of a human tumour in situ. Lancet 1983; 1(8339):1435–1436.
2. Negendank W. Studies of human tumors by MRS: a review. NMR Biomed 1992; 5(5):303–324.
3. Barker PB, Glickson JD, Bryan RN. In vivo magnetic resonance spectroscopy of human brain tumors. Top Magn Reson Imaging 1993; 5(1):32–45.
4. Tien RD, Lai PH, Smith JS, Lazeyras F. Single-voxel proton brain spectroscopy exam (PROBE/SV) in patients with primary brain tumors. AJR Am J Roentgenol 1996; 167(1):201–209.
5. Webb PG, Sailasuta N, Kohler SJ, Raidy T, Moats RA, Hurd RE. Automated single-voxel proton MRS: technical development and multisite verification. Magn Reson Med 1994; 31(4):365–373.
6. Nelson SJ. Imaging of brain tumors after therapy. Neuroimaging Clin N Am 1999; 9(4):801–819.
7. Matthews PM, Wylezinska M, Cadoux-Hudson T. Novel approaches to imaging brain tumors. Hematol Oncol Clin North Am 2001; 15(4):609–630.
8. Leclerc X, Huisman TA, Sorensen AG. The potential of proton magnetic resonance spectroscopy [(1)H-MRS] in the diagnosis and management of patients with brain tumors. Curr Opin Oncol 2002; 14(3):292–298.
9. Burtscher IM, Holtas S. Proton magnetic resonance spectroscopy in brain tumours: clinical applications. Neuroradiology 2001; 43(5):345–352.
10. Ronen SM, Leach MO. Imaging biochemistry: applications to breast cancer. Breast Cancer Res 2001; 3(1):36–40.
11. Katz-Brull R, Lavin PT, Lenkinski RE. Clinical utility of proton magnetic resonance spectroscopy in characterizing breast lesions. J Natl Cancer Inst 2002; 94(16): 1197–1203.
12. Kurhanewicz J, Swanson MG, Nelson SJ, Vigneron DB. Combined magnetic resonance imaging and spectroscopic imaging approach to molecular imaging of prostate cancer. J Magn Reson Imaging 2002; 16(4):451–463.
13. Swanson MG, Vigneron DB, Tran TK, Kurhanewicz J. Magnetic resonance imaging and spectroscopic imaging of prostate cancer. Cancer Invest 2001; 19(5):510–523.
14. Fulham MJ, Bizzi A, Dietz MJ, et al. Mapping of brain tumor metabolites with proton MR spectroscopic imaging: clinical relevance. Radiology 1992; 185(3):675–686.
15. Herholz K, Heindel W, Luyten PR, et al. In vivo imaging of glucose consumption and lactate concentration in human gliomas. Ann Neurol 1992; 31(3):319–327.
16. Ricci PE, Pitt A, Keller PJ, Coons SW, Heiserman JE. Effect of voxel position on single-voxel MR spectroscopy findings. AJNR Am J Neuroradiol 2000; 21(2):367–374.
17. Kurhanewicz J, Vigneron DB, Nelson SJ. Three-dimensional magnetic resonance spectroscopic imaging of brain and prostate cancer. Neoplasia 2000; 2(1–2):166–189.
18. Alger JR, Frank JA, Bizzi A, et al. Metabolism of human gliomas: assessment with H-1 MR spectroscopy and F-18 fluorodeoxyglucose PET. Radiology 1990; 177(3):633–641.
19. Danielsen ER, Michaelis T, Ross BD. Three methods of calibration in quantitative proton MR spectroscopy. J Magn Reson B 1995; 106(3):287–291.

20. Gupta RK, Cloughesy TF, Sinha U, et al. Relationships between choline magnetic resonance spectroscopy, apparent diffusion coefficient and quantitative histopathology in human glioma. J Neurooncol 2000; 50(3):215–226.
21. Meyerand ME, Pipas JM, Mamourian A, Tosteson TD, Dunn JF. Classification of Biopsy-Confirmed Brain Tumors Using Single-Voxel MR Spectroscopy. AJNR Am J Neuroradiol 1999; 20(1):117–123.
22. Isobe T, Matsumura A, Anno I, et al. Quantification of cerebral metabolites in glioma patients with proton MR spectroscopy using T2 relaxation time correction. Magn Reson Imaging 2002; 20(4):343–349.
23. Gillies RJ, Barry JA, Ross BD. In vitro and in vivo 13C and 31P NMR analyses of phosphocholine metabolism in rat glioma cells. Magn Reson Med 1994; 32(3):310–318.
24. Aiken NR, Gillies RJ. Phosphomonoester metabolism as a function of cell proliferative status and exogenous precursors. Anticancer Res 1996; 16(3B):1393–1397.
25. Katz-Brull R, Seger D, Rivenson-Segal D, Rushkin E, Degani H. Metabolic markers of breast cancer: enhanced choline metabolism and reduced choline-ether-phospholipid synthesis. Cancer Res 2002; 62(7):1966–1970.
26. Ackerstaff E, Pflug BR, Nelson JB, Bhujwalla ZM. Detection of increased choline compounds with proton nuclear magnetic resonance spectroscopy subsequent to malignant transformation of human prostatic epithelial cells. Cancer Res 2001; 61(9):3599–3603.
27. Sabatier J, Gilard V, Malet-Martino M, et al. Characterization of choline compounds with in vitro 1H magnetic resonance spectroscopy for the discrimination of primary brain tumors. Invest Radiol 1999; 34(3):230–235.
28. Tzika AA, Cheng LL, Goumnerova L, et al. Biochemical characterization of pediatric brain tumors by using in vivo and ex vivo magnetic resonance spectroscopy. J Neurosurg 2002; 96(6):1023–1031.
29. Cheng LL, Anthony DC, Comite AR, Black PM, Tzika AA, Gonzalez RG. Quantification of microheterogeneity in glioblastoma multiforme with ex vivo high-resolution magic-angle spinning (HRMAS) proton magnetic resonance spectroscopy. Neuro-oncol 2000; 2(2):87–95.
30. Nakagami K, Uchida T, Ohwada S, Koibuchi Y, Morishita Y. Increased Choline Kinase Activity in 1,2-Dimethylhydrazine-Induced Rat Colon Cancer. Jpn J Cancer Res 1999; 90(11):1212–1217.
31. Ramirez dM, Gutierrez R, Ramos MA, et al. Increased choline kinase activity in human breast carcinomas: clinical evidence for a potential novel antitumor strategy. Oncogene 2002; 21(27):4317–4322.
32. Ronen SM, Jackson LE, Beloueche M, Leach MO. Magnetic resonance detects changes in phosphocholine associated with ras activation and inhibition in NIH 3T3 Cells. Br J Cancer 2001; 84(5):691–696.
33. Podo F. Tumour phospholipid metabolism. NMR Biomed 1999; 12(7):413–439.
34. Jensen JE, Drost DJ, Menon RS, Williamson PC. In vivo brain (31)P-MRS: measuring the phospholipid resonances at 4 Tesla from small voxels. NMR Biomed 2002; 15(5):338–347.
35. Murphy-Boesch J, Stoyanova R, Srinivasan R, et al. Proton-decoupled 31P chemical shift imaging of the human brain in normal volunteers. NMR Biomed 1993; 6(3):173–180.
36. Li CW, Kuesel AC, Padavic-Shaller KA, et al. Metabolic characterization of human soft tissue sarcomas in vivo and in vitro using proton-decoupled phosphorus magnetic resonance spectroscopy. Cancer Res 1996; 56(13):2964–2972.
37. Gillies RJ, Raghunand N, Karczmar GS, Bhujwalla ZM. MRI of the tumor microenvironment. J Magn Reson Imaging 2002; 16(4):430–450.
38. Birken DL, Oldendorf WH. N-acetyl-l-aspartic acid: a literature review of a compound prominent in 1H-NMR spectroscopic studies of brain. Neurosci Biobehav Rev 1989; 13(1):23–31.

39. Urenjak J, Williams SR, Gadian DG, Noble M. Proton nuclear magnetic resonance spectroscopy unambiguously identifies different neural cell types. J Neurosci 1993; 13(3): 981–989.
40. Cecil KM, Schnall MD, Siegelman ES, Lenkinski RE. The evaluation of human breast lesions with magnetic resonance imaging and proton magnetic resonance spectroscopy. Breast Cancer Res Treat 2001; 68(1):45–54.
41. Kvistad KA, Bakken IJ, Gribbestad IS, et al. Characterization of neoplastic and normal human breast tissues with in vivo (1)H MR spectroscopy. J Magn Reson Imaging 1999; 10(2):159–164.
42. Kurhanewicz J, Vigneron DB, Nelson SJ, et al. Citrate as an in vivo marker to discriminate prostate cancer from benign prostatic hyperplasia and normal prostate peripheral zone: detection via localized proton spectroscopy. Urology 1995; 45(3):459–466.
43. Maintz D, Heindel W, Kugel H, Jaeger R, Lackner KJ. Phosphorus-31 MR spectroscopy of normal adult human brain and brain tumours. NMR Biomed 2002; 15(1):18–27.
44. Howe FA, Barton SJ, Cudlip SA, et al. Metabolic profiles of human brain tumors using quantitative in vivo 1H magnetic resonance spectroscopy. Magn Reson Med 2003; 49(2):223–232.
45. Negendank WG, Sauter R, Brown TR, et al. Proton magnetic resonance spectroscopy in patients with glial tumors: a multicenter study. J Neurosurg 1996; 84(3):449–458.
46. Preul MC, Caramanos Z, Collins DL, et al. Accurate, noninvasive diagnosis of human brain tumors by using proton magnetic resonance spectroscopy. Nat Med 1996; 2(3):323–325.
47. Dowling C, Bollen AW, Noworolski SM, et al. Preoperative proton MR spectroscopic imaging of brain tumors: correlation with histopathologic analysis of resection specimens. Am J Neuroradiol 2001;22(4):604 [Comment In: AJNR Am J Neuroradiol. 2001 Apr;22(4):597–8 UI: 21185634].
48. Bruhn H, Frahm J, Gyngell ML, et al. Noninvasive differentiation of tumors with use of localized H-1 MR spectroscopy in vivo: initial experience in patients with cerebral tumors. Radiology 1989; 172(2):541–548.
49. Preul MC, Caramanos Z, Leblanc R, Villemure JG, Arnold DL. Using pattern analysis of in vivo proton MRSI data to improve the diagnosis and surgical management of patients with brain tumors. NMR Biomed 1998; 11(4–5):192–200.
50. Butzen J, Prost R, Chetty V, et al. Discrimination between neoplastic and nonneoplastic brain lesions by use of proton MR spectroscopy: the limits of accuracy with a logistic regression model. AJNR Am.J Neuroradiol 2000; 21(7):1213–1219.
51. Pirzkall A, McKnight TR, Graves EE, et al. MR-spectroscopy guided target delineation for high-grade gliomas. Int J Radiat Oncol Biol Phys 2001; 50(4):915–928.
52. Preul MC, Leblanc R, Caramanos Z, Kasrai R, Narayanan S, Arnold DL. Magnetic resonance spectroscopy guided brain tumor resection: differentiation between recurrent glioma and radiation change in two diagnostically difficult cases. Can J Neurol Sci 1998; 25(1):13–22.
53. Hall WA, Martin A, Liu H, Truwit CL. Improving diagnostic yield in brain biopsy: coupling spectroscopic targeting with real-time needle placement. J Magn Reson Imaging 2001; 13(1):12–15.
54. Vigneron D, Bollen A, McDermott M, et al. Three-dimensional magnetic resonance spectroscopic imaging of histologically confirmed brain tumors. Magn Reson Imaging 2001; 19(1):89–101.
55. Tedeschi G, Lundbom N, Raman R, et al. Increased choline signal coinciding with malignant degeneration of cerebral gliomas: a serial proton magnetic resonance spectroscopy imaging study. J Neurosurg 1997; 87(4):516–524.
56. Wald LL, Nelson SJ, Day MR, et al. Serial proton magnetic resonance spectroscopy imaging of glioblastoma multiforme after brachytherapy. J Neurosurg 1997; 87(4):525–534.
57. Graves EE, Nelson SJ, Vigneron DB, et al. A preliminary study of the prognostic value of proton magnetic resonance spectroscopic imaging in gamma knife radiosurgery of recurrent malignant gliomas. Neurosurgery 2000; 46(2):319–326.

58. Graves EE, Nelson SJ, Vigneron DB, et al. Serial proton MR spectroscopic imaging of recurrent malignant gliomas after gamma knife radiosurgery. [Comment In: AJNR Am J Neuroradiol. 2001 Apr; 22(4):598–9 UI: 21185635]. AJNR Am J Neuroradiol 2001; 22(4):613–624.
59. Preul MC, Caramanos Z, Villemure JG, et al. Using proton magnetic resonance spectroscopic imaging to predict in vivo the response of recurrent malignant gliomas to tamoxifen chemotherapy. Neurosurgery 2000; 46(2)306–318.
60. Swanson MG, Vigneron DB, Tran TK, Kurhanewicz J. Magnetic resonance imaging and spectroscopic imaging of prostate cancer. Cancer Invest 1901; 19(5):510–523.

11

Dynamic MRI Techniques

Anwar R. Padhani
Mount Vernon Cancer Centre, London, U.K.

David J. Collins
Cancer Research UK Clinical Magnetic Resonance Research Group, Institute of Cancer Research and The Royal Marsden NHS Trust, Sutton, Surrey, U.K.

A Note from the Editors

D ynamic contrast enhanced magnetic resonance imaging (DCE-MRI) using small molecular weight gadolinium chelates enables non-invasive imaging characterization of tissue vascularity. Depending on the technique used, data reflecting tissue perfusion, microvessel permeability surface area product, and extracellular leakage space can be obtained. The authors of this chapter are experts in this field and show how insights into these physiological processes can be obtained from inspection of kinetic enhancement curves and by the application of complex compartmental modeling techniques. They compare and contrast DCE-MRI with functional CT in terms of technique and application. Potential clinical applications of DCE-MRI, which include screening for malignant disease, lesion characterization, monitoring lesion response to treatment and assessment of residual disease, and newer applications including pharmacodynamic assessments of antivascular anticancer drugs and predicting efficacy of treatment are mentioned to provide the appropriate clinical context. The authors point out that standardized approaches to measurement and robust analysis approaches are needed with appropriate validation if the technique is to "make it" in clinical environments.

INTRODUCTION

Angiogenesis, the sprouting of new capillaries from existing blood vessels, and vasculogenesis, the de novo generation of blood vessels are the two primary methods of vascular expansion by which nutrient supply to tissues is adjusted to match physiological needs. Pathological angiogenesis is critical for growth and metastasis of malignant tumors (1). Conventionally, the vascularity of tissues has been assessed directly by microvessel density (MVD) counting after immunostaining with variety of panendothelial antibodies (2). This technique requires extracted tissue material and so is unable to provide information on the functional state of the vasculature. More recently, indirect or surrogate methods such as blood levels of angiogenic factors and imaging methods have been used to assess neovasculature (3). Advantages of indirect methods include the fact that they can be quantitative, noninvasive, and can be performed with the tumor in situ, and in the case of imaging techniques, the functional status of the vasculature can be assessed. In this respect it is important to note that implanted tumor xenograft data show that there is a discrepancy between perfused and visible microvessels; a variable 20% to 85% of microvessels are perfused at any given time. This results in a difference between histological MVD and what is described as the "true or functional vascular density", which at least in part accounts for the discrepancy between imaging and histological assessments of vascularity (4).

IMAGING TISSUE VASCULARITY WITH MR IMAGING

Several imaging techniques are able to assess human tumors with respect to their angiogenic status, many of which are reviewed in this book. Magnetic resonance imaging (MRI) techniques with contrast media are classified by the type of contrast medium used; (i) low-molecular weight agents (less than 1 kDa) that rapidly diffuse in the extracellular fluid space (ECF agents), (ii) intermediate molecular weight contrast agents, (iii) large molecular agents (greater than 30 kDa) designed for prolonged intravascular retention [macromolecular contrast media (MMCM) or blood pool agents] (5), and (iv) agents intended to accumulate at sites of concentrated angiogenesis-mediating molecules (6). This chapter concentrates exclusively on noninvasive characterization of vasculature with dynamic contrast medium enhanced MRI (DCE-MRI) using low-molecular weight contrast agents, and explains how perfusion-related data can be extracted depending on the technique utilized (7–10). We also compare and contrast DCE-MRI with perfusion CT (functional multi-detector CT) in terms of technique and application.

MRI Contrast Agent Kinetics

When a bolus of paramagnetic, low-molecular weight contrast agent passes through a capillary bed, it is transiently confined within the vascular space. Concentrated contrast media within the vessels and in the immediate vicinity, cause magnetic field (B_o) inhomogeneities that result in a decrease in the signal intensity of surrounding tissues (susceptibility effects). In most tissues except the brain, testes, and retina, the contrast agent rapidly passes into the extravascular-extracellular space (EES, also called leakage space -v_e) at a rate determined by the blood flow (which determines contrast medium delivery), and the permeability and surface area of the microvessels

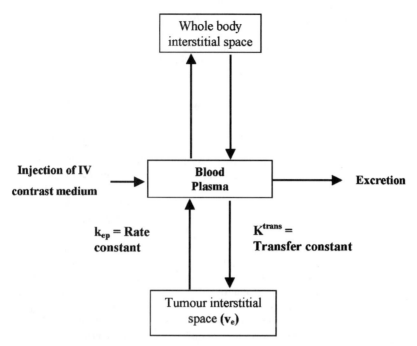

Figure 1 Body compartments accessed by low-molecular weight, gadolinium-containing contrast media injected intravenously.

(Fig. 1). When low molecular weight contrast agents are used, typically 12% to 45% of the contrast media leaks into the EES during the first pass in tumors (11). The transfer constant (K^{trans}) describes the transendothelial transport of the contrast medium. Three major factors determine the behavior of the contrast media during the first few minutes after injection; contrast medium delivery by blood perfusion, transport of contrast agent across vessel walls, and diffusion of contrast medium in the interstitial space. If the delivery of the contrast medium to a tissue is insufficient with respect to maintaining a high enough concentration to continually supply the extracellular space (flow-limited situations or where vascular permeability is greater than inflow), then perfusion will determine contrast agent distribution and K^{trans} approximates to tissue blood flow per unit volume (12); this is a situation commonly found in tumors and in many normal tissues. If transport out of the vasculature does not deplete intravascular contrast medium concentration (nonflow-limited situations), then K^{trans} approximates to permeability surface area product–PS. The latter circumstance occurs in some tumors that have a low blood supply such as lobular carcinoma, carcinoma in situ, and in some brain tumors (which have a largely intact blood–brain barrier), but can also occur in extracranial tumors usually after treatment (including chemotherapy and radiation), in fibrotic lesions and in some normal tissues.

As low-molecular weight contrast media do not cross cell membranes, the volume of distribution is effectively the EES (v_e). After a variable time, the contrast agent diffuses back into the vasculature (described by the rate constant or k_{ep}) from where it is excreted principally by the kidneys, although some contrast media have significant hepatic excretion. When capillary permeability is very high, the return of contrast medium is typically rapid resulting in faster washout as plasma contrast

Table 1 Comparison of T_2^*- and T_1-weighted DCE-MRI Techniques

	T_2^*W imaging (susceptibility methods)	T_1W imaging (relaxivity methods)
Tissue signal intensity change	Darkening	Enhancement
Duration of effect and optimal data acquisition	Seconds/subsecond	Minutes/2–25 sec
Magnitude of effect	Small	Larger
Optimal contrast medium dose	≥ 0.2 mmol/kg	0.1–0.2 mmol/kg
Quantification method used	Relative, more than absolute	Relative and absolute
Physiological property determining effects	Perfusion/blood volume	Perfusion, transendothelial permeability, capillary surface area, lesion leakage space
Kinetic parameters derived	Blood volume and flow, transit time	Transfer and rate constants, leakage space
Pathological correlates	Various, including tumor grade and microvessel density	Various, including microvessel density and VEGF expression
Clinical usage	Lesion characterization – breast, liver and brain	Lesion detection and characterization
	Noninvasive brain tumor grading	Improving accuracy of tumor staging
	Directing brain tumor biopsy	Predicting response to treatment
	Determining brain tumor prognosis	Monitoring response to treatment
	Monitoring treatment e.g., radiotherapy	Novel therapies including antiangiogenic drugs
		Detecting tumor relapse

Abbreviations: DCE-MRI, dynamic contrast medium enhanced magnetic resonance imaging; VEGF, vascular endothelial growth factor.

agent concentrations fall. Contrast medium elimination from very slow-exchange tissues, such as those with fibrosis and necrosis, occurs more slowly, and contrast media may occasionally be retained for a day or two.

MRI sequences can be designed to be sensitive to the vascular phase of contrast medium delivery (so-called T_2^* or susceptibility-based methods) which reflect on tissue perfusion and blood volume (13,14). T_1-weighted sequences are sensitive to the presence of diluted contrast medium in the EES and thus reflect microvessel perfusion, permeability, and extracellular leakage space volume (so-called T_1 or relaxivity-based methods). These two methods are compared in Table 1.

T_2^*-WEIGHTED DSC-MRI

Data Acquisition

Perfusion-weighted images can be obtained with "bolus-tracking techniques" that are sensitive to the passage of contrast material through a capillary bed (13,14).

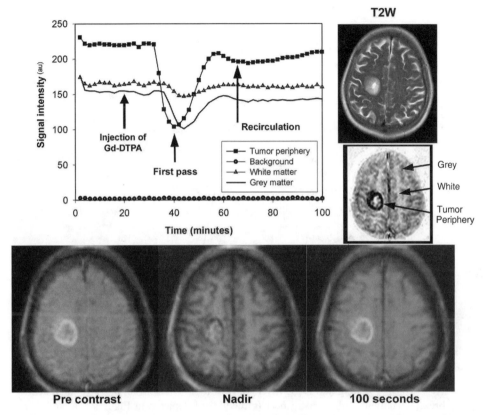

Figure 2 Typical T_2^*-weighted DCE-MRI study of a patient with a malignant astrocytoma. 30 mL of IV contrast Gd-DTPA was given after the 10th data point. First pass T_2^* susceptibility effects cause marked darkening of the tumor periphery. Darkening of the grey matter of the brain is greater than the less vascular white matter. The first pass and recirculation phases are indicated. Signal intensity changes for four regions of interest are shown in the insert [subtraction T_2^* image of the nadir point for the tumor regions of interest (ROI)]. An anatomic T_2-weighted image at the same slice position is also shown for reference.

A decrease in signal intensity of tissues caused by susceptibility occurs due to the presence of concentrated contrast media within vessels (Figs. 2 and 3). The degree of observed signal intensity loss is dependent on the type of sequence used, on vascular concentration of the contrast agent, and microvessel size and density (15). The signal to noise ratio (SNR) of dynamic susceptibility contrast-enhanced (DSC)-MR images can be enhanced by using higher doses of contrast medium (i.e., ≥ 0.2 mmol/kg body weight) (16).

The typical imaging strategy is to collect data using a fast imaging technique to produce a temporal resolution of approximately two seconds. During this short acquisition window it is usually possible to acquire multislice data at a matrix resolution of 128×128 or greater, depending on scanner specifications. High specification, echo-planar–capable MRI systems allow 5 to 15 slices to be acquired. However, echo-planar sequences have limited applications in extracranial tissues because of greater intrinsic sensitivity to susceptibility-inducing environments (e.g., highly concentrated contrast media and bowel gas/tissue boundaries), which can result in spatial misregistration of major vessels during the first passage of the contrast agent

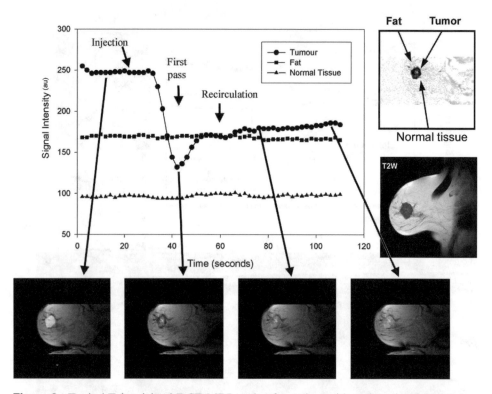

Figure 3 Typical T_2^*-weighted DCE-MRI study of a patient with an invasive ductal cancer of the breast. A patient with breast cancer (same patient depicted in Figures 5, 6, and 8) was given 22 ml of IV contrast Gd-DTPA after the 10th data point. First pass T_2^* susceptibility effects cause marked darkening of the tumor with no alteration in signal intensity of fibro-glandular breast parenchyma (normal tissue) or fat. The first pass and recirculation phases can clearly be seen. Insert shows a subtraction T_2^* image of the nadir point for the tumor regions of interest.

through the vessels (17). Standard spoiled gradient-echo sequences on conventional MRI systems can also characterize these effects but are usually limited to a single slice (Figs. 2 and 3). It has been noted that susceptibility-weighted, spin-echo sequences are more sensitive to capillary blood flow but the signals obtained are of lower magnitude compared with gradient-echo sequences, which incorporate signals from larger vessels (18). It is unclear whether there are significant advantages of using spin-echo sequences, but there are certainly significant costs in terms of SNR.

Quantification

Analysis of DSC-MRI data is based on the assumption that the contrast agent remains within the vascular space throughout the examination, acting as a blood pool marker. This assumption is untrue except in the brain where there is no contrast medium leakage due to the blood–brain barrier. The application of DSC-MRI was, therefore, initially limited to studies of normal brain, although modifications of the technique have subsequently allowed its use in enhancing tissues (see below).

The conventional approach to calculating blood flow uses the area under the contrast concentration curve as an estimate of blood volume within the pixel (BV), and the width of the contrast bolus as an estimate of the mean transit time (MTT).

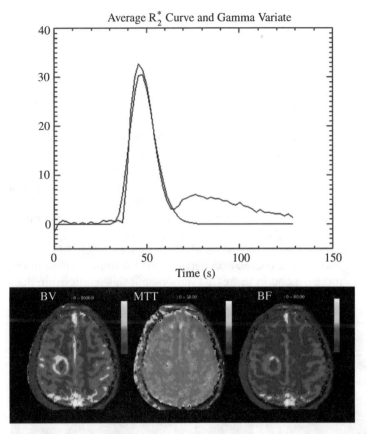

Figure 4 Model fitting of T_2^*-weighted data and parametric map formation. T_2^* signal intensity data from Figure 2 (tumor periphery) is converted into R_2^* ($1/T_2^*$) and then fitted with a gamma variate function. Parametric maps representing blood flow kinetics (rBF, rBV, MTT) are derived on a pixel-by-pixel basis. The computed values of rBV, rBF and MTT for this region of interest are 509, 21.3 arbitrary units, and 24 seconds. *Abbreviations*: rBV, relative blood volume; rBF, relative blood flow; MTT, mean transit time. (*See color insert for Fig. 4B.*)

MTT is the average time taken by the contrast agent to pass through the tissue being studied (Fig. 4) (13,14,19). Blood flow (BF) can be calculated by using the central volume theorem equation (BF = BV/MTT). The initial calculation of local contrast concentration from the observed signal change is straightforward as contrast concentration is linearly related to the T_2 rate changes (ΔR_2), which can be calculated using the relationship

$$\Delta R_2 = -\ln(S(t)/S(0))/TE$$

where $S(0)$ is the base line signal intensity, $S(t)$ is the pixel intensity at time t and TE is the echo time. This allows the transformation of signal intensity time course data to changing R_2.

The most robust parameter which can be extracted reliably from first pass techniques is BV, which is obtained from the integral of the data time series during the first pass of the contrast agent (20).

$$rCBV = \int_{t_0}^{t_e} \Delta R_2(t)dt \qquad (3)$$

where t_0 is the time of first arrival of contrast and t_e is the time at which ΔR_2 returns to baseline values. The MTT is then estimated from the width of the curve at half the maximum height [full width at half maximum (FWHM)].

In addition to the flow related parameters described above, it is also possible to calculate time to contrast medium arrival into a tissue (T_0), or more commonly, the time to peak (TTP) concentration. Additionally, an appreciation of the spatial distribution of tissue perfusion can be obtained by simple subtraction images taken at the nadir point (maximal signal attenuation). This easily obtained image has been strongly correlated with relative blood flow and volume in tumors (compare Fig. 2 with Fig. 4 and Fig. 3 with Fig. 5) (34,35). Subtraction analysis should only be done if there is a linear relationship between rBV and rBF; that is, when MTT is in a narrow range (Figs. 4 and 5). The correlation between the maximum signal intensity drop and rBV/rBF appears good in untreated tumors, but this relationship does

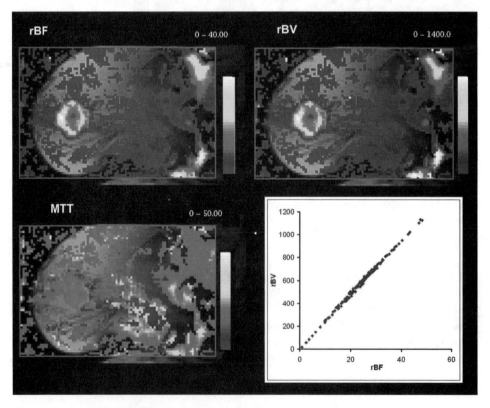

Figure 5 Parametric DCE-MRI images of an invasive ductal cancer of the breast. This is the same tumor illustrated in Figures 3, 6, and 8. Parametric images of rBV, rBF, MTT are shown. The graph shows that there is a linear correlation between blood volume and flow on a pixel level (the gradient of this line is the MTT; rBF = rBV/MTT). *Abbreviations*: rBV, relative blood volume; rBF, relative blood flow; MTT, mean transit time. (*See color insert.*)

not appear to be sustained following therapy (21). An additional parameter that can be derived from DSC-MRI data is the tortuosity index, which is the difference between the total time series integral and the integral of the gamma variate derived from the first pass (see below) (22). The tortuosity index reflects the abnormal retention of contrast material in the tumor vasculature. The tortuosity index can only be derived for brain tumors because there is no or little loss of compartmentalization of contrast medium bolus during the first pass. Absolute quantification of DSC-MRI parameters can be obtained by measuring the changing concentration of contrast agent in the feeding vessel, and in this way, quantified perfusion parameters in normal brain and of low grade gliomas have been obtained (23,24). Absolute quantification is not currently possible for evaluation of visceral tissues and tumors because of a number of limitations that are discussed below.

Limitations

There are a number of limitations of DSC-MRI techniques which include the effects of contrast medium recirculation, contrast medium leakage and subsequent tissue enhancement and bolus dispersion (7).

Analysis of the contrast bolus passage assumes that the bolus passes through the tissue, and that the signal intensity (i.e., concentration of contrast medium) then returns to zero. In practice, the contrast medium recirculates through the body and a second recirculation peak is always seen (Figs. 2 and 3). With bolus dispersion, the second peak is lower and broader than the first pass, and by the time of the third recirculation the intravascular contrast has mixed evenly throughout the blood volume. Measurement of kinetic parameters is, therefore, subjected to errors due to the presence of both first pass and recirculating contrast in the vessels during the later part of the bolus passage. One way of overcoming this limitation is to use an idealized model to the observed data (Fig. 4). This relies on the fact that the shape of the contrast concentration curve during the passage of the first bolus can be shown theoretically to always conform to a specific shape known as a gamma variate (25). The use of curve fitting also smoothes the data effectively reducing noise, and eliminates the contamination of the first pass bolus due to contrast agent recirculation.

Loss of contrast medium compartmentalization during the first pass into the interstitial space will cause aberrant signal intensity changes by the end of the experiment (either enhancement or failure of the signal intensity to return to baseline). Recirculation and contrast leakage into the extracellular space during the first pass of contrast medium are the principle causes of falsely lower blood volume values. Furthermore, the T_1 signal–enhancing effects of contrast medium leaking from blood vessels can counteract T_2^* signal–lowering effects. Quantitative imaging is thus most reliably used for normal brain and nonenhancing brain lesions because the contrast medium is completely or largely retained within the intravascular space.

Solutions for counteracting the T_1-enhancing effects of gadolinium chelates include optimization of sequences by using dual or multiecho sequences that minimize T_1 sensitivity and pre-dosing with contrast medium to saturate the leakage space (26). (i) The use of techniques with reduced T_1 sensitivity, such as low flip angle gradient-echo–based sequences, effectively removes relaxivity effects although some workers have observed residual effects in rapidly enhancing tumors (27,28). The major problem with this method is the lowering of SNR produced by the reduction in flip angle, although this can be partially compensated by increasing contrast agent doses. (ii) Another approach to reducing T_1 sensitivity is to use a dual echo technique in which the T_1-weighted first echo is used to correct the predominantly T_2-weighted second echo (26,29). The dual echo technique is technically challenging for most machines, and reducing the sampling time inevitably restricts the number of samples and therefore, the slices which can be obtained. (iii) The third approach is to use pre-enhancement with an additional dose of contrast agent. Saturating the extracellular space with contrast medium induces maximum T_1 shortening, and the arrival of further contrast medium given during the susceptibility experiment causes little additional relaxivity-based signal intensity responses. Recently, Johnson et al. (30), have shown that it is possible to pharmacokinetically model the first pass effect in the presence of leaking capillaries, and to obtain an estimate of blood volume, vascular transfer constant, and EES volume. Other solutions for overcoming some of these problems include the use of nongadolinium-susceptibility contrast agents based on the element dysprosium or ultrasmall, superparamagnetic iron oxide particles (USPIOs), which have strong T_2^* effects but weak T_1 effects (31,32). Preliminary results have indicated that dysprosium-based relative cerebral blood volume (rCBV) maps are superior to those obtained with gadolinium chelates (33,34). USPIOs designed for bolus injection have the advantage of being retained within the vascular space during the first pass owing to their larger size (35,36).

As noted above, the measurement of CBF requires an accurate estimation of MTT which is extracted from the width of the contrast bolus. The width of the contrast bolus is actually affected by a combination of the following three factors: (i) the width of the bolus at the tissue level [the arterial input function (AIF)], (ii) changes in bolus width due to regional alterations in flow related to nonlaminar flow (which arises from the presence of irregular caliber vessels), nondichotomous branching and high vascular permeability (which leads to increased blood viscosity from hemoconcentration), and variations in the hematocrit fraction as blood passes through a vascular bed, and (iii) physical bolus broadening due to dispersive effects which are unrelated to flow. Additionally, the width of the bolus is strongly affected by individual variations in injection technique, contrast dose, and cardiovascular functioning and structural architecture including upstream vascular stenoses.

Clinical Experience

Quantitative imaging is currently most reliable for normal brain and nonenhancing brain lesions because the contrast medium is retained within the intravascular space. DSC perfusion mapping techniques have progressively entered neurological practice (37–39). Clinical applications include characterization of tumor vascularity, follow-up of treatment response and the study of stroke (24,27,37,39–44). There is very little literature data on DSC-MRI outside the brain. Both Kuhl et al. (45) and Kvistad et al. (46) have qualitatively evaluated the value of DSC-MRI for characterizing breast lesions. Both studies showed strong decreases in signal intensity in malignant tissues, whereas susceptibility effects in fibroadenomas were minor. Quantitative DSC-MRI have been used to monitor the effects of chemotherapy in breast cancer. Ah-See et al. (47) have observed that rBV and rBF reduce with successful treatment, whereas no changes were seen in nonresponding tumors.

T_1-WEIGHTED DCE-MRI

Data Acquisition

Extracellular contrast media readily diffuse from the blood into the EES of tissues at a rate determined by tissue perfusion, permeability of the capillaries, and their surface area. Increases in $1/T_1$ relaxation rate resulting from the leakage of contrast media yields increases in tissue signal intensity. Most DCE-MRI studies employ 2D/3D T_1-weighted gradient-echo, saturation recovery/inversion recovery snapshot sequences (e.g., turboFLASH) or echoplanar sequences. Each of these techniques enable tissue T_1 relaxation rates to be estimated in a reasonably short period of time, and this allows quantification of tissue contrast medium concentration (48–52). The choice of the sequence and parameters used is dependent on the intrinsic advantages and disadvantages of the sequences, taking into account T_1 sensitivity, anatomical coverage, acquisition times, susceptibility to artefacts arising from magnetic field inhomogeneities, and accuracy for quantification. The amount of signal enhancement observed on T_1-weighted images is dependent on a number of physiological and physical factors. Physiological factors include tissue perfusion, capillary surface area, permeability to contrast agent, and volume of the extracellular leakage space. Physical factors include the native (or precontrast) T_1 relaxation rate of the tissue, contrast agent dose, rate of intracellular–extracellular water exchange, imaging sequence parameters used, and measurement gain and scaling factors.

   T_1-weighted kinetic enhancement curves have three distinct phases; the upslope, maximum enhancement, and washout (Figs. 6 and 7). It is generally recognized that the upslope is highly dependent on tissue perfusion and permeability, with perfusion predominating. Maximum enhancement is related to the total uptake concentration of the contrast medium in the interstitial space (with an additional vascular contribution), and washout rate is associated with tissue contrast agent concentration decrease and, thus, is strongly related to vascular permeability. If it is assumed that tissue enhancement has contributions from vascular and extravascular compartments (see two-compartment modelling below), then it is possible to separate these inputs mathematically using deconvolution techniques which is helpful for understanding the shape of kinetic curves (53,54). The dominant contribution of perfusion to the upslope of T_1-weighted DCE-MRI enhancement curves can be verified empirically by correlating T_1- and T_2^*-weighted DCE-MRI enhancement curves and corresponding kinetic pixel maps (Fig. 7) (26).

Quantification

Signal enhancements seen on T_1-weighted DCE-MRI can be assessed in two ways: by the analysis of signal intensity changes (semiquantitative), and/or by quantifying tissue T_1 relaxivity (R_1) or contrast agent concentration change using pharmacokinetic modeling techniques. Semiquantitative parameters describe signal intensity changes using a number of descriptors. These parameters include curve shape classification done visually, onset time (a number of definitions exist), gradient of the upslope of enhancement curves, maximum signal intensity, and washout gradient (combinations of these can also be found in the literature) (55,56). As the rate of enhancement has been shown to be important for improving the specificity of clinical diagnoses, so parameters that include a timing element are often used [e.g., maximum intensity time ratio (MITR)] and maximum focal enhancement

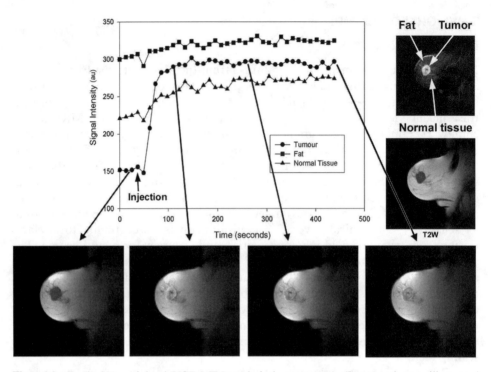

Figure 6 Typical T_1-weighted DCE-MRI study in breast tumor. (Same patient as illustrated in Figures 3, 5, and 8.) Data from serial T_1-weighted images obtained before and after the injection of 11 mL of Gd-DTPA given intravenously. Marked and sustained, early enhancement of the breast tumor is seen in the signal intensity time curves compared to the gradual enhancement of fibroglandular breast parenchyma and fat. The shape of the curve is in marked contrast to that seen on T_2^*-DCE-MRI in Figure 3. Insert shows an image obtained by subtracting the 100 seconds image from baseline.

at one minute (57–59). The uptake integral or initial area under the signal intensity (IAUC) or gadolinium contrast medium concentration (IAUGC) curve has been also been studied (60). IAUGC is a relatively robust and simple technique, which characterizes all enhancing regions without the problems associated with model fitting failures in pharmacokinetic models (see below). However, IAUGC does not have a simple relationship to the physiology parameters of interest (perfusion, permeability, and leakage space). Thus, semiquantitative parameters have a close, but complex and not well-defined link to underlying tissue physiology, but have the advantage of being relatively straightforward to calculate. Limitations of semiquantitative parameters include the fact that they are derived from signal intensity data that may not accurately reflect the changing contrast medium concentration in tissues, and that signal intensity data can be influenced by scanner settings (including gain and scaling factors). These factors limit the usefulness of semiquantitative parameters and make between-patient and between-system comparisons potentially problematic.

Quantitative techniques use pharmacokinetic modeling applied to changes in tissue contrast agent concentration or R_1. In general, it is not recommended that pharmacokinetic modeling be done on signal intensity data *unless* it is has been shown that there is a direct relationship between signal intensity and contrast agent concentration over the entire range expected in tissues. Signal intensity changes

Figure 7 Superimposing signal data from T_1- and T_2^*-weighted DCE-MRI on the same time scale. T_1-weighted subtraction (100 seconds postcontrast medium) DCE-MRI image from a patient with necrotic invasive ductal breast cancer. T_1- and T_2^*-weighted DCE-MRI curves for the four regions of interest (ROI) are superimposed on the same time scale. The zero point represents the point of injection of contrast medium for both studies, performed consecutively. The onset and short duration of early T_2^*-weighted DCE-MRI effects correspond precisely to the upslope on the T_1-weighted enhancement curves for ROI-1 and -2, confirming that the upslope has a significant vascular contribution. ROI-3 represents a small area where flow contribution is undetectable by T_2^*-weighted DCE-MRI. The corresponding T_1-weighted enhancement curve for ROI-3 is typical of one with low flow, and probably reflects an area where enhancement is mostly determined by tissue permeability and microvessel surface area. ROI-4 is necrotic and no flow is detected. Computed rBV and K^{trans} from these data are shown. Note modeling failures anteriorly in the transfer constant map. *Abbreviations:* rBV, relative blood volume; K^{trans}, transfer constant; (*See color insert.*)

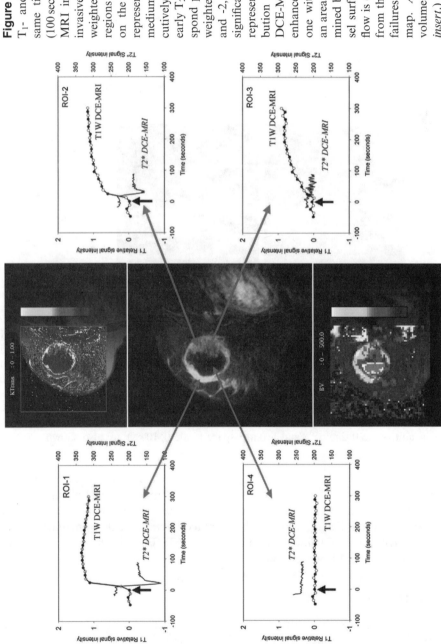

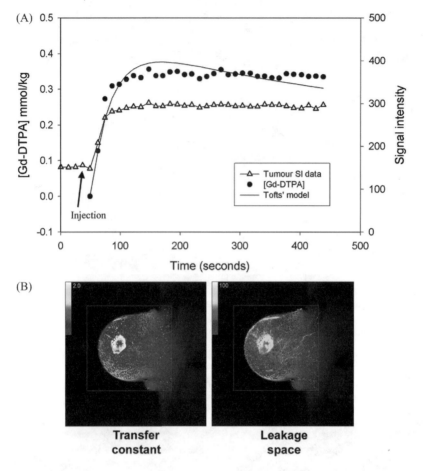

Figure 8 Converting signal intensity into contrast concentration and model fitting. Data obtained from the patient illustrated in Figures 3, 5, and 6. Contrast medium injection (11 mL of Gd-DTPA) took place after the third data point. Quantification of time signal intensity data (Δ) into contrast agent concentration ($\bullet$) is performed first, according to the. method described by Parker et al. (49). The model fitting procedure (continuous line) is done using the Tofts' model (62) with the standard Weinmann input function (68). Note that model fitting to contrast agent concentration data is not perfect. Calculated quantified parameters: transfer constant, $0.82\,\mathrm{min}^{-1}$; leakage space, 47%; rate constant, $1.74\,\mathrm{min}^{-1}$. Parametric transfer constant (scale $0-2\,\mathrm{min}^{-1}$) and leakage space (scale 0–100%) are also shown. (*See color insert.*)

observed during dynamic acquisition are used to estimate contrast agent concentration in vivo (48,49,52,61). Concentration-time curves are then mathematically fitted using one of a number of recognized pharmacokinetic models principally those of Tofts and Kermode (62) and Larsson and Tofts (63) (Fig. 8). This is also considered in detail in chapter 14 of this book.

Kinetic Modeling

As low-molecular weight contrast agents exchange between central and the extracellular space of tumors, the pharmacokinetic models used consist of two compartments:

the central blood plasma compartment and the tissue extracellular compartment. The rate equation describing the transport of the contrast agent between the two compartments is the following (12,64,65):

$$\frac{dC_t(t)}{dt} = K^{trans} C_p(t) - k_{ep} C_t(t)$$

where $C_t(t)$ is the tissue concentration, $C_p(t)$ is the plasma concentration, and K^{trans} and k_{ep} are volume rate constants for exchange between central and tissue compartments and vice versa, respectively, reflecting bulk tissue properties. Again following Tofts et al. (12) the extracellular extravascular space (v_e) is defined as

$$v_e = \frac{K^{trans}}{k_{ep}}$$

K^{trans} is considered within a general mixed perfusion and permeability condition to be equal to $E^*F^*rho(1\text{-}Hct)$, where E is the extraction fraction of the contrast tracer, F is blood flow, rho is tissue density, and Hct is the hematocrit. As already noted in the section on contrast agent kinetics, when flow is adequate and the rate of extraction E is small compared to supply, then K^{trans} is largely equal to the product of the capillary permeability and surface area. If the delivery of the contrast agent to tissue is insufficient, then blood perfusion is the dominant factor. However, it should be noted that in tissue regions with poor blood supply, low K^{trans} values can be obtained in regions where there would otherwise be high vessel permeability (66).

A major difficulty for quantitative DCE-MRI is the determination of the $C_p(t)$ required for model-based analysis. Measuring $C_p(t)$ (often called the arterial input function) directly using DCE-MRI requires measurement sequences, which yield signal intensity outputs that scale linearly over a large range of tissue and plasma concentrations. $C_p(t)$ has to be sampled in an artery at sufficient temporal resolution to accurately characterize the rapid change in tracer concentration following a bolus injection (ideally less than two seconds), which is currently impractical within the constraints of useful spatial image resolution. Further confounding factors in measurements of $C_p(t)$ are inflow artefacts and motion. There are also difficulties relating to water proton exchange kinetics within the blood plasma. It is generally assumed that gadolinium containing chelates interact sufficiently quickly with the plasma water protons to induce relaxation, which is directly proportional to chelate concentrations, but this assumption ignores the rate of exchange of water protons between the intra- and extracellular spaces in blood. It has been shown that substantial errors can occur when ignoring the effects of water exchange (67).

Several approaches have been utilized for obtaining or estimating $C_p(t)$ with an acceptance of the limitations described. The most common method of obtaining $C_p(t)$ is to use a general input function derived from real measurement of plasma concentration done in volunteers (68,69). An alternative method is to use a reference tissue from which an estimate of $C_p(t)$ can be derived from the Kety equation using the reference tissue concentration $C_t(t)$ data and known physiological parameters of the reference tissue (70,71). In practice, a polynomial function is fitted to the $C_t(t)$ curve from which the required derivative is obtained. The advantages of the reference tissue approach are that the temporal sampling can be relaxed, as the rate of change in tracer concentration in the reference tissue is not as rapid as in plasma, the size of the reference tissue sample can be large which improves the SNR of the $C_t(t)$ obtained and averages motion effects. The disadvantages are that clinical treatments may effect blood flow in reference tissues, and the implicit assumption that the reference tissue derived $C_p(t)$ is relevant to the tissues of interest (i.e., the tumor).

As already noted, model-based analysis of DCE-MRI data involves model fitting the individual pixel concentration time curves to a general solution to the Kety equation. If the plasma concentration $C_p(t)$ is described as the sum of two decaying exponentials, the following solution can be obtained

$$C_t(t) = D \cdot K^{trans} \cdot \sum_{i=1}^{2} a_i \cdot \frac{\left[e^{-\left(\frac{K^{trans}}{v_e}\right) \cdot (t-t_0)} - e^{-m_i \cdot (t-t_0)} \right]}{m_i - \left(\frac{K^{trans}}{v_e}\right)}$$

where D = dose of contrast medium, m_i are rate constants for elimination, and a_i are physiologically derived constants (68). Using this equation it is possible to fit individual pixel-derived time series data $C_t(t)$. The results of the fitting process can be used to generate parametric images (K^{trans}, v_e, k_{ep}) and these parametric images can be overlaid onto the source anatomical images. The advantage of individual fitted pixels is that the parametric images provide an indication of the heterogeneity of the distributions of model-based parameters. There are a number of extensions to the basic model described above. One major assumption in the generalized model of Tofts is that the tissue vascular fraction (v_p) is small and can be ignored; however, this is not necessarily the case in tumors. A solution which includes the vp contribution is widely used in radionuclear and computer tomography tracer kinetic studies, and has been shown to be useful in DCE-MRI in so-called first pass studies, in which the model is applied only for the first pass of the tracer through the circulatory system (65,72). It is important when applying this model to avoid recirculation effects of the tracer and to obtain a sufficient number of sample points within the first pass; a temporal resolution in the order of one second is ideal. Rapid data acquisition with a temporal resolution of one second per image can be achieved with sophisticated DCE-MRI measurements using data sharing (26). An advantage of the Patlak method (65) is the ease of computation of the model parameters as the model solution can be linear, which is computationally efficient to solve. The 'Patlak' solution is

$$C_t(t) = v_p \cdot C_p(t) + K^{trans} \cdot \int_0^t C_p(\tau) d\tau \quad Y = \frac{C_t(t)}{C_p(t)} \quad X = \frac{\int_0^t C_p(\tau) d\tau}{C_p(t)}$$

which is linearized by expressing the Patlak equation in terms of Y and X axes shown above. The Y intercept provides an estimate of v_p and the slope is K^{trans}. A disadvantage of this approach is that it is not possible to estimate v_e. Figure 9 shows parametric images derived from the application of the Patlak method and compares these with the application of the Larsson model to a T_1-weighted DCE-MRI dataset. For further detailed discussion on pharmacokinetic modeling techniques readers are directed to the review by Tofts (73) and chapter 14 of this book. A detailed analysis of the data acquisition methodology can be found in the review by Dale et al. (74).

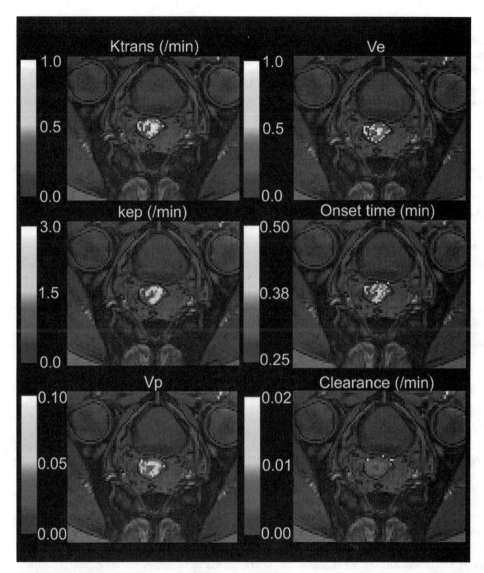

Figure 9 Application of multiple kinetic models to a DCE-MRI dataset A T_1-weighted DCE-MRI dataset (lasting 5 minutes) acquired every second in a patient with rectal cancer. The Larsson model was fitted and yields K^{trans}, v_e and k_{ep}. The Patlak solution applied to the first 60 seconds of enhancement yields permeability (clearance) and v_p. *Abbreviations*: K^{trans}, transfer constant; v_e, leakage space; k_{ep}, rate constant; v_p, fractional blood volume. (*See color insert.*)

Limitations

Quantitative parameters are more complicated to derive compared with those derived semiquantitatively which deters their use at the workbench. Difficulties arise from more complex data acquisition requirements and by the lack of commercially available software to analyze acquired data. The model chosen may not exactly fit the data obtained (Fig. 8) and each model makes a number of assumptions that may not be valid for every tissue or tumor type (12,73). From the above discussions, it is clear that there are uncertainties with regard to the reliability of kinetic parameter estimates derived from the application of tracer kinetic models to T_1-weighted DCE-MRI data (67,75,76). These derive from assumptions implicit in kinetic models and from those for the measurement of tissue contrast agent concentration (74). For example, the Tofts' model uses a standard description of the time varying blood concentration of contrast agent, and assumes that the supply of contrast medium is not flow limited, and that tissue blood volume contributes negligibly to signal intensity changes compared with that arising from contrast medium in the interstitial space (68). As already noted above, this is not universally true in extracranial tumors; Figure 7 depicts a good example where the vascular contribution to the T_1 tissue enhancement curve is obviously sizable in the anterior part of the tumor. Buckley (77) has suggested that the application of commonly accepted models and their respective model-based assumptions to DCE-MRI data, leads to systematic overestimation of K^{trans} in tumors. Thus, it is difficult to be certain about how accurately the model-based kinetic parameter estimates compare with the physiological parameters that they purport to measure, particularly as there is no reliable clinical gold standard.

Despite these complexities, it is important to remember that quantitative kinetic parameters can provide insights into underlying tissue pathophysiological processes that the semiquantitative descriptors cannot. If the time varying contrast agent concentration can be measured accurately, and the type, volume, and method of administration of the contrast agent are consistent, then it is possible to directly compare pharmacokinetic parameters acquired serially in a given patient and in different patients imaged at the same or different scanning sites. Furthermore, it is possible to use quantitative DCE-MRI as a tool for decision making as attested by extensive clinical experience (see below).

Validation

Recently Kiessling et al. (78) reported a strong positive correlation between microbubble-enhanced Doppler ultrasound and dynamic T_1-weighted DCE-MRI kinetic parameters. Previously, it has been shown that there is a near-linear correlation between microbubble velocity measured on Doppler ultrasound and red blood cell velocity (79). Both Lankester et al. (Lankester K, personal communication) and Ah-See et al. (80) have shown strong positive correlations between K^{trans} and relative blood flow (rBF) derived from T_1- and T_2^*-weighted DCE-MRI in pelvic and breast cancer respectively, but such a correlation has not been observed for rectal cancers (81).

Many studies have attempted to correlate tissue MR enhancement with immunohistochemical microvessel density (MVD) measurements in a variety of tumors. Some MRI studies have shown broad correlations between T_1 kinetic parameter estimates and MVD, whereas others have found no correlation (54,78,82–89). Recently vascular endothelial growth factor (VEGF), a potent vascular permeability and angiogenic factor, has been implicated as an additional explanatory factor that determines MR signal enhancement. Knopp et al. (90) reported that MRI vascular permeability to contrast media closely correlated with tissue VEGF expression in breast tumors, whereas Su et al. (54) and Ah-See et al. (91) did not do so. The importance of the role of VEGF in determining MR enhancement is supported by the spatial association of hyperpermeable capillaries detected by macromolecular contrast-enhanced MRI, and VEGF expression on histological specimens (92). Furthermore, the observation that T_1-weighted DCE-MRI measurements can detect changes in flow and permeability after the administration of anti-VEGF antibody and inhibitors of VEGF signaling in xenografts and in humans, lends weight to the important role played by VEGF in determining MR enhancement (93–99). Other tissue characteristics that have been correlated with T_1-weighted enhancement patterns include the degree of stromal cellularity and fibrosis, tissue oxygenation, and tumor proliferation (84,89,100–103).

Clinical Experience

Analysis of enhancement seen on T_1-weighted DCE-MRI is a valuable diagnostic tool in a number of clinical situations. The most established role is in lesion characterization, for example, in distinguishing benign from malignant breast and musculoskeletal lesions (55–59,104). In the brain, T_1 DCE-MRI can be used to noninvasively grade brain tumors (105–107). Dynamic T_1-weighted MRI studies have also been found to be of value in staging gynecological malignancies, and bladder and prostate cancers (108–111). DCE-MRI studies have also been found to be of value in detecting tumor relapse in the presence of fibrosis within treated tissues of the breast and pelvis (112–119). DCE-MRI is also able to predict response to or monitor the effects of a variety of treatments. These include neoadjuvant chemotherapy in bladder and breast cancers, and bone sarcomas (120–123). Other treatments that can be monitored include radiotherapy in rectal and cervix cancers, androgen deprivation in prostate cancer, and vascular embolization of uterine fibroids (124–131). Recently, DCE-MRI has been used to monitor the effects of antivascular, anticancer drugs (97–99,132–134). It is noteworthy that enhancement on DCE-MRI can be affected by most types of successful treatments. This reflects on the fact that tumor cell kill, no matter how it is achieved, ultimately results in vascular shut down, probably because of the loss of proangiogenic cytokine support which results in apoptosis of proliferating endothelial cells.

DCE-MRI VS. F-MDCT

As noted elsewhere in this book, functional multidetector CT (f-MDCT) (see Chap. 12) is also advocated for assessment of tumor vascularity, as this technique provides excellent anatomical imaging and reliable quantitative perfusion data, and is easily incorporated into routine examinations. However, differences in acquisition techniques, mathematical analysis, and measurement parameters, and the propensity to artifacts influence the choice of whether f-MDCT or DCE-MRI is used for angiogenesis assessments (135). Both CT and MRI techniques can provide qualitative and quantitative assessment of tumor vascularity; however, quantification by DCE-MRI is technically more challenging than f-MDCT because, as already noted, there is complex relationship between MR signal intensity and contrast agent concentration, particularly in large vessels. The relationship between contrast concentration and enhancement is straightforward with CT; there is a direct linear relationship between enhancement change and iodine concentration. For example, at 120 kV, an enhancement change of 25 HU is equivalent to 1 mg/mL of iodine (136). As a result, the arterial input, required for quantitative analysis, can be measured directly from an artery in the imaging volume. Thus, absolute quantification of perfusion is possible using f-MDCT and this has been hailed as the major advantage over DCE- MRI.

Functional MDCT techniques are most commonly sequential single-level acquisitions, though sequential volume acquisitions are technically possible with current technology. Tumor coverage with single-level techniques will depend on the number of detectors, but is currently between 2 and 4 cm. A wide variation in acquisition techniques are found in clinical practice; this in part is due to the differing commercial software available, which themselves impose strict data acquisition requirements. These software packages implement a variety of quantitative analysis methods, which include compartmental analysis, deconvolution, Patlak analysis, and the distributed parameter model. As with DCE-MRI, there remains a lack of consensus regarding the optimal acquisition technique, the type of analysis method and the kinetic parameter to use (137).

The choice between f-MDCT or DCE-MRI will be determined by several key factors including local availability and expertise, tumor site, desired perfusion parameter, and the need to reduce radiation burden. The widespread availability of MDCT may be a major determinant in future use. MDCT is already used extensively in oncology for diagnosis and therapeutic assessment. The availability of commercial software and the ability for direct quantification makes assessment straightforward; multicentre assessment is easily achievable, in comparison with DCE-MRI (where the quality assurance challenges are greater). To date no studies have compared the performance of f-MDCT and DCE-MRI in tumor assessment, though a recent study has compared the performance of f-MDCT and DCE-MRI in the evaluation of solitary pulmonary nodules; the authors concluded that there was no significant difference between the performances of both techniques (138).

There are anatomical regions where f-MDCT is preferable to DCE-MRI, mainly due to the presence of artifacts that would interfere with MRI evaluations. These include the upper abdomen, in particular the root of the visceral vessels (in the region of the pancreas and duodenum), the mediastinum, and at the pulmonary hila. Phase-encoded artifacts arising from vascular pulsatility and exaggerated by concentrated intravascular contrast medium, can render DCE-MRI uninterruptible in these anatomical areas. On the other hand, for brain examinations, MRI should be the preferred imaging modality as the radiation burden from MDCT, particularly in serial examinations, may become unacceptable. For anatomical sites such as lung or liver, where respiratory movement along the long axis of the body occurs, there is a requirement to minimize misregistration and resulting mathematical modeling failures. Breath-hold acquisitions typically in the order of 40 seconds are possible with the assistance of oxygen breathing. Multiple breath-holds acquisitions can be performed, for example, to assess liver tumor perfusion, though care must be taken to ensure that the same tumor level is examined during data acquisitions. Motion misregistration appears to be less of a problem for MRI, because motion can be compensated for by the use of navigator techniques (see below), or by imaging in the plane of motion and then using anatomical registration techniques prior to data analysis.

CHALLENGES FOR PERFUSION DCE-MRI

For DCE-MRI, it is recognized that high resolution and short imaging time are the competing examination strategies on current equipment and software. Higher temporal resolution imaging necessitates reduced spatial resolution, decreased anatomic coverage, or a combination of them. Accuracy in the parameters derived from

DCE-MRI, is dependent on the image acquisition rate as can be seen from the following expression

$$E = \sqrt{\sum_{i=1}^{N} \frac{\left(C_i^2 - c_i^2\right)^2}{N - P}}$$

where E is the error, N the number of sample data points, P the number of free parameters in the model, C_i is the contrast media concentration and c_i is the model estimate of the contrast media concentration (139). From this expression, we can immediately see that a small number of sample points N leads to large error estimates. High spatial resolution will by necessity reduce the number of data samples, leading to increased error estimates. Additionally, the finer the spatial resolution, the greater the need for accurate image registration as misregistration will result in increased motion-induced noise in the data. Conversely, a large number of data samples acquired at a high sampling rate reduces the error and enables more complex models with a greater number of free variables to be used in the model fitting process. Thus, compromises have to be made by trading temporal resolution against coverage and spatial resolution. Even though data collection procedures for quantitative examinations differ from those used in routine clinical practice; there is debate as to which technique(s) is/are best (66,140,141). To meet this need, the MRI community has met on a number of occasions and agreed on examination and analysis protocols, in order to enable DCE-MRI to be more completely validated and used in clinical trials. Both generic and organ-specific consensus methods for quantified, T_1-weighted DCE-MRI data collection can now be found (142–145).

A major source of variability in the DCE-MRI literature relates to the method of contrast administration. The dose and method of administration of contrast agent affects modeling procedures and clinical results. Typically, contrast agents are given either as a bolus or infusion (62,146). When a powered injector is used, reproducible injections are ensured. Short injection times are optimal for fast DCE-MRI imaging techniques, especially when evaluating lesions with high microvessel permeability for ECF contrast agents (147,148); but conversely, slower infusion methods may be better when the temporal resolution of the study is longer and volume coverage is being undertaken (140). The method of contrast medium administration also needs to be tailored to the sequence used and the sequence sensitivity to T_2^* and T_1 effects (149–151). Using injection rates of 5 mL/s can reduce the T_1 and T_2 relaxation times in blood to the order of 10 ms during the first pass of the contrast medium (152). Gradient-echo sequences using echo times of the order of 10 ms will be subject to significant T_2-related attenuation that will require correction in quantitative analysis methods. The current trend in DCE-MRI is to acquire data in 3D volumes; this requires the use of both short repetition times (TR) and short echo times (TE). The short TR requires that DCE-MRI data be acquired with a small nutation angle for excitation. This is for two reasons; to reduce the specific absorption rate of electromagnetic energy in the body (a safety reason) and to ensure that the signal obtained is related to the actual concentration of contrast medium. As a consequence of this, a number of precontrast measurements with differing nutation angles are required to obtain sufficient data for the calculation of the initial tissue relaxation rate (R_1). However, larger nutation angles also reduce the SNR of the measurement, which can be compensated for, in part by the SNR advantage of obtaining 3D volumes.

Another issue that needs to be addressed is that of data collection in body parts where there is a large degree of physiological movement such as the lungs and liver. The presence of motion can invalidate functional vascular parameter estimates, particularly for pixel-by-pixel analyses. Methods for overcoming/minimizing these effects include the application of navigator techniques, or imaging in the nonaxial plane using sequential breath-holds during data acquisition and subsequently registering the data prior to analysis (153,154). Unlike navigator techniques, the latter method has the advantage that a fixed time interval between measurements is maintained. Sophisticated image registration methods have also been used to eliminate misregistration and motion-induced noise in DCE-MRI studies in breast (155).

A practical question often asked is whether it is necessary to quantify imaging data, to answer important clinical questions. Simple morphologic and semiquantitative analyses seem to work well in the clinic. However, it is important to realize that semiquantitative diagnostic criteria cannot be applied simply from one center to another, particularly when different equipments and sequences are used. Quantification techniques aim to minimize errors that can result from the use of different equipment and imaging protocols. Quantification techniques also enable the derivation of kinetic parameters that are based on some understanding of physiological processes, and so can provide insights into tumor biology (see above). Quantification techniques are therefore preferred when evaluating antivascular, anticancer drugs (156). Quantification techniques rely on the fitting of the data acquired to a mathematical model. Experience shows that the model chosen may not fit the data acquired (modeling failures), and that apparently sensible kinetic values can be obtained even from noisy data. The causes of modeling failures are complex and often not well understood. Reasons include high vascular permeability (i.e., when the intravascular contrast medium concentration cannot be maintained due to markedly leaky vessels in the setting of limited blood flow), high tissue blood volumes (Fig. 7), multiple tissue compartments, and an incorrect or assumed arterial input function [some organs (liver and lung) and tumors have a dual blood supply (both arterial and venous) complicating modeling procedures]. Modeling failures would be reduced if the arterial input function (AIF) was measured and used to estimate kinetic parameters. Fitting of data with the Tofts' model can be improved if patient-derived vascular input functions are used as inputs in the pharmacokinetic model in place of the standard Weinmann coefficients (68). Reliable methods for measuring arterial input functions for routine DCE-MRI studies are now emerging (70–72,157,158). The use of uptake integrals (see quantification methods discussed above) for both T_1 and T_2^* data overcomes the issue of characterizing pixels which fail to fit a model.

Inevitably, the future will yield kinetic models of increasing sophistication; for example, the effects of variable proton exchange rates are yet to be incorporated into a model of contrast agent uptake. We do not have models that fit all data types, and more sophisticated models that provide insights into tissue compartment behavior are needed (12,149). It is probably true that modeling approaches are not always applied to suitable data in ways that are robust to overfitting, systematic errors, and noise. The application of more sophisticated models, available in the literature, requires superior scanning methods to achieve their full potential. The combination of 3 Tesla scanning and parallel imaging techniques will allow very rapid data acquisition of suitable SNR to permit increased accuracy and precision in quantitative DCE-MRI.

Analysis and presentation of imaging data needs to take into account the heterogeneity of tumor vascular characteristics. User-defined whole-tumor regions of interest (ROI) yield graphical outputs with good SNR, but lack spatial resolution and are prone to partial-volume averaging errors, and thus, are unable to evaluate tumor heterogeneity. As a result, whole-tumor ROIs may not reflect small areas of rapid change, and so may be insensitive to drug action. Many authors have commented that whole-tumor ROI assessment may be inappropriate, particularly, for the evaluation of malignant lesions where heterogeneous areas of enhancement are diagnostically important (27,52,59).

Pixel mapping has a number of advantages including the appreciation of heterogeneity of enhancement and removal of the need to selectively place user-defined ROIs. The risk of missing important diagnostic information, and of creating ROIs that contain more than one tissue type, is reduced. Important advantages of pixel mapping are being able to spatially map tumor vascular characteristics and to be able to probe the relationship between different kinetic parameters. Such displays provide unique insights into tumor structure, function, and response to treatment. Pixel mapping techniques have the disadvantages of having poor SNR ratios and require specialist software for their generation. Whilst visual appreciation of heterogeneity is improved by pixel mapping displays, quantification of the same can be more difficult. Recently, histogram and principal components analysis, and fractal approaches have been used to quantify the heterogeneity of tumors for comparative and longitudinal studies, for monitoring the effects of treatment, and to show the regression or development of angiogenic hot spots (126,159–161).

CONCLUSIONS

Both, functional MDCT and DCE-MRI are advocated as techniques for assessment of tumor vascularity as they provide excellent anatomical imaging, reliable quantitative perfusion data, and are easily incorporated into routine examinations. However, differences in acquisition techniques, mathematical analysis, measurement parameters, and propensity to artifacts influence the choice of imaging modality. Depending on the technique used, physiological insights into tissue perfusion, micro-vessel-permeability surface area product, and extracellular leakage space can be non-invasively obtained. Angiogenesis imaging techniques potentially have widespread clinical applications and their recent development has been spurred on by the development of antivascular, anticancer approaches. A realistic appraisal of the strengths and limitations of the techniques is required, and a number of challenges must be met if they are to enter into widespread clinical practice. Such developments will be essential for multicenter trials where it will be necessary to establish effective cross-site standardization of measurements and evaluation.

ACKNOWLEDGMENTS

We are grateful to Dr. Jane Taylor and Simon Walker-Samuel for their assistance in the preparation of the illustrative material for this review. Parametric calculations and images were produced by Magnetic Resonance Imaging Software (MRIW) developed at the Institute of Cancer Research, Royal Marsden Hospital, London. The support of Cancer Research UK and the Childwick Trust who support the work of the Clinical Magnetic Resonance Research Group at the Royal Marsden Hospital and at the Paul Strickland Scanner Centre, Mount Vernon Hospital respectively is gratefully acknowledged.

REFERENCES

1. Folkman J. Angiogenesis in cancer, vascular, rheumatoid and other disease. Nat Med 1995; 1:27–31.
2. Vermeulen PB, Gasparini G, Fox SB, et al. Quantification of angiogenesis in solid human tumours: an international consensus on the methodology and criteria of evaluation. Eur J Cancer 1996; 32A(14):2474–2484.
3. Kerckhaert OA, Voest EE. The prognostic and diagnostic value of circulating angiogenic factors in cancer patients. In: Voest EE, D'Amore PA, eds. Tumor Angiogenesis and Microcirculation. New York: Marcel Dekker, Inc., 2001:487–500.
4. Endrich B, Vaupel P. The role of microcirculation in the treatment of malignant tumors: facts and fiction. In: Molls M, Vaupel P, eds. Blood Perfusion and Microenvironment Of Human Tumors. Berlin: Springer-Verlag, 1998:19–39.
5. Brasch R, Turetschek K. MRI characterization of tumors and grading angiogenesis using macromolecular contrast media: status report. Eur J Radiol 2000; 34(3): 148–155.
6. Weissleder R, Mahmood U. Molecular imaging. Radiology 2001; 219(2):316–333.
7. Jackson A. Analysis of dynamic contrast enhanced MRI. Br J Radiol 2004; 77(Spec No 2):S154–S166.
8. Collins DJ, Padhani AR. Dynamic magnetic resonance imaging of tumor perfusion. Approaches and biomedical challenges. IEEE Eng Med Biol Mag 2004; 23(5):65–83.
9. Choyke PL, Dwyer AJ, Knopp MV. Functional tumor imaging with dynamic contrast-enhanced magnetic resonance imaging. J Magn Reson Imaging 2003; 17(5):509–520.
10. Parker GJ, Tofts PS. Pharmacokinetic analysis of neoplasms using contrast-enhanced dynamic magnetic resonance imaging. Top Magn Reson Imaging 1999; 10(2): 130–142.
11. Daldrup HE, Shames DM, Husseini W, Wendland MF, Okuhata Y, Brasch RC. Quantification of the extraction fraction for gadopentetate across breast cancer capillaries. Magn Reson Med 1998; 40(4):537–543.
12. Tofts PS, Brix G, Buckley DL, et al. Estimating kinetic parameters from dynamic contrast-enhanced T(1)-weighted MRI of a diffusable tracer: standardized quantities and symbols. J Magn Reson Imaging 1999; 10(3):223–232.
13. Barbier EL, Lamalle L, Decorps M. Methodology of brain perfusion imaging. J Magn Reson Imaging 2001; 13(4):496–520.
14. Sorensen AG, Tievsky AL, Ostergaard L, Weisskoff RM, Rosen BR. Contrast agents in functional MR imaging. J Magn Reson Imaging 1997; 7(1):47–55.
15. Dennie J, Mandeville JB, Boxerman JL, Packard SD, Rosen BR, Weisskoff RM. NMR imaging of changes in vascular morphology due to tumor angiogenesis. Magn Reson Med 1998; 40(6):793–799.
16. Bruening R, Berchtenbreiter C, Holzknecht N, et al. Effects of three different doses of a bolus injection of gadodiamide: assessment of regional cerebral blood volume maps in a blinded reader study. AJNR Am J Neuroradiol 2000; 21(9):1603–1610.
17. Rausch M, Scheffler K, Rudin M, Radu EW. Analysis of input functions from different arterial branches with gamma variate functions and cluster analysis for quantitative blood volume measurements. Magn Reson Imaging 2000; 18(10):1235–1243.
18. Simonsen CZ, Ostergaard L, Smith DF, Vestergaard-Poulsen P, Gyldensted C. Comparison of gradient- and spin-echo imaging: CBF, CBV, and MTT measurements by bolus tracking. J Magn Reson Imaging 2000; 12(3):411–416.

19. Rosen BR, Belliveau JW, Buchbinder BR, et al. Contrast agents and cerebral hemodynamics. Magn Reson Med 1991; 19(2):285–292.

20. Ostergaard L, Sorensen AG, Kwong KK, Weisskoff RM, Gyldensted C, Rosen BR. High resolution measurement of cerebral blood flow using intravascular tracer bolus passages. Part II: Experimental comparison and preliminary results. Magn Reson Med 1996; 36(5):726–736.

21. Taylor NJ, Ah-See WM-L, Stirling JJ, et al. Pre- and post-chemotherapy comparisons of calculated rBV and rBF with signal intensity drop on T2* dynamic contrast enhanced MRI of breast cancers. In: International Society of Magnetic Resonance in Medicine, 13th Scientific Meeting; Miami, FL.2005:91.

22. Jackson A, Kassner A, Zhu XP, Li KL. Reproducibility of T2* blood volume and vascular tortuosity maps in cerebral gliomas. J Magn Reson Imaging 2001; 14(5): 510–516.

23. Wenz F, Rempp K, Brix G, et al. Age dependency of the regional cerebral blood volume (rCBV) measured with dynamic susceptibility contrast MR imaging (DSC). Magn Reson Imaging 1996; 14(2):157–162.

24. Wenz F, Rempp K, Hess T, et al. Effect of radiation on blood volume in low-grade astrocytomas and normal brain tissue: quantification with dynamic susceptibility contrast MR imaging. AJR Am J Roentgenol 1996; 166(1):187–193.

25. Davenport R. The derivation of the gamma-variate relationship for tracer dilution curves. J Nucl Med 1983; 24(10):945–948.

26. d'Arcy JA, Collins DJ, Rowland IJ, Padhani AR, Leach MO. Applications of sliding window reconstruction with cartesian sampling for dynamic contrast enhanced MRI. NMR Biomed 2002; 15(2):174–183.

27. Aronen HJ, Gazit IE, Louis DN, et al. Cerebral blood volume maps of gliomas: comparison with tumor grade and histologic findings. Radiology 1994; 191(1):41–51.

28. Maeda M, Maley JE, Crosby DL, et al. Application of contrast agents in the evaluation of stroke: conventional MR and echo-planar MR imaging. J Magn Reson Imaging 1997; 7(1):23–28.

29. Miyati T, Banno T, Mase M, et al. Dual dynamic contrast-enhanced MR imaging. J Magn Reson Imaging 1997; 7(1):230–235.

30. Johnson G, Wetzel SG, Cha S, Babb J, Tofts PS. Measuring blood volume and vascular transfer constant from dynamic, T(2)*-weighted contrast-enhanced MRI. Magn Reson Med 2004; 51(5):961–968.

31. Moseley ME, Vexler Z, Asgari HS, et al. Comparison of Gd- and Dy-chelates for T2 contrast-enhanced imaging. Magn Reson Med 1991; 22(2):259–264.

32. Reimer P, Schuierer G, Balzer T, Peters PE. Application of a superparamagnetic iron oxide (Resovist) for MR imaging of human cerebral blood volume. Magn Reson Med 1995; 34(5):694–697.

33. Lev MH, Kulke SF, Sorensen AG, et al. Contrast-to-noise ratio in functional MRI of relative cerebral blood volume with sprodiamide injection. J Magn Reson Imaging 1997; 7(3):523–527.

34. De La Paz RL, Ott IL, Paola T. Recurrent brain tumour versus radiation necrosis: comparison of MR relative cerebral blood volume maps and FDG-PET. Radiology 1995; 197(P):169.

35. Forsting M, Reith W, Dorfler A, von Kummer R, Hacke W, Sartor K. MRI in acute cerebral ischaemia: perfusion imaging with superparamagnetic iron oxide in a rat model. Neuroradiology 1994; 36(1):23–26.

36. Bjornerud A, Johansson LO, Ahlstrom HK. Renal T(*)(2) perfusion using an iron oxide nanoparticle contrast agent-influence of T(1) relaxation on the first-pass response. Magn Reson Med 2002; 47(2):298–304.

37. Cha S, Lu S, Johnson G, Knopp EA. Dynamic susceptibility contrast MR imaging: correlation of signal intensity changes with cerebral blood volume measurements. J Magn Reson Imaging 2000; 11(2):114–119.

38. Maeda M, Itoh S, Kimura H, et al. Tumor vascularity in the brain: evaluation with dynamic susceptibility-contrast MR imaging. Radiology 1993; 189(1):233–238.

39. Siegal T, Rubinstein R, Tzuk-Shina T, Gomori JM. Utility of relative cerebral blood volume mapping derived from perfusion magnetic resonance imaging in the routine follow up of brain tumors. J Neurosurg 1997; 86(1):22–27.

40. Barbier EL, den Boer JA, Peters AR, Rozeboom AR, Sau J, Bonmartin A. A model of the dual effect of gadopentetate dimeglumine on dynamic brain MR images. J Magn Reson Imaging 1999; 10(3):242–253.

41. Hacklander T, Reichenbach JR, Modder U. Comparison of cerebral blood volume measurements using the T1 and T2* methods in normal human brains and brain tumors. J Comput Assist Tomogr 1997; 21(6):857–866.

42. Sugahara T, Korogi Y, Shigematsu Y, et al. Value of dynamic susceptibility contrast magnetic resonance imaging in the evaluation of intracranial tumors. Top Magn Reson Imaging 1999; 10(2):114–124.

43. Ostergaard L, Hochberg FH, Rabinov JD, et al. Early changes measured by magnetic resonance imaging in cerebral blood flow, blood volume, and blood-brain barrier permeability following dexamethasone treatment in patients with brain tumors. J Neurosurg 1999; 90(2):300–305.

44. Sorensen AG, Copen WA, Ostergaard L, et al. Hyperacute stroke: simultaneous measurement of relative cerebral blood volume, relative cerebral blood flow, and mean tissue transit time. Radiology 1999; 210(2):519–527.

45. Kuhl CK, Bieling H, Gieseke J, et al. Breast neoplasms: T2* susceptibility-contrast, first-pass perfusion MR imaging. Radiology 1997; 202(1):87–95.

46. Kvistad KA, Lundgren S, Fjosne HE, Smenes E, Smethurst HB, Haraldseth O. Differentiating benign and malignant breast lesions with T2*-weighted first pass perfusion imaging. Acta Radiol 1999; 40(1):45–51.

47. Ah-See MW, Makris A, Taylor NJ, et al. Multi-functional magnetic resonance imaging predicts for clinico-pathological response to neoadjuvant chemotherapy in primary breast cancer. In: 26th Annual San Antonio Breast Cancer Symposium, San Antonio; 2003:252.

48. Wang HZ, Riederer SJ, Lee JN. Optimizing the precision in T1 relaxation estimation using limited flip angles. Magn Reson Med 1987; 5(5):399–416.

49. Parker GJ, Barker GJ, Tofts PS. Accurate multislice gradient echo T(1) measurement in the presence of non-ideal RF pulse shape and RF field nonuniformity. Magn Reson Med 2001; 45(5):838–845.

50. Larsson HB, Stubgaard M, Frederiksen JL, Jensen M, Henriksen O, Paulson OB. Quantitation of blood-brain barrier defect by magnetic resonance imaging and gadolinium-DTPA in patients with multiple sclerosis and brain tumors. Magn Reson Med 1990; 16(1):117–131.

51. Gowland P, Mansfield P, Bullock P, Stehling M, Worthington B, Firth J. Dynamic studies of gadolinium uptake in brain tumors using inversion-recovery echo-planar imaging. Magn Reson Med 1992; 26(2):241–258.

52. Parker GJ, Suckling J, Tanner SF, et al. Probing tumor microvascularity by measurement, analysis and display of contrast agent uptake kinetics. J Magn Reson Imaging 1997; 7(3):564–574.

53. Su MY, Jao JC, Nalcioglu O. Measurement of vascular volume fraction and blood-tissue permeability constants with a pharmacokinetic model: studies in rat muscle tumors with dynamic Gd-DTPA enhanced MRI. Magn Reson Med 1994; 32(6):714–724.

54. Su MY, Cheung YC, Fruehauf JP, et al. Correlation of dynamic contrast enhancement MRI parameters with microvessel density and VEGF for assessment of angiogenesis in breast cancer. J Magn Reson Imaging 2003; 18(4):467–477.

55. Kuhl CK, Mielcareck P, Klaschik S, et al. Dynamic breast MR imaging: are signal intensity time course data useful for differential diagnosis of enhancing lesions? Radiology 1999; 211(1):101–110.

56. Daniel BL, Yen YF, Glover GH, et al. Breast disease: dynamic spiral MR imaging. Radiology 1998; 209(2):499–509.

57. Flickinger FW, Allison JD, Sherry RM, Wright JC. Differentiation of benign from malignant breast masses by time-intensity evaluation of contrast enhanced MRI. Magn Reson Imaging 1993; 11(5):617–620.

58. Kaiser WA, Zeitler E. MR imaging of the breast: fast imaging sequences with and without Gd-DTPA. Preliminary observations. Radiology 1989; 170(3 Part 1):681–686.

59. Gribbestad IS, Nilsen G, Fjosne HE, Kvinnsland S, Haugen OA, Rinck PA. Comparative signal intensity measurements in dynamic gadolinium-enhanced MR mammography. J Magn Reson Imaging 1994; 4(3):477–480.

60. Evelhoch JL. Key factors in the acquisition of contrast kinetic data for oncology. J Magn Reson Imaging 1999; 10(3):254–259.

61. Parker GJ, Baustert I, Tanner SF, Leach MO. Improving image quality and T(1) measurements using saturation recovery turboFLASH with an approximate K-space normalisation filter. Magn Reson Imaging 2000; 18(2):157–167.

62. Tofts PS, Kermode AG. Measurement of the blood-brain barrier permeability and leakage space using dynamic MR imaging. 1. Fundamental concepts. Magn Reson Med 1991; 17(2):357–367.

63. Larsson HB, Tofts PS. Measurement of blood-brain barrier permeability using dynamic Gd-DTPA scanning – a comparison of methods. Magn Reson Med 1992; 24(1):174–176.

64. Kety SS. The theory and applications of the exchange of inert gas at the lungs and tissues. Pharmacol Rev 1951; 3:1–41.

65. Patlak CS, Blasberg RG, Fenstermacher JD. Graphical evaluation of blood-to-brain transfer constants from multiple-time uptake data. J Cereb Blood Flow Metab 1983; 3(1):1–7.

66. Degani H, Gusis V, Weinstein D, Fields S, Strano S. Mapping pathophysiological features of breast tumors by MRI at high spatial resolution. Nat Med 1997; 3(7):780–782.

67. Landis CS, Li X, Telang FW, et al. Determination of the MRI contrast agent concentration time course in vivo following bolus injection: effect of equilibrium transcytolemmal water exchange. Magn Reson Med 2000; 44(4):563–574.

68. Weinmann HJ, Laniado M, Mutzel W. Pharmacokinetics of GdDTPA/dimeglumine after intravenous injection into healthy volunteers. Physiol Chem Phys Med NMR 1984; 16(2):167–172.

69. Fritz-Hansen T, Rostrup E, Ring PB, Larsson HB. Quantification of gadolinium-DTPA concentrations for different inversion times using an IR-turbo flash pulse sequence: a study on optimizing multislice perfusion imaging. Magn Reson Imaging 1998; 16(8):893–899.

70. Kovar DA, Lewis M, Karczmar GS. A new method for imaging perfusion and contrast extraction fraction: input functions derived from reference tissues. J Magn Reson Imaging 1998; 8(5):1126–1134.

71. Yang C, Karczmar GS, Medved M, Stadler WM. Estimating the arterial input function using two reference tissues in dynamic contrast-enhanced MRI studies: fundamental concepts and simulations. Magn Reson Med 2004; 52(5):1110–1117.

72. Li KL, Zhu XP, Waterton J, Jackson A. Improved 3D quantitative mapping of blood volume and endothelial permeability in brain tumors. J Magn Reson Imaging 2000; 12(2):347–357.

73. Tofts PS. Modeling tracer kinetics in dynamic Gd-DTPA MR imaging. J Magn Reson Imaging 1997; 7(1):91–101.

74. Dale BM, Jesberger JA, Lewin JS, Hillenbrand CM, Duerk JL. Determining and optimizing the precision of quantitative measurements of perfusion from dynamic contrast enhanced MRI. J Magn Reson Imaging 2003; 18(5):575–584.

75. Tofts PS, Berkowitz B, Schnall MD. Quantitative analysis of dynamic Gd-DTPA enhancement in breast tumors using a permeability model. Magn Reson Med 1995; 33(4):564–568.

76. Buckley DL. Transcytolemmal water exchange and its affect on the determination of contrast agent concentration in vivo. Magn Reson Med 2002; 47(2):420–421.

77. Buckley DL. Uncertainty in the analysis of tracer kinetics using dynamic contrast-enhanced T(1)-weighted MRI. Magn Reson Med 2002; 47(3):601–606.

78. Kiessling F, Krix M, Heilmann M, et al. Comparing dynamic parameters of tumor vascularization in nude mice revealed by magnetic resonance imaging and contrast-enhanced intermittent power Doppler sonography. Invest Radiol 2003; 38(8):516–524.

79. Cosgrove D, Eckersley R, Blomley M, Harvey C. Quantification of blood flow. Eur Radiol 2001; 11(8):1338–1344.

80. Ah-See MW, Padhani AR, Taylor NJ, et al. Evaluation of VEGF expression within breast cancer biopsies & tumour microvasculature assessment by multi-functional dynamic contrast-enhanced MRI. In: The 4th European Breast Cancer Conference (EBCC-4); Hamburg, Germany; 2004.

81. Atkin G, Taylor NJ, Daley FM, et al. An investigation of DCE-MRI as a non-invasive measure of angiogenesis in rectal cancer. In: Proceedings of the International Society of Magnetic Resonance in Medicine, 12th Scientific meeting, Kyoto, 2004:1976.

82. Stomper PC, Winston JS, Herman S, Klippenstein DL, Arredondo MA, Blumenson LE. Angiogenesis and dynamic MR imaging gadolinium enhancement of malignant and benign breast lesions. Breast Cancer Res Treat 1997; 45(1):39–46.

83. Hawighorst H, Knapstein PG, Weikel W, et al. Angiogenesis of uterine cervical carcinoma: characterization by pharmacokinetic magnetic resonance parameters and histological microvessel density with correlation to lymphatic involvement. Cancer Res 1997; 57(21):4777–4786.

84. Tynninen O, Aronen HJ, Ruhala M, et al. MRI enhancement and microvascular density in gliomas. Correlation with tumor cell proliferation. Invest Radiol 1999; 34(6): 427–434.

85. Buckley DL, Drew PJ, Mussurakis S, Monson JR, Horsman A. Microvessel density of invasive breast cancer assessed by dynamic Gd-DTPA enhanced MRI. J Magn Reson Imaging 1997; 7(3):461–464.

86. Schlemmer HP, Merkle J, Grobholz R, et al. Can pre-operative contrast-enhanced dynamic MR imaging for prostate cancer predict microvessel density in prostatectomy specimens? Eur Radiol 2003; 14(2):309–317.

87. Carriero A, Ambrossini R, Mattei PA, Angelucci D, Bonomo L. Magnetic resonance of the breast: correlation between enhancement patterns and microvessel density in malignant tumors. J Exp Clin Cancer Res 2002; 21(suppl 3):83–87.

88. Hulka CA, Edmister WB, Smith BL, et al. Dynamic echo-planar imaging of the breast: experience in diagnosing breast carcinoma and correlation with tumor angiogenesis. Radiology 1997; 205(3):837–842.

89. Cooper RA, Carrington BM, Loncaster JA, et al. Tumour oxygenation levels correlate with dynamic contrast-enhanced magnetic resonance imaging parameters in carcinoma of the cervix. Radiother Oncol 2000; 57(1):53–59.

90. Knopp MV, Weiss E, Sinn HP, et al. Pathophysiologic basis of contrast enhancement in breast tumors. J Magn Reson Imaging 1999; 10(3):260–266.

91. Ah-See MW, Padhani AR, Taylor NJ, et al. Tumour microvasculature assessment by dynamic contrast-enhanced MRI fails to correlate with VEGF expression in breast cancer biopsies. In: British Cancer Research Meeting, Manchester. Br J Cancer 2004: S16 #5.4.

92. Bhujwalla ZM, Artemov D, Natarajan K, Ackerstaff E, Solaiyappan M. Vascular differences detected by MRI for metastatic versus nonmetastatic breast and prostate cancer xenografts. Neoplasia 2001; 3(2):143–153.

93. Pham CD, Roberts TP, van Bruggen N, et al. Magnetic resonance imaging detects suppression of tumor vascular permeability after administration of antibody to vascular endothelial growth factor. Cancer Invest 1998; 16(4):225–230.

94. Gossmann A, Helbich TH, Kuriyama N, et al. Dynamic contrast-enhanced magnetic resonance imaging as a surrogate marker of tumor response to anti-angiogenic therapy in a xenograft model of glioblastoma multiforme. J Magn Reson Imaging 2002; 15(3): 233–240.

95. Checkley D, Tessier JJ, Kendrew J, Waterton JC, Wedge SR. Use of dynamic contrast-enhanced MRI to evaluate acute treatment with ZD6474, a VEGF signaling inhibitor, in PC-3 prostate tumours. Br J Cancer 2003; 89(10):1889–1895.

96. Turetschek K, Preda A, Floyd E, et al. MRI monitoring of tumor response following angiogenesis inhibition in an experimental human breast cancer model. Eur J Nucl Med Mol Imaging 2003; 30(3):448–455.

97. Morgan B, Thomas AL, Drevs J, et al. Dynamic contrast-enhanced magnetic resonance imaging as a biomarker for the pharmacological response of PTK787/ZK 222584, an inhibitor of the vascular endothelial growth factor receptor tyrosine kinases, in patients with advanced colorectal cancer and liver metastases: results from two phase I studies. J Clin Oncol 2003; 21(21):3955–3964.

98. Jayson GC, Zweit J, Jackson A, et al. Molecular imaging and biological evaluation of HuMV833 anti-VEGF antibody: implications for trial design of antiangiogenic antibodies. J Natl Cancer Inst 2002; 94(19):1484–1493.

99. Yung WK, Friedman H, Conrad C, et al. A phase I trial of single-agent PTK 787/ZK 222584 (PTK/ZK), an oral VEGFR tyrosine kinase inhibitor, in patients with recurrent glioblastoma multiforme. In: ASCO; 2003; Chicago; 2003:395.

100. Matsubayashi R, Matsuo Y, Edakuni G, Satoh T, Tokunaga O, Kudo S. Breast masses with peripheral rim enhancement on dynamic contrast-enhanced MR images: correlation of MR findings with histologic features and expression of growth factors. Radiology 2000; 217(3):841–848.

101. Yamashita Y, Baba T, Baba Y, et al. Dynamic contrast-enhanced MR imaging of uterine cervical cancer: pharmacokinetic analysis with histopathologic correlation and its importance in predicting the outcome of radiation therapy. Radiology 2000; 216(3):803–809.

102. Lyng H, Vorren AO, Sundfor K, et al. Assessment of tumor oxygenation in human cervical carcinoma by use of dynamic Gd-DTPA-enhanced MR imaging. J Magn Reson Imaging 2001; 14(6):750–756.

103. Konouchi H, Asaumi J, Yanagi Y, et al. Evaluation of tumor proliferation using dynamic contrast enhanced-MRI of oral cavity and oropharyngeal squamous cell carcinoma. Oral Oncol 2003; 39(3):290–295.

104. van der Woude HJ, Verstraete KL, Hogendoorn PC, Taminiau AH, Hermans J, Bloem JL. Musculoskeletal tumors: does fast dynamic contrast-enhanced subtraction MR imaging contribute to the characterization? Radiology 1998; 208(3):821–828.

105. Ludemann L, Hamm B, Zimmer C. Pharmacokinetic analysis of glioma compartments with dynamic Gd-DTPA-enhanced magnetic resonance imaging. Magn Reson Imaging 2000; 18:1201–1214.

106. Roberts HC, Roberts TP, Bollen AW, Ley S, Brasch RC, Dillon WP. Correlation of microvascular permeability derived from dynamic contrast-enhanced MR imaging with histologic grade and tumor labeling index: a study in human brain tumors. Acad Radiol 2001; 8(5):384–391.

107. Roberts HC, Roberts TP, Brasch RC, Dillon WP. Quantitative measurement of microvascular permeability in human brain tumors achieved using dynamic contrast-enhanced MR imaging: correlation with histologic grade. AJNR Am J Neuroradiol 2000; 21(5):891–899.

108. Liu PF, Krestin GP, Huch RA, Gohde SC, Caduff RF, Debatin JF. MRI of the uterus, uterine cervix, and vagina: diagnostic performance of dynamic contrast-enhanced fast

multiplanar gradient-echo imaging in comparison with fast spin-echo T2-weighted pulse imaging. Eur Radiol 1998; 8(8):1433–1440.

109. Barentsz JO, Jager GJ, van Vierzen PB, et al. Staging urinary bladder cancer after trans-urethral biopsy: value of fast dynamic contrast-enhanced MR imaging. Radiology 1996; 201(1):185–193.

110. Jager GJ, Ruijter ET, van de Kaa CA, et al. Dynamic TurboFLASH subtraction technique for contrast-enhanced MR imaging of the prostate: correlation with histopathologic results. Radiology 1997; 203(3):645–652.

111. Huch Boni RA, Boner JA, Lutolf UM, Trinkler F, Pestalozzi DM, Krestin GP. Contrast-enhanced endorectal coil MRI in local staging of prostate carcinoma. J Comput Assist Tomogr 1995; 19(2):232–237.

112. Gilles R, Guinebretiere JM, Shapeero LG, et al. Assessment of breast cancer recurrence with contrast-enhanced subtraction MR imaging: preliminary results in 26 patients. Radiology 1993; 188(2):473–478.

113. Kerslake RW, Fox JN, Carleton PJ, et al. Dynamic contrast-enhanced and fat sup-pressed magnetic resonance imaging in suspected recurrent carcinoma of the breast: preliminary experience. Br J Radiol 1994; 67(804):1158–1168.

114. Mussurakis S, Buckley DL, Bowsley SJ, et al. Dynamic contrast-enhanced magnetic resonance imaging of the breast combined with pharmacokinetic analysis of gadolinium-DTPA uptake in the diagnosis of local recurrence of early stage breast carcinoma. Invest Radiol 1995; 30(11):650–662.

115. Kinkel K, Tardivon AA, Soyer P, et al. Dynamic contrast-enhanced subtraction versus T2-weighted spin-echo MR imaging in the follow-up of colorectal neoplasm: a prospective study of 41 patients. Radiology 1996; 200(2):453–458.

116. Hawnaur JM, Zhu XP, Hutchinson CE. Quantitative dynamic contrast enhanced MRI of recurrent pelvic masses in patients treated for cancer. Br J Radiol 1998; 71(851):1136–1142.

117. Dao TH, Rahmouni A, Campana F, Laurent M, Asselain B, Fourquet A. Tumor recurrence versus fibrosis in the irradiated breast: differentiation with dynamic gadolinium-enhanced MR imaging. Radiology 1993; 187(3):751–755.

118. Heywang-Kobrunner SH, Schlegel A, Beck R, et al. Contrast-enhanced MRI of the breast after limited surgery and radiation therapy. J Comput Assist Tomogr 1993; 17(6):891–900.

119. Blomqvist L, Fransson P, Hindmarsh T. The pelvis after surgery and radio-chemotherapy for rectal cancer studied with Gd-DTPA-enhanced fast dynamic MR imaging. Eur Radiol 1998; 8(5):781–787.

120. Barentsz JO, Berger-Hartog O, Witjes JA, et al. Evaluation of chemotherapy in advanced urinary bladder cancer with fast dynamic contrast-enhanced MR imaging. Radiology 1998; 207(3):791–797.

121. Reddick WE, Taylor JS, Fletcher BD. Dynamic MR imaging (DEMRI) of microcirculation in bone sarcoma. J Magn Reson Imaging 1999; 10(3):277–285.

122. van der Woude HJ, Bloem JL, Verstraete KL, Taminiau AH, Nooy MA, Hogendoorn PC. Osteosarcoma and Ewing's sarcoma after neoadjuvant chemotherapy: value of dynamic MR imaging in detecting viable tumor before surgery. Am J Roentgenol 1995; 165(3):593–598.

123. Knopp MV, Brix G, Junkermann HJ, Sinn HP. MR mammography with pharmacokinetic mapping for monitoring of breast cancer treatment during neoadjuvant therapy. Magn Reson Imaging Clin N Am 1994; 2(4):633–658.

124. Devries AF, Griebel J, Kremser C, et al. Tumor microcirculation evaluated by dynamic magnetic resonance imaging predicts therapy outcome for primary rectal carcinoma. Cancer Res 2001; 61(6):2513–2516.

125. de Vries A, Griebel J, Kremser C, et al. Monitoring of tumor microcirculation during fractionated radiation therapy in patients with rectal carcinoma: preliminary results and implications for therapy. Radiology 2000; 217(2):385–391.

126. Mayr NA, Yuh WT, Arnholt JC, et al. Pixel analysis of MR perfusion imaging in predicting radiation therapy outcome in cervical cancer. J Magn Reson Imaging 2000; 12(6):1027–1033.

127. George ML, Dzik-Jurasz AS, Padhani AR, et al. Non-invasive methods of assessing angiogenesis and their value in predicting response to treatment in colorectal cancer. Br J Surg 2001; 88(12):1628–1636.

128. Padhani AR, MacVicar AD, Gapinski CJ, et al. Effects of androgen deprivation on prostatic morphology and vascular permeability evaluated with MR imaging. Radiology 2001; 218(2):365–374.

129. Burn PR, McCall JM, Chinn RJ, Vashisht A, Smith JR, Healy JC. Uterine fibroleiomyoma: MR imaging appearances before and after embolization of uterine arteries. Radiology 2000; 214(3):729–734.

130. Jha RC, Ascher SM, Imaoka I, Spies JB. Symptomatic fibroleiomyomata: MR imaging of the uterus before and after uterine arterial embolization. Radiology 2000; 217(1): 228–235.

131. Li W, Brophy DP, Chen Q, Edelman RR, Prasad PV. Semiquantitative assessment of uterine perfusion using first pass dynamic contrast-enhanced MR imaging for patients treated with uterine fibroid embolization. J Magn Reson Imaging 2000; 12(6): 1004–1008.

132. Galbraith SM, Maxwell RJ, Lodge MA, et al. Combretastatin A4 phosphate has tumor antivascular activity in rat and man as demonstrated by dynamic magnetic resonance imaging. J Clin Oncol 2003; 21(15):2831–2842.

133. Galbraith SM, Rustin GJ, Lodge MA, et al. Effects of 5,6-dimethylxanthenone-4-acetic acid on human tumor microcirculation assessed by dynamic contrast-enhanced magnetic resonance imaging. J Clin Oncol 2002; 20(18):3826–3840.

134. Galbraith SM, Maxwell RJ, Lodge MA, et al. Combretastatin A4 Phosphate has tumor antivascular activity in rat and man as demonstrated by dynamic magnetic resonance imaging. J Clin Oncol 2003; 21(15):2831–2842.

135. Goh V, Padhani AR. Imaging tumor angiogenesis: functional assessment using MDCT or MRI? Abdom Imaging 2005 (in press).

136. Dawson P. Contrast agents as tracers. In: Miles KA, Dawson P, Hayball MP, eds. Functional Computed Tomography. Oxford, UK: Isis Medical Media, 1997:29–45.

137. Miles KA. Perfusion CT for the assessment of tumour vascularity: which protocol? Br J Radiol 2003; 76(Spec No 1):S36–S42.

138. Kim JH, Kim HJ, Lee KH, Kim KH, Lee HL. Solitary pulmonary nodules: a comparative study evaluated with contrast-enhanced dynamic MR imaging and CT. J Comput Assist Tomogr 2004; 28(6):766–775.

139. Vincensini D, Dedieu V, Renou JP, Otal P, Joffre F. Measurements of extracellular volume fraction and capillary permeability in tissues using dynamic spin-lattice relaxometry: studies in rabbit muscles. Magn Reson Imaging 2003; 21(2):85–93.

140. Hoffmann U, Brix G, Knopp MV, Hess T, Lorenz WJ. Pharmacokinetic mapping of the breast: a new method for dynamic MR mammography. Magn Reson Med 1995; 33(4):506–514.

141. den Boer JA, Hoenderop RK, Smink J, et al. Pharmacokinetic analysis of Gd-DTPA enhancement in dynamic three-dimensional MRI of breast lesions. J Magn Reson Imaging 1997; 7(4):702–715.

142. Leach MO, Brindle KM, Evelhoch JL, et al. Assessment of antiangiogenic and antivascular therapeutics using MRI: recommendations for appropriate methodology for clinical trials. Br J Radiol 2003; 76(Spec No 1):S87–S91.

143. Brasch RC, Li KC, Husband JE, et al. In vivo monitoring of tumor angiogenesis with MR imaging. Acad Radiol 2000; 7(10):812–823.

144. Evelhoch J, Brown T, Chenevert T, et al. Consensus recommendation for acquisition of dynamic contrast-enhanced MRI data in oncology. In: Proceedings of the International Society of Magnetic Resonance in Medicine, Denver, Colarado, 2000:1439.

145. Brown J, Buckley D, Coulthard A, et al. Magnetic resonance imaging screening in women at genetic risk of breast cancer: imaging and analysis protocol for the UK multi-centre study. UK MRI Breast Screening Study Advisory Group. Magn Reson Imaging 2000; 18(7):765–776.

146. Brix G, Semmler W, Port R, Schad LR, Layer G, Lorenz WJ. Pharmacokinetic parameters in CNS Gd-DTPA enhanced MR imaging. J Comput Assist Tomogr 1991; 15(4):621–628.

147. Henderson E, Rutt BK, Lee TY. Temporal sampling requirements for the tracer kinetics modeling of breast disease. Magn Reson Imaging 1998; 16(9):1057–1073.

148. Tofts PS, Berkowitz BA. Measurement of capillary permeability from the Gd enhancement curve: a comparison of bolus and constant infusion injection methods. Magn Reson Imaging 1994; 12(1):81–91.

149. Port RE, Knopp MV, Hoffmann U, Milker-Zabel S, Brix G. Multicompartment analysis of gadolinium chelate kinetics: blood-tissue exchange in mammary tumors as monitored by dynamic MR imaging. J Magn Reson Imaging 1999; 10(3):233–241.

150. Ludemann L, Hamm B, Zimmer C. Pharmacokinetic analysis of glioma compartments with dynamic Gd-DTPA-enhanced magnetic resonance imaging. Magn Reson Imaging 2000; 18(10):1201–1214.

151. Roberts TP. Physiologic measurements by contrast-enhanced MR imaging: expectations and limitations. J Magn Reson Imaging 1997; 7(1):82–90.

152. Shetty AN, Bis KG, Kirsch M, Weintraub J, Laub G. Contrast-enhanced breath-hold three-dimensional magnetic resonance angiography in the evaluation of renal arteries: optimization of technique and pitfalls. J Magn Reson Imaging 2000; 12(6): 912–923.

153. Taylor NJ, Lankester KJ, Stirling JJ, et al. Application of navigator techniques to breath-hold DCE-MRI studies of the liver. In: Proceedings of the International Society of Magnetic Resonance in Medicine, 11th Scientific meeting, Toronto, 2003:1306.

154. Noseworthy MD, Sussman MS, Haider M, Baruchel S. Dynamic contrast enhanced liver MRI using a motion tracking algorithm. In: Proceedings of the International Society of Magnetic Resonance in Medicine, Glasgow, Scotland, 2001:2240.

155. Tanner C, Schnabel JA, Degenhard A, et al. Validation of volume preserving non rigid registration: application to contrast enhanced MR mammography. In: Proceedings of MICCAI'02: Springer Verlag, 2002:307–314.

156. Leach MO, Brindle KM, Evelhoch JL, et al. Assessment of anti-angiogenic and anti-vascular therapeutics using Magnetic Resonance Imaging: recommendations for appropriate methodology for clinical trials. In: American Association for Cancer Research, Washington D.C., 2003:504.

157. Fritz-Hansen T, Rostrup E, Larsson HB, Sondergaard L, Ring P, Henriksen O. Measurement of the arterial concentration of Gd-DTPA using MRI: a step toward quantitative perfusion imaging. Magn Reson Med 1996; 36(2):225–231.

158. Rijpkema M, Kaanders JH, Joosten FB, van der Kogel AJ, Heerschap A. Method for quantitative mapping of dynamic MRI contrast agent uptake in human tumors. J Magn Reson Imaging 2001; 14(4):457–463.

159. Hayes C, Padhani AR, Leach MO. Assessing changes in tumour vascular function using dynamic contrast-enhanced magnetic resonance imaging. NMR Biomed 2002; 15(2):154–163.

160. Zhu XP, Li KL, Checkley DR, et al. Quantification of endothelial permeability, leakage space, and blood volume in brain tumors using combined T1 and T2* contrast-enhanced dynamic MR imaging. J Magn Reson Imaging 2000; 11(6):575–585.

161. Collins D, Walker S, Dzik-Jurasz AS, Leach MO. Fractal analysis of parametric images derived from dynamic contrast enhanced MRI data in-vivo: methods for describing dispersion in parametric data. In: Proceedings of the International Society of Magnetic Resonance in Medicine, Toronto, 2003:1269.

12

Functional Computed Tomography

Ken Miles

Brighton and Sussex Medical School, Falmer, Brighton, U.K.

A Note from the Editors

---

*T*he main aspect of tumor biology that can be assessed by functional computed tomography (CT) is the assessment of vasculature. The pioneer of this technique explains how the evolution of CT systems and analysis software now enables functional CT to be incorporated into routine patient examinations. Major constraints are discussed, including the limited volume of tissue that can be examined, susceptibility to motion artifacts particularly for lung and liver evaluations, and radiation exposure because the need to minimize photon noise is paramount. It is the linear relationship between measurements of X-ray attenuation by CT (HU) and concentration of iodination contrast medium that is fundamental to the quantification of attenuation-time data. Application of single compartment models to the data enables tissue perfusion to be determined. Two-compartment model analysis enables the determination of other vascular characteristics including blood volume, capillary permeability, and extra-vascular-extracellular leakage space. Potential clinical applications of functional CT are discussed, including lung lesion characterization and detection of occult liver metastases in patients with colorectal cancer. Monitoring responses to conventional treatments including chemotherapy and radiation as well as new anti-angiogenesis treatments are important applications. The assessment of activity of residual disease at the end of definitive therapy and patient prognostication are additional promising clinical areas in need of research. Clinical data to date show that in brain applications, it is the permeability component that provides the greatest discriminate power. In extra-cranial applications of functional CT, it is the differences in tissue perfusion that appears most important. Ongoing technical developments including hardware improvements will enable increased anatomical coverage; reduced radiation dose will occur by modulation of exposure according to body shape and with improved detector technology. These developments together with the introduction of combination PET/CT systems will improve the mapping of metabolism to tissue perfusion (demand and supply), which should enable an improved understanding of tumor biology and the nature of response to therapy.

245

INTRODUCTION

Since its introduction by Godfrey Hounsfield in 1971, computed tomography (CT) has largely been recognized as a powerful imaging tool for demonstrating internal anatomy. However, CT also has the ability to quantify physiological processes, as was first shown in 1980 when Axel (1) published a methodology for the determination of cerebral blood flow by rapid-sequence CT. At that time, the speed of image acquisition and data processing of conventional CT systems was too slow for the technique to become widely accepted. Thus, throughout the 1980s, use of CT to quantify physiological processes was largely confined to studies of myocardial and renal blood flow using electron-beam CT systems, restricting its application to research only (2,3). The development of faster, spiral CT systems in the 1990s enabled the development of methodologies that could measure tissue perfusion and other physiological processes on conventional CT systems that were widely available (4). Interest in this area has been stimulated further, by the introduction of multislice CT and by the release of commercial perfusion CT software from a number of major equipment manufacturers. The first reported assessment of tumor physiology by conventional spiral CT was in 1993, which was a study of hepatic perfusion, including patients with metastases (5). This chapter aims to describe the current capabilities of CT in the assessment of tumor physiology, to describe the technique's advantages and limitations, and to identify future potential developments.

FUNCTIONAL CT AND TUMOR PHYSIOLOGY

The main aspect of tumor biology that is accessible with CT is the physiology of the tumor vasculature. CT measurements of perfusion and other aspects of vascular physiology can therefore provide a noninvasive imaging marker for tumor angiogenesis in vivo. Angiogenesis has emerged as an important topic within oncology not only because tumors are dependent on vascularization for their ability to grow and metastasize, but also because angiogenesis is a potential target for anticancer therapeutic agents. Angiogenesis in turn, reflects the genetic phenotype of the tumor. For instance, p53 oncogene expression has been linked to angiogenesis (6). Thus, perfusion CT has the potential to indirectly evaluate tumor gene expression.

CT can assess vascular physiology by measuring the temporal changes in X-ray attenuation that occur in major blood vessels and tissues after intravenous administration of conventional iodinated X-ray contrast agents. The measured increase in attenuation, quantified in Hounsfield units (HU), is proportional to the concentration of iodine; 1mg/mL being approximately equivalent to 25 HU. From a series of images acquired over time[a], it is possible to derive time-attenuation curves that depict temporal changes in iodine concentration within the tissues and vascular system, thus enabling the contrast agent to be used as a physiological indicator. The pharmacokinetic properties of the contrast agent will determine the physiological processes available for study. The behavior of X-ray contrast agents in vivo approximates a two-compartmental model with intravascular and extravascular components and hence, with suitable physiological modeling, it is possible to measure perfusion, relative blood volume, vascular permeability, and relative

---

[a] Such an image series is sometimes referred to as "dynamic contrast enhanced CT."

Table 1 Semiquantitative and Absolute Physiological Parameters That Can Be Derived by Functional CT

Semi quantitative parameters	Absolute physiological parameters
Enhancement rate	Perfusion including hepatic arterial, portal and HPI
Peak tissue enhancement	Standardized perfusion value
Time to peak enhancement	Mean transit time
Area of tissue enhancement curve	Relative blood volume
Wash-out rate	Capillary permeability
	Relative extravascular volume (leakage space)

Note: The semiquantitative parameters have been aligned with their nearest physiological equivalent.
Abbreviation: HPI, hepatic perfusion index.

extravascular volume (sometimes referred to as "leakage space") (Table 1) (7). Even without physiological modeling, simple enhancement characteristics will reflect vascular physiology. In particular, the maximal enhancement within a tumor, when corrected for dose of contrast agent and patient's weight, provides an estimate of the ratio of tumor perfusion to mean perfusion throughout the body, dubbed as the standardized perfusion value (SPV) (8). The term "functional CT" can be applied to any of these semiquantitative or absolute measurements acquired using CT.

Tumor angiogenesis is morphologically characterized by increased numbers of small blood vessels. This increased microvessel density (MVD) translates in vivo to increased tumor perfusion and blood volume. Tumor microvessels also have incomplete basement membranes that are abnormally leaky to circulating molecules, resulting in increased permeability and size of the extravascular space. Thus, the physiological parameters captured by functional CT can provide correlates for the microvascular changes of angiogenesis. Indeed, peak tumor-enhancement has been shown to correlate with histological measurements of MVD in lung and renal cancer and with the expression of vascular endothelial growth factor (VEGF) in lung cancer (9–11).

PHYSIOLOGICAL MODELS

The methods most commonly used to quantify vascular physiology by analysis of temporal changes in contrast enhancement on CT, have been developed from compartmental analysis and linear systems theory (deconvolution). In either case, time-attenuation data is required not only from the tissue of interest but also from the vascular system. Pixel-by-pixel analysis enables generation of quantified parametric images, often color-coded, to display intratumoral variations in perfusion or other physiological aspects. Commercial software developers have adopted both methods. For example, Siemens and Picker use compartmental analysis while General Electric have implemented a linear systems approach. The methods are summarized below, with a full description available elsewhere (7).

Compartmental Analysis

A one-compartmental model is used for measurement of tumor perfusion while a two-compartmental analysis allows determination of blood volume, capillary permeability, and leakage space.

The one-compartmental model applies the Fick principle to data obtained during the first pass of contrast. If the organ concentration of contrast material is measured before any contrast agent leaves the organ of interest, then tissue blood flow per unit volume (F/V), i.e., perfusion, can be determined by:

$$\frac{F}{V} = \frac{[dC_t/dt(\max)]}{C_a(\max)} \tag{1}$$

or

$$\frac{F}{V} = \frac{C_t(\max)}{\int_0^t C_a(t)dt} \tag{2}$$

where C_t and C_a are the tissue and arterial concentrations, respectively, of the contrast material at any time (t). For (Eq. (1)), dC_t/dt (max) is derived from the maximal slope of the tissue concentration–time curve and C_a (max) from the peak height of the arterial curve. This technique was first applied to CT by Miles (12), and is sometimes called the "slope method". For (Eq. (2)), $C_t(\max)$ is the peak height of the tissue curve and $\int_0^t C_a(t)\,dt$ is the area under the arterial curve corrected for recirculation using a gamma variate fit. This implementation is also known as the Mullani–Gould method (13).

The two-compartmental model is mathematically given by:

$$Q(t) = V_b.C_a(t) + K^{\text{trans}}.\int_0^t C_a(u)e^{-(K^{\text{trans}}/Ve)(t-u)}du \tag{3}$$

where $Q(t)$ is the quantity of contrast material in the tissue of interest, V_b the relative blood volume, $C_a(t)$ the arterial concentration at time (t), K^{trans} the tissue permeability, and V_e the relative volume of the extravascular space or leakage space. $Q(t)$ and $C_a(t)$ are determined by the tissue and arterial concentration–time curves, respectively. To derive values for all the three physiological parameters, the equation must be solved iteratively. Alternatively, if it is assumed that back flux of contrast medium from extravascular to intravascular compartments is negligible for the first 60 to 120 seconds after contrast medium administration, Patlak analysis can be used to measure capillary permeability and relative blood volume.

Linear Systems Approach (Deconvolution)

The mathematical process of deconvolution, applied to the arterial and tissue concentration–time curves, can determine the impulse residue function (IRF) for the tissue of interest, where the IRF is a theoretical tissue curve that could be obtained from an instantaneous arterial input. The tissue concentration (C_t) of contrast medium at any time (t) is given by:

$$C_t(t) = F/V .[C_a(t) * R(t)] = C_a(t) * F/V . R(t) \tag{4}$$

where $R(t)$ is the IRF and $*$ denotes the convolution operator [other symbols as for Eqs. (1–3)]. To simplify the calculation, the IRF can be constrained in its shape to comprise a plateau followed by a single exponential decay. The height of the flow corrected IRF will give the tissue perfusion (F/V), and the area under the curve will determine the relative blood volume. This approach can also be extended to include a measurement of capillary permeability by use of a distributed parameter model. This method essentially uses curve stripping to separate the IRF into flow and permeability components.

TECHNICAL VALIDATION AND REPRODUCIBILITY

Perfusion CT methods have typically been validated against either microsphere methods in animals studies or stable xenon-washout methods and O^{15}-water positron-emission tomography (PET) in humans. The Mullani–Gould formulation has been validated against microspheres in canine myocardial studies, and the slope method has been successfully validated in humans and animals for abdominal organs and the brain (3,5,14–18). The deconvolution method has been validated against microspheres in normal brain tissue and cerebral tumors, and against stable xenon–CT in human cerebral studies (19–21). Permeability being fundamentally dependent on the molecular size and charge of the physiological indicator used, its measurements have proved hard to validate.

Reproducibility of CT measurements of perfusion has been assessed in a number of studies. The only tumor-specific study that evaluated the reproducibility of the deconvolution method as applied to brain tumors, reports a variability of 13% (21). Repeated cerebral perfusion studies in normal animals have shown variations ranging between 26% and 35% when using small regions of interest, and with greater variability in white matter (21,22). Using the slope method to measure cerebral perfusion in humans, Gillard et al. (23) found little variability in repeated CT studies in seven patients, performed 24 hours apart ($r = 0.88$). The data produced a variability of 13% when reanalyzed using the GE deconvolution software (Griffiths MR 2002, personal communication). Reproducibility is an important issue when considering the use of perfusion CT to monitor the effects of therapeutic interventions. In comparison to the variability reported above, reductions in perfusion due to antiangiogenesis drug therapy range from 30% to greater than 90% (24,25).

Interoperator reproducibility has proved to be good with a correlation coefficient (r-value) of 0.94 with an interoperator variability of 8% as reported by Griffiths for splenic perfusion calculated using the slope method (preliminary PhD submission, Queensland University of Technology, 1999). Similar interoperator results were reported by Blomley et al. (16) for peak aortic CT number ($r^2 = 0.99$) and liver slope values ($r^2 = 0.83$) using the slope method and electron beam CT.

Preliminary investigations of the comparability of perfusion values from the slope method and deconvolution method in lung nodule, spleen, and normal brain have showed good correlations ($r = 0.86$, $r = 0.90$, and $r = 0.79$; Griffiths MR, 2001 personal communication). The slope method tended to produce lower perfusion values than the deconvolution method but further cross calibration studies are required.

CLINICAL VALIDATION AND APPLICATIONS IN ONCOLOGY

The most appropriate parameter for any particular tumor application is yet to be determined. In general, permeability measurements are most applicable to the brain because permeability levels within tumors are considerably higher in comparison to the almost impermeable blood-brain barrier, whereas tumor perfusion values are often close to those of the normal cerebral cortex. In other body regions, the differences in permeability between malignant and normal tissues are lower and measurements of tumor perfusion and blood volume are often more appropriate. In liver, functional CT can quantify hepatic arterial and portal perfusion separately (8). For both primary and secondary liver tumors, new vessels are derived almost exclusively from the arterial system and hence arterial values may be most relevant for hepatic mass lesions. However, micrometastatic disease within the liver is associated with alterations in hepatic portal perfusion, even when the tumor burden is very low (e.g., 0.5 mm metastases) (26).

The use of functional CT to characterize solitary pulmonary nodules (SPNs) illustrates the diagnostic capability of the technique, exploiting the differences in MVD between benign and malignant lesions. Using a variety of techniques, several studies have measured peak enhancement, perfusion, or other functional CT parameters in SPNs and have consistently shown sensitivity and specificity values of 88–100% and 36–85%, respectively, for the detection of malignancy (8,27–29). The lower specificity reflects the fact that some inflammatory lesions exhibit high enhancement and perfusion values; low values within a nodule are highly predictive for benignity and may be cost saving by avoiding additional investigations such as fine needle aspiration or fluorodeoxyglucose PET (FDG-PET) (30).

CT measurements of hepatic perfusion and enhancement can improve the staging of cancer by inferring the presence of hepatic micrometastases, a phenomenon that may account for the fact that many patients with an apparently normal liver as found by conventional staging investigations subsequently develop overt metastases in the next 18–24 months. Increased hepatic parenchymal enhancement during dual-phase spiral CT with increased arterial phase enhancement has been shown to herald the subsequent development of overt lesions and occult hepatic metastases have also been identified as areas of high perfusion on CT-derived images of hepatic perfusion (31–34) . Nodal staging may also be improved by quantifying contrast enhancement within nodes. Malignant nodes in gastric cancer have been shown to enhance more avidly reflecting increased perfusion as a result of tumor-associated angiogenesis (35).

The recognized association between greater tumor angiogenesis and a poorer prognosis is reflected by the ability of functional CT to stratify risk for patients with cancer. Functional CT parameters are frequently more abnormal in tumors of higher grade or advanced stage and among patients with shortened survival. High-grade gliomas demonstrate increased blood volume and heterogeneity on blood volume images, and CT perfusion values above 0.5 mL/min/mL in lymphoma masses have been shown to imply high- or intermediate-grade tumor (Fig. 1) (36,37). Lung tumors of more advanced stage have demonstrated higher CT perfusion values (38); CT measurements of perfusion in head and neck cancers are significantly different between tumors with a favorable and an unfavorable outcome following radiotherapy (39). Survival of patients with hepatic metastases appears to correlate with hepatic perfusion measured by CT. Increased arterial perfusion, particularly in the periphery of the lesion, is associated with longer survival (40). Furthermore, preliminary data from patients with metastatic colon cancer suggest that low portal perfusion throughout the liver (i.e., below 0.3 mL/min/mL) is associated with progressive disease and a poor response to chemotherapy (36,41). Risk stratification is an emerging aspect of cancer care, with the potential to individualize

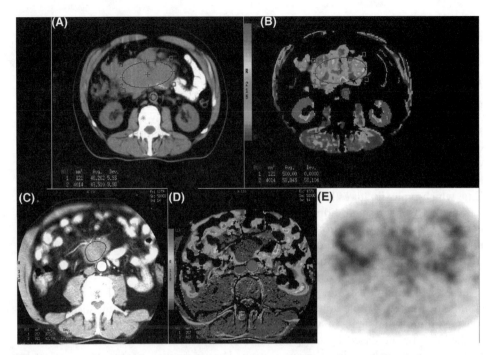

Figure 1 Perfusion CT in lymphoma. *Top row*: The mass seen on conventional CT (**A**) demonstrates perfusion values greater than 50 mL/min/mL on functional CT (**B**), implying active intermediate-/high-grade lymphoma. *Bottom row*: In another patient, conventional CT (**C**), demonstrates a residual mass following lymphoma chemotherapy. Perfusion CT (**D**) shows low perfusion (9 mL/min/mL) implying inactive disease as is confirmed by low FDG uptake on PET (**E**). (*See color insert.*)

the patient's treatment by matching the therapy to the tumor biology. Patients with aggressive tumors may be suitable for additional treatment, or invasive local treatments could be withheld when unlikely to be of benefit. The use of functional CT to predict tumor behavior in vivo could avoid the biopsy-sampling error that may occur due to tumor heterogeneity when using histological markers of aggression. Imaging assessments may also be of value when biopsy is difficult (e.g., brain tumors), or as an alternative to repeated biopsy when there is a propensity for tumor biology to change with time.

Studies that have used functional CT to measure changes in tumor vascular physiology following chemotherapy or radiotherapy illustrate potential for the technique to monitor cancer therapy. Such studies include the measurement of changes in the permeability of cerebral glioma in response to steroid therapy and to the bradykinin analogue RMP-7, reductions in tumor perfusion following successful lymphoma chemotherapy (Fig. 1), and during treatment of metastatic colon cancer with BW12C (37,42–44). Radiotherapy-induced changes in tumor perfusion and permeability have been reported by Harvey et al. (45,46). An important consideration when monitoring the effects of therapeutic agents upon tumor perfusion is the possibility that the drug will induce generalized vascular response whereby a change in total cardiac output can alter the perfusion within a tumor with no change in microvascular density. The SPV, which normalizes the tumor perfusion to mean whole-perfusion as given by the cardiac output (l/min) per kilogram body weight, will remain unaffected by a change in cardiac output alone and may therefore be more suitable for therapeutic monitoring than perfusion measurements.

ADVANTAGES AND LIMITATIONS

A major advantage of functional CT is that it can be readily incorporated into existing CT protocols that remain the mainstay for the staging and follow-up of patients with cancer. The technique requires no more than a conventional CT scanner and standard contrast agents and the additional data acquisition adds only a few minutes to the normal time of examination. Commercial software has simplified data processing, which typically takes less than 10 minutes, and can yield multiple physiological parameters from a single administration of contrast agent. The linear relationship between measured attenuation and concentration of contrast agents makes the absolute quantification of physiological parameters relatively simple, and the physiological information obtained can be displayed as parametric maps with high spatial resolution.

A significant constraint upon the application of functional CT to assess perfusion is the limited sample volume available for study. Even with multislice scanners, the maximum axial field of view is of the order of 20 mm. The volume of tissue studied can be increased by using multiple spiral acquisitions or by "toggling" the scan back and forth during the acquisition. However, such protocols are offset by reduced temporal resolution to one image every five seconds, as compared to as short as every 0.5–1 second for some protocols without table movement (47).

Movement of the patient during acquisition of the image sequence can create significant problems for functional CT, particularly while imaging organs such as the lung or liver, that are subject to respiratory motion. Motion artifacts can be minimized by acquiring images during quiet respiration while instructing the patient to carefully avoid deep breaths. Protocols that utilize respiratory gating are under development but may increase the time between image acquisitions when used. Some software packages have adopted image registration methods to make correction for motion within the image plane.

The radiation exposure associated with functional CT is a disadvantage relative to techniques such as ultrasound and magnetic resonance imaging that do not use ionizing radiation. However, the radiation burden (1–5 mSv depending upon body region examined) is relatively low, especially in the context of oncology where many patients undergo radiotherapy. Acquisition protocols must balance the radiation exposure against the benefit of increased image frequency. Rapid acquisitions of every 0.5–1 second usually adopt lower beam intensities (e.g., 50–100 mAs) but at the expense of increased photon noise within each individual image. The slope method for determination of perfusion [Eq. (1)] is particularly prone to errors from photon noise. Thus, greater beam intensities (e.g., 200–400 mAs) but reduced image frequency (every 2 to 3 seconds) are preferable when using this method. Administering more contrast agent, preferably at a greater concentration rather than increased volume, can also reduce the effects of photon noise. Determination of perfusion by compartmental analysis assumes the condition that none of the contrast bolus has left the tissue of interest at the time of measurement. For tissues with short vascular transit times, larger volumes of contrast agent and longer bolus times may result in failure to meet this assumed condition, leading to underestimation of perfusion, particularly when using the Mullani–Gould method [Eq. (2)].

FUTURE DEVELOPMENTS

Technical developments that would advance functional CT include more sophisticated CT technologies that vary the X-ray exposure during the scan rotation, thus reducing the radiation dose associated with repeated volume acquisitions. Development of new contrast agents with longer intravascular residence time may also overcome some of the complexities of physiological modeling required for conventional contrast agents that exhibit two-compartmental pharmacokinetics.

The recent introduction of integrated PET/CT systems affords the particularly exciting prospect of combining perfusion CT data with FDG-PET in a single examination while minimizing image misregistration. Perfusion CT measurements can be combined with PET measurements of FDG uptake, in a number of ways. Incorporating CT perfusion measurements into kinetic analysis of FDG uptake enables determination of FDG extraction fraction. The standardized uptake value (SUV) to quantify FDG uptake in PET has a derivation similar to the SPV proposed for functional CT in which, both parameters are normalized to whole body measurements. Thus, SUV and SPV can be used additively and the ratio of SUV to SPV provide an index of FDG extraction. Tumor perfusion and glucose metabolism are aspects of tumor function with a complex interaction. SUV measurements in lung nodules have shown correlations with peak enhancement and SPV on CT (8,48). Despite the fact that both angiogenesis and increased glucose metabolism are common phenotypic expressions of cancer cells, the relationship between these two processes is more complex than a simple correlation. Although acquired on different systems, preliminary experience of combining perfusion CT and FDG-PET has shown that the sum of SUV and SPV correlated with staging of lung cancer more closely than either parameter taken alone (Fig. 2) (49). Tumors frequently exhibit a ''burst'' of angiogenesis before periods of accelerated growth, and thus by evaluating the balance between metabolic demand (FDG uptake) and supply (perfusion), combined perfusion CT/FDG-PET measurements may provide an assessment of tumor aggression. Indeed, in the above

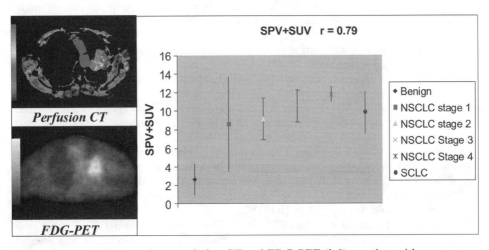

Figure 2 Combined data from perfusion CT and FDG-PET (*left*) correlate with tumor stage in lung cancer (*right*). *Abbreviations*: SPV, standardized perfusion value; SUV, standardized uptake value. (*See color insert.*)

combined study, the most advanced cancers (i.e., stage 4) exhibited a relative excess of perfusion (49).

Combined perfusion CT/FDG-PET measurements may also be of advantage for therapeutic monitoring. For example, tumor metabolism and perfusion may become uncoupled during antiangiogenesis therapy and hence combined perfusion CT/FDG-PET could enable quantitative assessment of the contribution that reduced perfusion makes toward an apparent metabolic response (24).

SUMMARY

Functional CT redefines CT as a technique that can depict vascular physiology of tumors in addition to detailed anatomy with the potential to provide in vivo markers of tumor angiogenesis. The accumulated data on technical validation and clinical application at this time have reached a critical mass sufficient for the equipment manufacturers to offer perfusion CT software packages commercially. Functional CT is readily incorporated into the patient's routine CT examination, and clinical experience has identified roles for the technique in cancer diagnosis, staging, risk stratification, and therapeutic monitoring. Using integrated PET/CT systems to combine perfusion CT with FDG-PET creates opportunities for advanced characterization of tumor biology.

REFERENCES

1. Axel L. Cerebral blood flow determination by rapid-sequence computed tomography: theoretical analysis. Radiology 1980; 137:679.
2. Jaschke W, Sievers RS, Lipton MJ, Cogan MG. Cine-CT computed tomographic assessment of regional renal blood flow. Acta Radiologica 1989; 31:77–81.
3. Wolfkiel CJ, Ferguson JL, Chomka EV, et al. Measurement of myocardial blood flow by ultrafast computed tomography. Circulation 1987; 76:1262–1273.
4. Miles KA, Hayball MP, Dixon AK. Colour Perfusion Imaging: a new application of computed tomography. Lancet 1991; 337:643–645.
5. Miles KA, Hayball MP, Dixon AK. Functional images of hepatic perfusion obtained with dynamic computed tomography. Radiology 1993; 188:405–411.
6. Fontanini G, Vignati S, Lucchi M, et al. Neoangiogenesis and p53 protein in lung cancer: their prognostic role and their relation with vascular endothelial growth factor (VEGF) expression. Br J Cancer 1997; 75:1295–1301.
7. Miles KA, Charnsangavej C, Lee F, Fishman E, Horton K, Lee T-Y. Application of CT in the investigation of angiogenesis in oncology. Acad Radiol 2000; 7:840–850.
8. Miles KA, Griffiths MR, Fuentes MA. Standardized perfusion value: universal CT contrast enhancement scale that correlates with FDG PET in lung nodules. Radiology 2001; 220:548–553.
9. Swensen SJ, Brown LR, Colby TV, Weaver AL, Midthun DE. Lung nodule enhancement at CT: prospective findings. Radiology 1996; 201:447–455.
10. Tateishi U, Nishihara H, Watanabe S, Morikawa T, Abe K, Miyasaka K. Tumor angiogenesis and dynamic CT in lung adenocarcinoma: radiologic-pathologic correlation. J Comput Assist Tomogr 2001; 25:23–27.
11. Jinzaki M, Tanimoto A, Mukai M, et al. Double-phase helical CT of small renal parenchymal neoplasms: correlation with pathologic findings and tumor angiogenesis. J Comput Assist Tomogr 2000; 24:835–842.
12. Miles KA. Measurement of tissue perfusion by dynamic computed tomography. Br J Radiol 1991; 64:409–412.

13. Mullani N, Gould KL. First pass measurements of regional blood flow using external detectors. J Nucl Med 1983; 24:577–581.
14. Rumberger JA, Feiring AJ, Lipton MJ, Higgins CB, Ell SR, Marcus ML. Use of ultra-fast computed tomography to quantitate regional myocardial perfusion: a preliminary report. J Am Coll Cardiol 1987; 9:59–69.
15. Gould RG, Lipton MJ, McNamara MT, Sievers RE, Koshold S, Higgins CB. Measurement of regional myocardial blood flow in dogs by ultrafast CT. Invest Radiol 1988; 23:348–353.
16. Blomley MJ, Coulden R, Bufkin CRT, Lipton MJ, Dawson P. Contrast-bolus dynamic computed tomography for the measurement of solid organ perfusion. Invest Radiol 1993; 28(suppl 5):S72–S77.
17. Hattori H, Miyoshi T, Okada J, Yoshikawa K, Arimizu N, Hattori N. Tumor blood flow measured using dynamic computed tomography. Invest Radiol 1994; 29:873–876.
18. Gillard JH, Minhas PS, Hayball MP, et al. Assessment of quantitative computed tomographic cerebral perfusion imaging with H2(15)O positron emission tomography. Neurol Res 2000; 22:457–464.
19. Cenic A, Nabavi DG, Craen RA, Gelb AW, Lee TY. Dynamic CT measurement of cerebral blood flow: a validation study. Am J Neuroradiol 1999; 20:63–73.
20. Wintermark M, Thiran JP, Maeder P, Schnyder P, Meuli R. Simultaneous measurement of regional cerebral blood flow by perfusion CT and stable xenon CT: a validation study. Am J Neuroradiol 2001; 22:905–914.
21. Cenic A, Nabavi DG, Craen RA, Gelb AW, Lee TY. A CT method to measure hemodynamics in brain tumors: validation and application to cerebral blood flow maps. Am J Neuroradiol 2000; 21:462–470.
22. Nabavi DG, Cenic A, Dool J, et al. Quantitative assessment of cerebral hemodynamics using CT: stability, accuracy, and precision studies in dogs. J Comput Assist Tomogr 1999; 23:506–515.
23. Gillard JH, Antoun NM, Burnet NG, Pickard JD. Reproducibility of quantitative CT perfusion imaging. Br J Radiol 2001; 74:552–555.
24. Mullani N, Herbst R, Abbruzzese J, et al. Antiangiogenic treatment with endostatin results in uncoupling of blood flow and glucose metabolism in human tumors. Clin Positron Imaging 2000; 3:151.
25. Maxwell RJ, Wilson J, Prise VE, Vojnovic B, Rustin GJ, Lodge MA, Tozer GM. Evaluation of the anti-vascular effects of combretastatin in rodent tumours by dynamic contrast enhanced MRI. NMR Biomed 2002; 15:89–98.
26. Cuenod CA, Leconte I, Siauve N, et al. Early changes in liver perfusion caused by occult metastases in rats: detection with quantitative CT. Radiology 2001; 218:556–561.
27. Swensen SJ, Viggiano RW, Midthun DE, et al. Lung nodule enhancement at CT: multi-center study. Radiology 2000; 214:73–80.
28. Zhang M, Kono M. Solitary pulmonary nodules: evaluation of blood flow patterns with dynamic CT. Radiology 1997; 205:471–478.
29. Yamashita K, Matsunobe S, Tsuda T, Nemoto T, et al. Solitary pulmonary nodules: preliminary study of evaluation with incremental dynamic CT. Radiology 1995; 194:399–405.
30. Comber LA, Keith CJ, Griffiths MR, Miles KA. Solitary pulmonary nodules: impact of quantitative contrast enhanced CT on the cost-effectiveness of FDG-PET. Clin Radiol 2003; 58:706–711.
31. Platt JF, Francis IR, Ellis JH, Reige KA. Liver metastases: early detection based on abnormal contrast material enhancement at dual-phase helical CT. Radiology 1997; 205:49–53.
32. Sheafor DH, Killius JS, Paulson EK, DeLong DM, Foti AM, Nelson RC. Hepatic parenchymal enhancement during triple-phase helical CT: can it be used to predict which patients with breast cancer will develop hepatic metastases? Radiology 2000; 214:875–880.

33. Leggett DA, Kelley BB, Bunce IH, Miles KA. Colorectal cancer: diagnostic potential of CT measurements of hepatic perfusion and implications for contrast enhancement protocols. Radiology 1997; 205:716–720.

34. Dugdale, PE, Miles, KA. Hepatic metastases: the value of quantitative assessment of contrast enhancement on computed tomography. Eur J Radiol 1999; 30:206–213.

35. Fukuya T, Honda H, Hayashi T, et al. Lymph-node metastases: efficacy of detection with helical CT in patients with gastric cancer. Radiology 1995; 197:705–711.

36. Leggett DAC, Miles KA, Kelley BB. Blood-brain barrier and blood volume imaging of cerebral glioma using functional CT: a pictorial review. Australasian Radiology 1998; 42:335–340.

37. Dugdale PE, Miles KA, Kelley BB, Bunce IH, Leggett DAC. CT measurements of perfusion and permeability within lymphoma masses: relationship to grade, activity and chemotherapeutic response. J Comput Tomogr 1999; 23:540–547.

38. Miles KA, Sommerfeld NWB, Griffiths M. CT measurement of perfusion within lung masses: correlation with tumour stage and FDG-PET. Imaging, Oncology & Science, Birmingham UK, 2000:Abstract No. 357.

39. Hermans R, Lambin P, Van den Bogaert W, Haustermans K, Van der Goten A, Baert AL. Non-invasive tumour perfusion measurement by dynamic CT: preliminary results. Radiother Oncol 1997; 44:159–162.

40. Miles KA, Leggett DA, Kelley BB, Hayball MP, Sinnatamby R, Bunce I. In vivo assessment of neovascularization of liver metastases using perfusion CT. Br J Radiol 1998; 71:276–281.

41. Sommerfeld N, Miles K, Dugdale P, Leggett D, Bunce I. Colorectal cancer: progressive disease is associated with altered liver perfusion on functional CT. 50th Annual Meeting of the Royal Australia & New Zealand College of Radiologists, 1999.

42. Yeung WT, Lee TY, Del Maestro RF, Kozak R, Bennett J, Brown T. Effect of steroids on iopamidol blood-brain transfer constant and plasma volume in brain tumors measured with X-ray computed tomography. J Neurooncol 1994; 18:53–60.

43. Ford J, Miles K, Hayball M, Bearcroft P, Bleehan N, Osborn C. A simplified method for measurement of blood-brain barrier permeability using CT: Preliminary results and the effect of RMP-7. In: Faulkner K, et al., eds. Quantitative Imaging in Oncology. London: British Institute of Radiology, 1996:1–5.

44. Falk SJ, Ramsay JR, Ward R, Miles K, Dixon AK, Bleehen NM. BW12C perturbs normal and tumour tissue oxygenation and blood flow in man. Radiother Oncol 1994; 32:210–217.

45. Harvey C, Dooher A, Morgan J, Blomley M, Dawson P. Imaging of tumour therapy responses by dynamic CT. Eur J Radiol 1999; 30:221–226.

46. Harvey CJ, Blomley MJ, Dawson P, et al. Functional CT imaging of the acute hyperemic response to radiation therapy of the prostate gland: early experience. J Comput Assist Tomogr 2001; 25:43–49.

47. Roberts HC, Roberts TP, Smith WS, Lee TJ, Fischbein NJ, Dillon WP. Multisection dynamic CT perfusion for acute cerebral ischemia: the "toggling-table" technique. Am J Neuroradiol 2001; 22:1077–1080.

48. Tateishi U, Nishihara H, Tsukamoto E, Morikawa T, Tamaki N, Miyasaka K. Lung tumours evaluated with FDG-PET and dynamic CT: the relationship between vascular density and glucose metabolism. J Comput Assist Tomogr 2002; 26:185–190.

49. Miles KA, Griffiths MR, Comber L, Keith CJ, Fuentes M. Functional imaging of cancer: combining perfusion CT with FDG-PET. Cancer Imaging 2002; 3:17–18.

13

BOLD Imaging of Tumors

Simon P. Robinson
Division of Basic Medical Sciences, St. George's, University of London, London, U.K.

A Note from the Editors

*I*n this chapter, one of the key researchers who has scientifically
assessed intrinsic-susceptibility contrast (BOLD) MRI in
tumors, describes how gradient recalled echo images, sensitive
to endogenous paramagnetic deoxyhemoglobin within tumor blood
vessels can be utilized to assess tumor oxygenation, angiogenesis,
and response to antivascular therapies. The author explains how the
transverse MRI relaxation rate R_2^* of tissue can be quantified and
why synthetic R_2^* maps are free of contributions from blood flow.
The use of tumor R_2^* as a sensitive index of tissue oxygenation, and
the evaluation of tumor vascular maturation and function by
measuring changes in R_2^* in response to hypercapnia and hyperoxia,
is subsequently explained. Finally, the use of R_2^* as a biomarker
of response to antivascular therapy is discussed. The primary
advantage of BOLD MRI techniques for the assessement of tumors
is the high temporal and spatial resolution afforded by ^1H MRI, and
that there is no need to administer contrast material. Measurements
can thus be repeated as needed with almost no limitation. Major
limitations of BOLD MRI are low contrast-to-noise ratio in the
images obtained, and clinical studies with vasomodulation using
carbogen (95% O_2/5% CO_2) are technically challenging with a
high failure rate.

INTRODUCTION

The functional and morphological characteristics of tumor vasculature are critical determinants of tumor growth, metastatic potential, and therapeutic response (1,2). For example, tumors require a nutritive blood supply in order to proliferate, and high vascular density has been linked to poor prognosis (3–5). A functional tumor blood supply also dictates the potential to improve tumor oxygenation for optimizing radiotherapy, or for delivering chemotherapeutic agents to the tumor cells. In addition, the tumor vasculature itself has now become an attractive target for antiangiogenic and antivascular therapies (6).

Methods for assessing the tumor vascular status, especially with noninvasive techniques such as magnetic resonance imaging (MRI), are continually being sought to optimize information about tumor pathophysiology (7,8). The ultimate aim is the identification, development, and validation of quantitative clinical MRI indices associated with tumor blood vasculature to assist in planning of individual patient treatment protocols. In addition, these parameters are finding roles as biomarkers in clinical trials of anticancer therapies directed at tumor blood vessels.

The most common functional application of MRI in clinical oncology is dynamic contrast-enhanced (DCE) MRI using the exogenously administered contrast agent gadopentetate dimeglumine (Gd-DTPA), and this is discussed elsewhere in this book. The focus of this chapter is to highlight the potential utility of blood oxygenation level dependent (BOLD) MRI. Throughout this chapter, the term BOLD MRI will be used interchangeably with intrinsic-susceptibility contrast MRI, to acknowledge the primary source of BOLD MRI contrast, endogenous deoxyhemoglobin.

INTRINSIC-SUSCEPTIBILITY CONTRAST MRI

Deoxyhaemoglobin, which is paramagnetic, creates susceptibility variations in the magnetic field increasing the magnetic resonance transverse relaxation rate [R_2^* ($=1/T_2^*$)] of water in blood and in the tissue surrounding blood vessels. MRI methods, such as the gradient recalled echo (GRE) sequence, are sensitive to R_2^* and thus sensitive to blood deoxyhemoglobin levels. Deoxyhemoglobin therefore acts as an intrinsic BOLD contrast agent. BOLD MRI is now routinely used for functional imaging of cognitive function in the brain (9,10), and the methodology is now being used to investigate parameters related to tumor vasculature such as perfusion, blood oxygenation, blood-vessel development, remodeling, and function.

The earliest BOLD MRI studies of tumors demonstrated large decreases in the signal intensity of R_2^*-weighted images of a range of different rodent tumors when the host was given a high oxygen content gas to inhale, usually either 100% oxygen or carbogen (95% O_2/5% CO_2) (11,12). This image intensity decrease is consistent with a reduction in R_2^* because of a decrease in the tissue concentration of deoxyhemoglobin being replaced by well-oxygenated blood, and suggests improved tissue oxygenation which is the therapeutic basis of tumor radiosensitization by oxygen or carbogen breathing. Numerous studies have since demonstrated either oxygen or carbogen-induced decreases in R_2^*-weighted GRE MRI intensity in rodent tumors, and this approach has been translated into the clinic to study human tumors (13–27). Other studies have utilized intrinsic-susceptibility MRI to investigate the effects of other modifiers of the tumor microenvironment such as nicotinamide, hydralazine, angiotensin, calcitonin gene-related peptide (CGRP), the calcium-channel blocker diltiazem, and nitric oxide donors (16,28–32).

The interpretation of the BOLD MRI response to carbogen is complex, and there are several possible mechanisms responsible for the image intensity decrease (33). The primary mechanism is expected to be caused by alterations in the deoxyhemoglobin concentration of tumor blood vessels. A decrease in R_2^*-weighted image intensity will occur if the blood becomes more oxygenated, thereby reducing the amount of para-magnetic deoxyhemoglobin. However, a decrease in the deoxyhemoglobin content

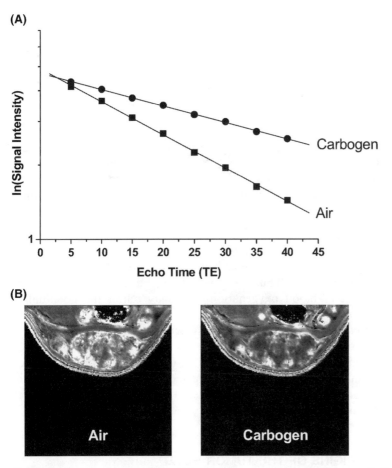

Figure 1 Multi-gradient echo MRI. **(A)** The transverse relaxation rate R_2^* can be determined from signal intensity measurements made at increasing echo times (TE). The plot ln(signal intensity) versus echo time yields a linear graph, the slope of which determines R_2^*. A decrease in the slope implies an increase in the p_aO_2 of blood, as occurs with carbogen (95% O_2/5% CO_2) breathing. As the oxygenation of hemoglobin is proportional to the arterial blood p_aO_2, and therefore in equilibrium with tissue pO_2, measurements of tumor R_2^* should provide a sensitive index of tissue oxygenation. **(B)** Calculated R_2^* maps obtained from a transplanted GH3 pro-lactinoma grown subcutaneously in the flank of a rat while the host breathed air and subse-quently carbogen. Intense regions (relatively fast R_2^*) in the initial air-breathing R_2^* map are consistent with the presence of deoxyhemoglobin, while dark areas (relatively slow R_2^*) are con-sistent with the presence of oxyhemoglobin. Carbogen challenge results in a clear decrease in R_2^* over most of the tumor, indicating a decrease in deoxyhemoglobin.

of tissue will also occur if there is an increase in tumor blood flow, thereby reducing the fraction of oxygen extracted from the blood. To overcome the disadvantage that changes in blood oxygenation and blood flow are not separately distinguished in R_2^*-weighted images acquired at a single echo time, a multi-GRE (MGRE) imaging sequence can be used, from which R_2^* maps can be synthesized. This approach decouples the effects of carbogen-induced changes in blood oxygenation from changes in blood flow, affords quantitative measurements of the tissue transverse relaxation rate R_2^*, and facilitates the interpretation of response to modifiers of the tumor microenvironment (Fig. 1).

The contribution of blood deoxyhemoglobin to the R_2^* relaxation rate of the surrounding tissue can be written as (33):

$$R_2^*(= 1/T_2^*) = R_2^*_{tissue} + R_2^*_{blood} = R_2^*_{tissue} + k \cdot V \cdot (1 - Y) \tag{1}$$

where, k is a constant, V is the blood volume, and Y the tumor blood oxygen saturation, or:

$$R_2^* = R_2^*_{tissue} + k'[dHb] \tag{2}$$

where, [dHb] is the concentration of deoxyhemoglobin in the tissue and R_2^* tissue is assumed to be a static component that is dependent on the structure and content of the tissue. Thus the baseline R_2^* contains a component that depends on the tumor tissue deoxyhemoglobin content ([dHb]), which is a function of the vascular volume of the tumor actively perfused by erythrocytes.

The carbogen-induced change in R_2^* (ΔR_2^*) can be defined by:

$$\Delta R_2^* = \Delta R_2^*_{tissue} + \Delta R_2^*_{blood} = k'\Delta[dHb] \tag{3}$$

where, Δ[dHb] is the change in tissue deoxyhemoglobin concentration caused by challenge with 95% O_2/5% CO_2. Thus ΔR_2^* is determined by both the vascular volume and the change in blood oxygenation, and may reflect the potential to enhance oxygen delivery to the tumor.

Several studies have shown quantitative carbogen-induced decreases in R_2^* in subcutaneous rodent models and, more recently, rat intracranial tumors (33–36). MGRE MRI has been implemented on standard clinical MRI instruments. Good reproducibility of human tumor baseline R_2^* maps has been demonstrated and the quantification of R_2^* and carbogen-induced changes in R_2^* of human head and neck cancers has been demonstrated (37,38).

PHYSIOLOGICAL ORIGINS OF THE TUMOR BOLD MRI RESPONSE TO CARBOGEN

Large differences in the BOLD MRI response to carbogen breathing have been observed between different experimental rodent tumor models. For example, carbogen has been shown to cause large decreases in R_2^* of transplanted rat GH3 prolactinomas, whereas in murine radiation-induced fibrosarcomas (RIF-1) a very small and transient signal increase was observed (14,19). Wide variations have also been observed in the R_2^*-weighted image response of human tumors to carbogen challenge (26,27). In addition to these large intertumoral variations, there is a wide intratumoral heterogeneity in the observed image intensity changes. This heterogeneity of response is interesting, as it suggests that the methodology is interrogating the distribution and function of structurally and functionally abnormal tumor vasculature.

A detailed study of two transplantable rodent tumor models which exhibited extremes of response to carbogen breathing, the GH3 prolactinoma and the RIF-1 , has shed more light on the physiological origins responsible for the varying BOLD MRI responses to carbogen (39). The average basal R_2^*, quantified by MGRE MRI, was significantly faster for the GH3 prolactinoma [$89 \pm 8\,s^{-1}$] compared to the RIF-1 [$58 \pm 4\,s^{-1}$], and the GH3 prolactinoma also showed a large decrease in R_2^* with carbogen breathing ($-23 \pm 4\,s^{-1}$), whereas the RIF-1 response to carbogen was negligible [$1 \pm 1\,s^{-1}$].

The two tumor types were subsequently investigated using susceptibility con-trast-enhanced MRI and immunohistochemistry. Intravascular contrast agents such as ultrasmall superparamagnetic iron oxide (USPIO) particles act similarly to deoxy-hemoglobin as a contrast agent, but are much more powerful in creating magnetic susceptibility variations close to blood vessels, inducing an increase in the transverse relaxation rates R_2^* and R_2 of water in the surrounding tissue (40). Changes in tissue R_2^* caused by USPIOs are dependent on the blood volume, hence an estimate of blood volume can be made by measuring the absolute changes in R_2^* following administration of USPIO. The blood volume of the GH3 prolactinoma was three-fold greater than the RIF-1 (8% vs. 2%). This correlated with a three-fold higher perfused vascular fraction of the GH3 prolactinoma (93%) compared to the RIF-1 (37%), assessed by fluorescence microscopy of tumor uptake of the perfusion marker Hoechst 33342.

In addition to estimating tumor blood volume, the ratio of the changes in tissue R_2^* and R_2 caused by USPIO are dependent on capillary size (40,41). The ratio $\Delta R_2^*/\Delta R_2$ was used to derive estimates of the average microvessel size, and showed that the capillary diameter in the GH3 prolactinoma was of the order of 14 to 21 µm, compared to 5 to 11 µm in the RIF-1 fibrosarcoma.

Both tumor blood volume and capillary size appear to be important determi-nants of the hemodynamic BOLD MRI response to carbogen. If the vascular archi-tecture of the GH3 prolactinoma and RIF-1 were similar, it might be expected that both tumor types would show a similar MRI response to a vascular challenge that altered blood susceptibility, such as by administration of a USPIO contrast agent or by altering the endogenous deoxyhemoglobin with carbogen breathing. Both tumor types showed a significant change in transverse relaxation rates after USPIO administration, and which was three-fold greater in the GH3 prolactinoma (39). On this basis, the carbogen-induced decrease in R_2^* of the RIF-1 would have been expected to be of the order ca. 8 s^{-1}. However, the RIF-1 response to carbogen breath-ing was negligible, suggesting that it has a different vascular architecture to the GH3 prolactinoma, possible differences being a lower fractional blood volume and a smal-ler, more tortuous vascular morphology. These studies show that the magnitude of the ΔR_2^* response to carbogen is determined by both the tumor blood volume and capil-lary size. As the blood volume of the RIF-1 fibrosarcoma is one-quarter that of the GH3 prolactinoma, the response to carbogen would be accordingly reduced. In addition, the small capillary diameter (and hence reduced hematocrit) would hinder erythrocyte accessibility (the source of intrinsic-susceptibility contrast)—additional reasons for the lack of R_2^* change in the RIF-1 with carbogen breathing. Thus the BOLD MRI technique, coupled with carbogen challenge, is interrogating both the tumor blood volume and the functionality of tumor vasculature (i.e., erythrocyte delivery).

INTRINSIC-SUSCEPTIBILITY CONTRAST MRI AND TUMOR OXYGENATION

A noninvasive method for measuring the heterogeneous distribution of hypoxia in a tumor would be of considerable use in the clinic. One approach that has been used to measure rodent tumor pO_2 noninvasively is ^{19}F nuclear magnetic resonance (NMR) oximetry, where exogenous perfluorocarbons are used as oxygen sensors (42). This approach affords absolute measurements of tumor pO_2, but suffers by only being able to sample a small proportion of the tumor. Furthermore, no perfluorocarbon has so far been approved for routine clinical use. ^1H MRI methods, in particular BOLD MRI, with their high temporal and spatial resolution, offer an alternative approach to interrogate tumour hypoxia.

As the oxygenation of hemoglobin is proportional to the arterial blood p_aO_2, and therefore in equilibrium with tissue pO_2, measurements of tumor R_2^* should provide a sensitive index of tissue oxygenation. The relationship of R_2^*-weighted image response and tumor pO_2 has been investigated by invasive Eppendorf histography with carbogen breathing and showed a weak correlation (15). A stronger correlation of carbogen-induced decreases in R_2^* with tumor oxygen tension, measured by oxygen microelectrodes, has been observed in rat mammary carcinomas (22). Recently, carbogen-induced decreases in R_2^* of rat intracranial gliomas were shown to correlate with an increase in pO_2 measured by electron paramagnetic resonance (EPR) oximetry (36). Simultaneous measurements of tumor R_2^* and pO_2 have been achieved using an MR-compatible fibre-optic (OxyLite, Oxford Optronix) pO_2 sensor (35,43). An additional example of simultaneous measurements of R_2^* and pO_2 is shown in Figure 2. These studies demonstrated that the R_2^* signal response to carbogen is temporally correlated with changes in tumor pO_2, but there was no correlation between absolute R_2^* and pO_2. Taken together, these data suggest that BOLD MRI can be used to assess changes in tumor oxygenation and provide good evidence that a carbogen-induced decrease in R_2^* is indicative of increased tissue oxygenation, but that measurements of R_2^* may have to be combined with additional techniques such as the OxyLite to provide absolute tumor pO_2 measurements in vivo.

As described earlier, carbogen increases blood oxygenation, and the magnitude of the change in tumor R_2^* is dependent on blood volume, which itself is a determinant of the hypoxic fraction (17,39). BOLD MRI has been shown to correctly predict the relative effects of radiosensitizers on tumor hypoxic fraction (23). One preclinical study sought to test the hypothesis that the baseline tumor R_2^* and carbogen-induced ΔR_2^* measured prior to radiotherapy were prognostic for treatment outcome. Before irradiation, tumor R_2^* was quantified whilst the host breathed air and subsequently carbogen, and correlated with the subsequent tumor growth inhibition in response to ionizing radiation. Overall, tumors which exhibited a significantly faster baseline R_2^* and a significantly greater carbogen-induced ΔR_2^* were more responsive to radiotherapy (44).

MGRE MRI has been used to quantify R_2^* and carbogen-induced changes in R_2^* of human head and neck cancers prior to entering the accelerated radiotherapy with carbogen and nicotinamide (ARCON) regime (38). In this limited study, all the eleven patients studied showed a carbogen-induced tumor ΔR_2^* (statistically significant in seven) prior to ARCON therapy. ARCON treatment has been shown to be highly effective in head and neck cancer. Consistent with this, all eleven patients imaged subsequently showed a low tumor recurrence rate after a considerable follow up time (M. Rijpkema, personal communication, 2003). A preliminary

(A)

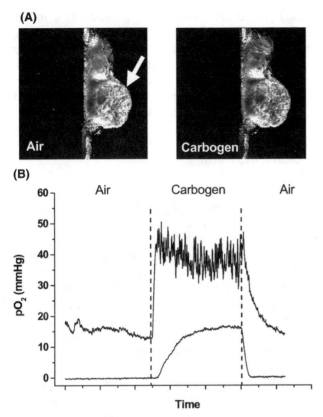

Figure 2 Simultaneous measurements of tumor R_2^* and pO_2. **(A)** Calculated R_2^* maps obtained from a transplanted GH3 prolactinoma grown in the flank of rat whilst the host breathed air and subsequently carbogen. Again, breathing carbogen results in a decrease in R_2^* over the tumor, indicating a decrease in deoxyhemoglobin. For these experiments MRI was performed using a quadrature volume coil with the rats lying supine to facilitate access and positioning of the fibre-optic pO_2 sensors, hence the different orientation and poorer signal-to-noise of the R_2^* maps compared to those in Figure 1. **(B)** Temporal traces obtained from the same GH3 prolactinoma from two MR-compatible fibre-optic pO_2 sensors inserted into the tumor. For this tumor, two very different initial pO_2 readings during air breathing were recorded, reflecting tissue heterogeneity. Upon switching to carbogen breathing an increase in tissue pO_2 was observed at both locations, whist resumption of air breathing resulted in recovery of pO_2 to baseline. Note also that the upper trace, which is reporting a higher initial pO_2 and greater ΔpO_2 with carbogen breathing than the lower trace, is also noisier, and maybe positioned proximal to a tumor blood vessel. Overall, the carbogen-induced changes in tumor R_2^* are temporally correlated with changes in pO_2, and provide good evidence that a carbogen-induced decrease in R_2^* is indicative of increased tissue oxygenation.

clinical study on hypoxia in prostate cancer has compared tumor R_2^* (measured by MGRE MRI) and blood volume (measured by DCE MRI) with tissue sections immunohistochemically stained for the hypoxia probe pimonidazole (45). Overall, tumors exhibiting a relatively fast R_2^* stained positive for pimonidazole, while those tumors with slow R_2^* stained negative. Tumor R_2^* alone gave the highest sensitivity and specificity, which was reduced with inclusion of the blood volume data. These two limited studies support the concept of using tumor R_2^* as a surrogate marker of hypoxia in the clinic.

Taken together, these data highlight the potential prognostic value in the measurement of tumor R_2^* and carbogen-induced ΔR_2^* to predict radiotherapeutic response. From equations 2 and 3 (see earlier), it is clear that both R_2^* (vascular volume) and ΔR_2^* (perfused fraction) are determinants of tumor radioresponsiveness. It has been hypothesized that tumors with a measurable blood volume and a relatively fast basal R_2^* may be relatively hypoxic compared to a similar tumor exhibiting a slower basal R_2^* (36,37), and recent preclinical studies are supportive of this concept (46).

INTRINSIC-SUSCEPTIBILITY CONTRAST MRI AND TUMOR ANGIOGENESIS

As previously highlighted (Eq. (2)), the baseline tumor R_2^* contains a component that depends on the tumor tissue deoxyhemoglobin content, which itself is a function of the vascular volume of the tumor which is actively perfused by erythrocytes. Thus the intrinsic R_2^* contrast produced by deoxyhemoglobin in tumor capillaries can be used as a probe for tumor blood volume and hence for angiogenesis. Intrinsic-susceptibility MRI permits repeated measurements of the same tumor with time and does not require administration of exogenous contrast agents. The method has no dependence on vascular permeability and can thus be used to interrogate tumor systems where permeability and angiogenesis are unassociated. A number of studies have utilized intrinsic-susceptibility contrast MRI as a rapid, quantitative non invasive approach for studying tumor angiogenesis.

The pioneering work of Neeman et al., realized and demonstrated the use of intrinsic-susceptibility contrast MRI to monitor tumor angiogenesis. This approach has been used to monitor, for example, the kinetics of tumor growth and neovascularization in a model system of implanted multicellular spheroids, vascular oscillations in the angiogenic response during the dormant phase of spheroid growth, tumor growth induced by proximal wounds, increased angiogenesis in ovarian tumors grown in ovariectomized hypergonadotrophic mice, and also to follow the suppression of angiogenesis induced by halofuginone, an inhibitor of collagen type I synthesis (47–52). Large hemodynamic responses of tumors expressing high levels of Met tyrosine kinase growth factor receptor following administration of its ligand, hepatocyte growth factor, have been measured by intrinsic-susceptibility MRI (53). Met is an important factor in the pathogenesis of a number of epithelial cancers, and this study highlights the potential of intrinsic-susceptibility MRI to monitor Met activity in vivo.

Intrinsic-susceptibility MRI of tumors derived from either wild type HEPA-1 hepatoma cells or cells deficient in hypoxia inducible factor-1β (HIF-1β) showed no significant difference in R_2^* and hence vascular development, and this was validated by immunohistochemistry (54). The absence of a difference suggested that deficiency in HIF-1β had little effect on tumor vascularity. In another study, R_2^* was significantly faster in tumors derived from mutant C6 glioma cells (clone D27) genetically engineered to constitutively overexpress dimethylarginine dimethylaminohydrolase (DDAH), compared to C6 wild type (55). This correlated with an increased uptake of the perfusion marker Hoechst 33342 and demonstrates that overexpression of DDAH, which metabolises the endogenous inhibitors of NO synthesis, results in increased neovascularization in vivo.

Another example and validation of intrinsic-susceptibility MRI for the assessment of tumor vascular development is shown in Figure 3, in which measurements of tumor R_2^* obtained from methyl nitrosourea (MNU)-induced rat mammary adenocarcinomas were correlated with Hoechst 33342 uptake.

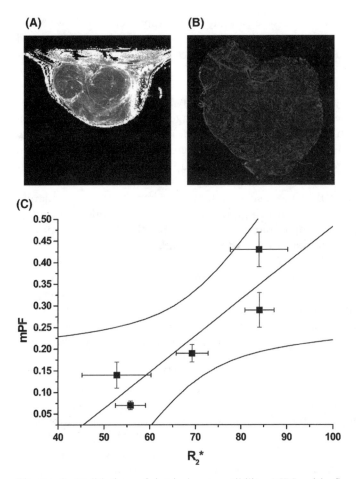

Figure 3 Validation of intrinsic-susceptibility MRI with fluorescence microscopy. (**A**) Calculated R_2^* map obtained from a rat mammary adenocarcinoma, induced by the injection of MNU. Such tumors arise from the transformation of a single cell and thus arguably give rise to tumors with a range of histopathologies more akin to the clinical situation. MGRE MRI was perfomed on five MNU-induced tumors and R_2^* maps obtained from five contiguous slices through each tumor. (**B**) After MRI, the rats were injected with 15 mg/kg of the perfusion marker Hoechst 33342 via the tail vein and, one minute later, sacrificed by cervical dislocation and the tumors were rapidly excised and frozen in liquid nitrogen. As Hoechst 33342 is only allowed to circulate for one minute, it only stains the nuclei of endothelial cells and cells immediately adjacent to tumor blood vessels which are perfused at the time of injection, and hence delineates functional tumor vasculature. Five frozen sections from each tumor were subsequently cut approximately in the same planes as for MRI, and fluorescence signals of whole tumor sections recorded using a motorized scanning stage on a fluorescence microscope. (**C**) Fluorescent particles were detected above a constant threshold, and the area of the tumor section with Hoechst 33342 fluorescence determined and expressed as a percentage of the area of the whole tumor section (mean perfused fraction, mPF). This was then correlated with the R_2^* measurements obtained from the same tumors, giving a linear fit with a significant correlation coefficient $r = 0.89$ ($p = 0.04$). These data thus demonstrate that the intrinsic R_2^* contrast produced by deoxyhemoglobin in tumor capillaries can be used as a probe for tumor blood volume. *Abbreviations*: MNU, methyl nitrosourea; MGRE, multi-gradient recalled echo. (*see colour insert for Fig. 3B.*)

An extension of the intrinsic-susceptibility MRI approach which was also demonstrated by Neeman et al. was to assess tumor blood vessel maturation and function by measuring changes in R_2^*-weighted images of tumors during hypercapnia (5% CO_2/95% air) and subsequently hyperoxia (5% CO_2/95% O_2), respectively. Mature blood vessels containing pericytes and smooth muscle cells would be expected to either vasodilate with hypercapnia or counteract any hyperoxia-induced vasoconstriction, resulting in a decrease in R_2^*. Signal changes in response to hyperoxia would be expected in all functional blood vessels as described earlier, also resulting in a decrease in R_2^*. The differential responses to hypercapnia and hyperoxia, which affords more contrast-to-noise, can thus be used to map tumor blood vessel maturation and function. This approach has been utilized to investigate the role of vascular endothelial growth factor (VEGF) as a survival factor for immature neovasculature in C6 gliomas derived from cells in which production of VEGF is under the control of a tetracycline-inducible promoter, and demonstrated that this MRI methodology could predict vascular susceptibility to VEGF withdrawal, based on the maturation status of the tumor vasculature (20,56). Importantly, the intrinsic-susceptibility MRI inferences on vascular maturation and function in this tumor system have been subsequently validated by immunohistochemical staining for α-actin, a marker specifically for vascular smooth muscle, and by intravital microscopy, which showed hypercapnia-induced vasoconstriction in mature blood vessels, the resulting decrease in blood volume causing an increase in R_2^* consistent with reduced deoxyhemoglobin (56,57).

A similar MRI approach has been previously used to investigate the role of hypoxia-inducible factor (HIF)-1α in tumor angiogenesis, in which reduced vascular functionality was measured in HIF-1α deficient tumors, demonstrating that hypoxia provides an important signal for tumor angiogenesis (58). A reduction in both vascular vasodilation and function, measured by intrinsic-susceptibility MRI, was also found in von Hippel-Lindau related paraganglioma xenografts grown in mice after treatment with the antiangiogenic agent linomide, consistent with suppression of VEGF expression (59). Conversely, intrinsic-susceptibility MRI has been used to demonstrate an increase in tumor blood vessel density and function caused by cell surface localization and secretion of the proangiogenic and prometastatic enzyme heparanase (60).

The maturation and functional state of blood vessels within tumors derived either from C6 wild type cells or clone D27 cells, genetically engineered to constitutively overexpress DDAH, has also been assessed by measuring the ΔR_2^* in response to hypercapnia and hyperoxia, respectively (61). Small decreases in R_2^* were identified within the periphery of both tumor types in response to hypercapnia and hyperoxia, and in this system there was no significant difference in either response between the C6 wild type and D27 gliomas. This contrasted with susceptibility-contrast MRI measurements and tumor uptake of Hoechst 33342, which demonstrated an increased blood volume and number of perfused blood vessels in the D27 tumors overexpressing DDAH.

INTRINSIC-SUSCEPTIBILITY CONTRAST MRI AND TUMOR RESPONSE TO ANTIVASCULAR THERAPY

Novel anticancer therapies are being developed to exploit differences between normal and tumor endothelium, with the aim of selectively targeting the destruction of tumor endothelium while leaving normal blood vessels relatively unaffected (6). As many of

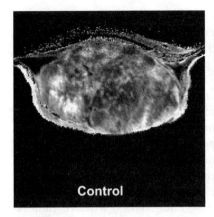 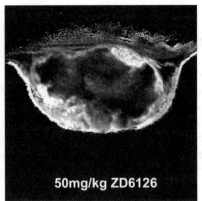

Figure 4 Tumor response to antivascular therapy. Calculated R_2^* maps obtained from a transplanted GH3 prolactinoma, grown subcutaneously in the flank of a rat prior to and 24 hours posttreatment with 50 mg/kg of the vascular targeting agent ZD6126. The hypothesis was that following treatment with ZD6126, hemoglobin within erythrocytes would deoxygenate, resulting in an increase in tumor R_2^*. However, this was not supported by the data, which showed a decrease in R_2^* after treatment, and which correlated with the induction of massive central necrosis (62). Note also the regions around the edge of the tumor showing relatively fast R_2^* posttreatment, consistent with a remaining viable rim of tissue, a common histopathological observation in response to this class of therapeutic agent.

these therapies are cytostatic, their clinical development requires the development and validation of quantitative biomarkers which are associated with tumor blood vasculature and its response, and that can be translated to the clinical use.

One study has investigated the use of intrinsic-susceptibility MRI to assess the efficacy of ZD6126 in rodent tumors (62). ZD6126 is a vascular targeting agent that causes the selective destruction of tumor blood vessels, cessation of tumor blood flow, death of tumor cells because of nutrient starvation, and massive tumor necrosis (63). The hypothesis was the following treatment with ZD6126, hemoglobin within erythrocytes would deoxygenate, resulting in an increase in tumor R_2^*. However, this hypothesis was not supported by the data, which showed a dose-dependent decrease in R_2^* 24 hours after treatment (Fig. 4), and correlated with massive central necrosis assessed histologically.

The decrease in tumor R_2^* observed at this time point could be because of one of the several factors. An agglomeration of deoxygenated, coagulated erythrocytes into localized tumor regions could decrease the magnetic field inhomogeneity, decreasing R_2^*. In addition, (i) vessel collapse before necrosis would decrease the blood volume, and (ii) the formation of edema which may be more fluid than viable tissue, would both cause R_2^* to decrease. Further work is required to elucidate the mechanisms responsible; yet a change in tumor R_2^* may prove to be a simple and convenient alternative end point for detecting acute changes induced by antivascular therapies.

LIMITATIONS AND FUTURE OF INTRINSIC-SUSCEPTIBILITY CONTRAST MRI

With respect to tumor oxygenation, it was recently highlighted that the variability and hence interpretation of R_2^* between different tumor types may be a confounding factor in the utility of intrinsic susceptibility contrast MRI as a prognostic index for radiotherapy in the clinic, but that within a tumor type this variability may be less and may relate to tumor pO_2 (36). The site of the tumor and subsequent ability to optimize the magnetic field (shim) will also strongly influence the basal R_2^*, particularly in the case of head and neck cancers (M. Rijpkema, personal communication, 2003). Such variability of R_2^* is also highlighted in Figure 3, measured from a panel of MNU-induced mammary carcinomas, a rodent tumor model arguably more representative of human cancers in which the tumor arises from the transformation of a single cell and exhibit a heterogeneous range of histopathologies.

The detection of BOLD MRI effects in tumors is based on the assumption that the water resonance has a homogeneous Lorentzian lineshape, and that changes in deoxyhemoglobin and hence R_2^* of this line are spectrally homogeneous. An alternative methodology, high spectral and spatial resolution (HiSS) MRI of tumors, has demonstrated that the water resonance within each voxel is complex and often contains multiple resolvable components (24). In such situations where each of these spectral components can respond differently to, for example, carbogen, the changes in BOLD contrast can be difficult to detect, accurately measure, and interpret. HiSS MRI, which has been implemented in the clinic (64), can detect these spectrally inhomogeneous R_2^* effects of endogenous contrast agents such as deoxyhaemoglobin, which reflect subvoxelar microenvironments and which may be missed by BOLD MRI. However, it has yet to be shown if measurements of tumour R_2^* by HiSS MRI yield superior prognostic value over those obtained by BOLD MRI.

It is intriguing to speculate that the radioresponsiveness of tumors could be graded by their basal R_2^* and carbogen-induced ΔR_2^*. The measurement of tumor R_2^* and ΔR_2^* prior to treatment may contribute to the success of radiotherapeutic response in the clinic and may ultimately prove prognostic, and in this context initial clinical studies appear promising (38,45).

Basal measurements of R_2^* appear to correlate with tumor blood volume and angiogenic potential (47–55) (Fig. 3). However, rodent tumor ΔR_2^* responses to hypercapnia and hyperoxia measured by intrinsic-susceptibility MRI are inherently small, primarily a consequence of the reduced contrast to noise ratio. In addition, the ability of 6 μm murine erythrocytes, the primary source of changes in R_2^* intrinsic contrast, to traverse similarly sized capillaries will be limited, which would abrogate the hypercapnic or hyperoxic response (39). This would explain why, for example, contrary to the hyperoxic ΔR_2^* response, a higher proportion of functional vasculature was measured in clone D27 tumors by uptake of the perfusion marker Hoechst 33342 (55,61).

A more rigorous evaluation of the effects and dynamics of an angiogenic growth factor on vascular remodeling assessed by intrinsic-susceptibility MRI is afforded in a tumor system where the angiogenic growth factor of interest is under inducible control, rather than being constitutively overexpressed, and hence where each tumor acts as its own control, maximizing statistical power. This has been elegantly demonstrated in several studies utilizing a C6 cell line in which production of VEGF is under the control of a tetracycline-inducible promoter (20,56,57). This approach is extremely powerful for preclinical studies of tumor angiogenesis in detecting differences in vascular morphology within a tumor system expressing a well-defined phenotypic difference in vivo, but the reduced contrast to noise ratio may preclude the extension of this specific approach to the clinic, particularly its use as a probe for vascular maturation.

With respect to antivascular therapies such as ZD6126, changes in tumor R_2^* are clearly complex and require further validation, but may also provide a useful alternative biomarker of response (65).

SUMMARY

Taken together these current results strongly suggest that intrinsic-susceptibility MRI is interrogating both the functionality of tumor vasculature (delivery of erythrocytes) and tumor blood volume. The combination of intrinsic-susceptibility MRI with contrast-enhanced and diffusion-weighted MRI should provide detailed maps of tumor vascular architecture and function. Since the hemodynamic and morphological characteristics of tumor vasculature are critical determinants of tumor growth, angiogenesis, metastatic potential, and therapeutic response, intrinsic-susceptibility MRI measures of R_2^* and ΔR_2^* may be sensitive and robust enough to provide clinical indices of tumor pathophysiology, such as grade and radioresponsiveness.

ACKNOWLEDGMENTS

This work was supported by The Royal Society and Cancer Research U.K., [CRC] grant SP 1971/0701. SPR is thankful to Franklyn Howe, Mark Rijpkema, and John Griffiths for valuable discussions.

REFERENCES

1. Molls M, Vaupel P. Blood perfusion and microenvironment of human tumors. Implications for Clinical Radiooncology. Berlin: Springer-Verlag, 1998.
2. Carmeliet P, Jain RK. Angiogenesis in cancer and other diseases. Nature 2000; 407: 249–257.
3. Weidner N, Folkman J, Pozza F, et al. Tumor angiogenesis: a new significant and independent prognostic indicator in early-stage breast carcinoma. J Natl Cancer Inst 1992; 84: 1875–1887.
4. Fox SB, Leek RD, Weekes MP, Whitehouse RM, Gatter KC, Harris AL. Quantitation and prognostic value of breast cancer angiogenesis: comparison of microvessel density, Chalkley count, and computer image analysis. J Pathol 1995; 177:275–283.
5. Cooper RA, Wilks DP, Logue J, et al. High tumor angiogenesis is associated with poorer survival in carcinoma of the cervix treated with radiotherapy. Clin Cancer Res 1998; 4:2795–2800.
6. Chaplin DJ, Dougherty GJ. Tumour vasculature as a target for cancer therapy. Br J Cancer 1999; 80(suppl 1):57–64.
7. Gillies RJ, Bhujwalla ZM, Evelhoch JL, et al. Applications of magnetic resonance in model systems: tumor biology and physiology. Neoplasia 2000; 2:139–151.
8. Gillies RJ, Raghunand N, Karczmar GS, Bhujwalla ZM. MRI of the tumor microenvironment. J Magn Reson Imag 2002; 16:430–450.
9. Ogawa S, Lee TM, Nayak AS, Glynn P. Oxygenation-sensitive contrast in magnetic resonance image of rodent brain at high magnetic fields. Magn Reson Med 1990; 14:68–78.
10. Ogawa S, Menon RS, Kim SG, Ugurbil K. On the characteristics of functional magnetic resonance imaging of the brain. Annu Rev Biophys Biomol Struct 1998; 27:447–474.
11. Karczmar GS, River JN, Li J, Vijayakumar S, Goldman Z, Lewis MZ. Effects of hyperoxia on T_2^* and resonance frequency weighted magnetic resonance images of rodent tumours. NMR Biomed 1994; 7:3–11.
12. Robinson SP, Howe FA, Griffiths JR. Noninvasive monitoring of carbogen-induced changes in tumor blood flow and oxygenation by functional magnetic resonance imaging. Int J Radiat Oncol Biol Phys 1995; 33:855–859.

13. Kuperman VY, River JN, Lewis MZ, Lubich LM, Karczmar GS. Changes in T_2^*-weighted images during hyperoxia differentiate tumors from normal tissues. Magn Reson Med 1995; 33:318–325.

14. Robinson SP, Rodrigues LM, Ojugo ASE, McSheehy PMJ, Howe FA, Griffiths JR. The response to carbogen breathing in experimental tumour models monitored by gradient-recalled magnetic resonance imaging. Br J Cancer 1997; 75:1000–1006.

15. Robinson SP, Collingridge DR, Rodrigues LM, Howe FA, Chaplin DJ, Griffiths JR. Tumour response to hypercapnia and hyperoxia monitored by FLOOD magnetic resonance imaging. NMR Biomed 1999; 12:98–106.

16. Howe FA, Robinson SP, Griffiths JR. Modification of tumor perfusion and oxygenation monitored by gradient recalled echo MRI and 31P MRS. NMR Biomed 1996; 9: 208–216.

17. Howe FA, Robinson SP, Rodrigues LM, Griffiths JR. Flow oxygenation dependent (FLOOD) contrast MR imaging to monitor the response of rat tumours to carbogen breathing. Magn Reson Imag 1999; 17:1307–1318.

18. Oikawa H, Al-Hallaq HA, Lewis MZ, River JN, Kovar DA, Karczmar GS. Spectroscopic imaging of the water resonance with short repetition time to study tumor response to hyperoxia. Magn Reson Med 1997; 38:27–32.

19. Zaim-Wadghiri Y, O'Hara JA, Grinberg O, Meyerand ME, Swartz HM, Dunn JF. NMR and EPR studies of BOLD contrast and oxygenation in tumors: measurement of pO_2 and T_2^* response after carbogen breathing (abstr). Proceedings of the International Society for Magnetic Resonance in Medicine 1997; 2082.

20. Abramovitch R, Frenkiel D, Neeman M. Analysis of subcutaneous angiogenesis by gradient echo magnetic resonance imaging. Magn Reson Med 1998; 39:813–824.

21. Peller M, Weissfloch L, Stehling MK, et al. Oxygen-induced MR signal changes in murine tumors. Magn Reson Imag 16; 7:799–809.

22. Al-Hallaq HA, River JN, Zamora M, Oikawa H, Karczmar GS. Correlation of magnetic resonance and oxygen microelectrode measurements of carbogen-induced changes in tumor oxygenation. Int J Radiat Oncol Biol Phys 1998; 41:151–159.

23. Al-Hallaq HA, Zamora M, Fish BL, Farrell A, Moulder JE, Karczmar GS. MRI measurements correctly predict the relative effects of tumor oxygenating agents on hypoxic fraction in rodent BA1112 tumors. Int J Rad Oncol Biol Phys 2000; 47: 481–488.

24. Al-Hallaq HA, Fan X, Zamora M, River JN, Moulder JE, Karczmar GS. Spectrally inhomogeneous BOLD contrast changes detected in rodent tumors with high spectral and spatial resolution. NMR Biomed 2002; 15:28–36.

25. Landuyt W, Hermans R, Bosmans H, et al. BOLD contrast fMRI of whole rodent tumour during air or carbogen breathing using echo-planar imaging at 1.5T. Eur Radiol 2001; 11:2332–2340.

26. Griffiths JR, Taylor NJ, Howe FA, et al. The response of human tumors to carbogen breathing, monitored by gradient-recalled echo magnetic resonance imaging. Int J Radiat Oncol Biol Phys 1997; 39:697–701.

27. Taylor NJ, Baddeley H, Goodchild KA, et al. BOLD MRI of human tumour oxygenation during carbogen breathing. J Magn Reson Imaging 2001; 14:156–163.

28. Robinson SP, Howe FA, Stubbs M, Griffiths JR. Effects of nicotinamide and carbogen on tumour oxygenation, blood flow, energetics and blood glucose levels. Br J Cancer 2000; 82:2007–2014.

29. Muruganandham M, Kasiviswanathan A, Jagannathan NR, Raghunathan P, Jain PC, Jain V. Diltiazem enhances tumor blood flow: MRI study in a murine tumor. Int J Radiat Oncol Biol Phys 1999; 43:413–421.

30. Jordan BF, Misson P, Demeure R, Baudelet C, Beghein N, Gallez B. Changes in tumor oxygenation/perfusion induced by the NO donor isosorbide dinitrate, in comparison with carbogen: monitoring by EPR and MRI. Int J Radiat Oncol Biol Phys 2000; 48: 565–570.

31. Robinson SP, Howe FA, Griffiths JR. Tumour response to the nitric oxide donor SIN-1 monitored by GRE MRI and 31P MRS. Proceedings of the International Society for Magnetic Resonance in Medicine 1997; 1092.

32. Lankester KJ, Hill SA, Tozer GM, Maxwell RJ. BOLD-MRI responses to vasoactive agents: influence of vessel maturity. Proceedings of the International Society for Magnetic Resonance in Medicine Workshop on In Vivo Functional and Molecular Assessment of Cancer, Santa Cruz, USA, 2002:18.

33. Howe FA, Robinson SP, McIntyre DJO, Stubbs M, Griffiths JR. Issues in flow and oxygenation dependent contrast (FLOOD) imaging of tumours. NMR Biomed 2001; 7: 497–506.

34. Robinson SP, Rodrigues LM, Howe FA, Stubbs M, Griffiths JR. Effects of different levels of hypercapnic hyperoxia on tumour R_2^* and arterial blood gases. Magn Reson Imag 2001; 19:161–166.

35. Baudelet C, Gallez B. How does blood oxygen level-dependent (BOLD) contrast correlate with oxygen partial pressure (pO_2) inside tumors? Magn Reson Med 2002; 48:980–986.

36. Dunn JF, O'Hara JA, Zain-Wadghiri Y, et al. Changes in oxygenation of intracranial tumors with carbogen: a BOLD MRI and EPR oximetry study. J Magn Reson Imag 2002; 16:511–521.

37. Taylor NJ, Lankester KJ, Stirling JJ, Rustin GJS, Hoskin PJ, Padhani AR. Reproducibility of human tumour R_2^* maps obtained from BOLD images. Proceedings of the International Society for Magnetic Resonance in Medicine 2002; 2065.

38. Rijpkema M, Kaanders JHAM, Joosten FBM, van der Kogel AJ, Heerschap A. Effects of breathing a hyperoxic hypercapnic gas mixture on blood oxygenation and vascularity of head and neck tumors as measured by MRI. Int J Radiat Oncol Biol Phys 2002; 53:1185–1191.

39. Robinson SP, Rijken PFJW, Howe FA, et al. Tumour vascular architecture and function evaluated by non-invasive susceptibility MRI methods and immunohistochemistry. J Magn Reson Imag 2003; 17:445–454.

40. Dennie J, Mandeville JB, Boxerman JL, Packard SD, Rosen BR, Weisskoff RM. NMR imaging of changes in vascular morphology due to tumor angiogenesis. Magn Reson Med 1998; 40:793–799.

41. Tropres I, Grimault S, Vaeth A, et al. Vessel size imaging. Magn Reson Med 2001; 45: 397–408.

42. Hunjan S, Zhao D, Constantinescu A, Hahn EW, Antich PP, Mason RP. Tumor oximetry: demonstration of an enhanced dynamic mapping procedure using fluorine-19 echo planar magnetic resonance imaging in the Dunning prostate R3327-AT1 rat tumor. Int J Radiat Oncol Biol Phys 2001; 49:1097–1108.

43. Maxwell RJ, Robinson SP, McIntyre DJO, Griffiths JR, Young WK, Vojnovic B. Simultaneous measurement of gradient-echo ^{1}H MR images and pO_2 using a fibre-optic oxygen sensor in rodent tumours and their response to carbogen breathing. Proceedings of the International Society for Magnetic Resonance in Medicine 1998; 1665.

44. Rodrigues LM, Howe FA, Griffiths JR, Robinson SP. Tumor R_2^* is a prognostic indicator of acute radiotherapeutic response in rodent tumors. J Magn Reson Imaging. 2004; 19:482–488.

45. Taylor NJ, Carnell DM, Smith RE, et al. Evaluation of prostate gland hypoxia with quantified BOLD MRI: initial results from a correlated histological study. Proceedings of the International Society for Magnetic Resonance in Medicine 2003; 531.

46. Kostourou V, Troy H, Murray JF, Cullis ER, Whitley GS, Griffiths JR, Robinson SP. Overexpression of dimethylarginine dimethylaminohydrolase enhances tumour hypoxia: an insight into the relationship of hypoxia and angiogenesis in vivo. Neoplasia 2004; 6:401–411.

47. Abramovitch R, Meir G, Neeman M. Neovascularization induced growth of implanted C6 glioma multicellular spheroids: magnetic resonance microimaging. Cancer Res 1995; 55:1956–1962.

48. Gilead A, Neeman M. Dynamic remodeling of the vascular bed precedes tumor growth: MLS ovarian carcinoma spheroids implanted in nude mice. Neoplasia 1999; 1:226–230.

49. Abramovitch R, Marikovsky M, Meir G, Neeman M. Stimulation of tumour angiogenesis by proximal wounds: spatial and temporal analysis by MRI. Br J Cancer 1998; 77: 440–447.

50. Schiffenbauer YS, Abramovitch R, Meir G, et al. Loss of ovarian function promotes angiogenesis in human ovarian carcinoma. Proc Natl Acas Sci 1997; 94:13,203–13,208.

51. Abramovitch R, Dafni H, Neeman M, Nagler A, Pines M. Inhibition of neovascularization and tumor growth, and facilitation of wound repair, by halofuginone, an inhibitor of collagen type I synthesis. Neoplasia 1999; 1:321–329.

52. Gross DJ, Reibstein I, Weiss L, et al. Treatment with halofuginone results in marked growth inhibition of a von Hippel-Lindau pheochromocytoma in vivo. Clin Cancer Res 2003; 9:3788–3793.

53. Shaharabany M, Abramovitch R, Kushnir T, et al. In vivo molecular imaging of met tyrosine kinase growth factor receptor activity in normal organs breast tumors. Cancer Res 2001; 61:4873–4878.

54. Griffiths JR, McSheehy PM, Robinson SP, et al. Metabolic changes detected by in vivo magnetic resonance studies of HEPA-1 wild-type tumors and tumors deficient in hypoxia-inducible-factor-1β (HIF-1β): evidence of an anabolic role for the HIF-1 pathway. Cancer Res 2002; 62:688–695.

55. Kostourou V, Robinson SP, Cartwright JE, Whitley GS. Dimethylarginine dimethylaminohydrolase I enhances tumour growth and angiogenesis. Br J Cancer 2002; 87:673–680.

56. Abramovitch R, Dafni H, Smouha E, Benjamin LE, Neeman M. In vivo prediction of vascular susceptibility to vascular endothelial growth factor withdrawal: magnetic resonance imaging of C6 rat glioma in nude mice. Cancer Res 1999; 59:5012–5016.

57. Neeman M, Dafni H, Bukhari O, Braun RD, Dewhirst MW. In vivo BOLD contrast MRI mapping of subcutaneous vascular function and maturation: validation by intravital microscopy. Magn Reson Med 2001; 45:887–898.

58. Carmeliet P, Dor Y, Herbert J-M, et al. Role of HIF-1α in hypoxia-mediated apoptosis, cell proliferation and tumour angiogenesis. Nature 1998; 394:485–490.

59. Gross DJ, Reibstein I, Weiss L, et al. The antiangiogenic agent linomide inhibits the growth rate of von Hippel-Lindau paraganglioma xenografts to mice. Clin Cancer Res 1999; 5:3669–3675.

60. Goldshmidt O, Zcharia E, Abramovitch R, et al. Cell surface expression and secretion of heparanase markedly promote tumor angiogenesis and metastasis. Proc Natl Acad Sci 2002; 99:10,031–10,036.

61. Kostourou V, Robinson SP, Whitley GS, Griffiths JR. Effects of overexpression of dimethylarginine dimethylaminohydrolase on tumour angiogenesis assessed by susceptibility magnetic resonance imaging. Cancer Res 2003; 63:4960–4966.

62. Robinson SP, McIntyre DJO, Checkley D, et al. Tumour dose response to the antivascular agent ZD6126 assessed by magnetic resonance imaging. Br J Cancer 2003; 88:1592–1597.

63. Blakey DC, Westwood FR, Walker M, et al. Anti-tumour activity of the novel vascular targeting agent ZD6126 in a panel of tumor models. Clin Cancer Res 2002; 8:1974–1983.

64. Du W, Du YP, Bick U, et al. Breast MR imaging with high spectral and spatial resolutions: preliminary experience. Radiology 2002; 224:577–585.

65. Robinson SP, Kalber TL, Howe FA, et al. Acute tumor response to ZD6126 assessed by intrinsic-susceptibility magnetic resonance imaging. Neoplasia 2005; 7:466–474.

14
Pharmacokinetic Modeling of Dynamic Contrast Enhanced MRI in Cancer

Peter L. Choyke
Molecular Imaging Program, National Cancer Institute, Bethesda, Maryland, U.S.A.

David Thomassen and Andrew J. Dwyer
Diagnostic Radiology Department, National Institutes of Health, Bethesda, Maryland, U.S.A.

A Note from the Editors

*P*harmacokinetic modeling has become a standard method of analyzing dynamic contrast enhanced imaging. The models produce terms, called rate constants, that suggest specific physiologic meanings with regard to blood flow and vessel permeability. The origin of these rate constants is somewhat mysterious to the non-expert who is the most likely consumer of these data. The purpose of this chapter is to explain the basics of the two compartment model and its mathematical structure. Several different models, each based on different sets of assumptions, are presented and compared as well as competing methods of analysis. The goal is to demystify the pharmacokinetic model so that both its positive features and its limitations can be better understood.

Angiogenesis, the remodeling and recruitment of established blood vessels, is necessary for tumors to grow beyond a few millimeters in diameter (1). Before they become angiogenic, tumors rely on host vessels to supply needed nutrients and oxygen through diffusion and convection, but to grow beyond the diffusion limit, new blood vessels must be recruited. Angiogenic blood vessels not only supply the needed oxygen, nutrient, and extracellular matrix to sustain tumor growth, but also serve as conduits for metabolic waste and hematogenous metastases.

Tumor blood vessels differ anatomically and functionally from normal vessels. They tend to have chaotic and inefficient capillary architecture with frequent shunt vessels and blind ending channels (2). Thus, angiogenic vessels can be inefficient both in delivering nutrient and in siphoning off metabolites. Moreover, because of fenestrations in the endothelial surfaces, basement membranes, and pericytes covering the outer surface of the vessel, neovessels are frequently more permeable than normal vessels (2).

These characteristics are exploited for diagnostic purposes in dynamic contrast enhanced (DCE) imaging studies. The observation that tumor vascularity differs from normal tissue vascularity was first made clinically by catheter angiography using intra-arterial iodinated contrast media. Tumors demonstrated a hypervascularity and a "tumor blush" on angiograms that were unresponsive to pharmacological doses of the potent vasoconstrictor, epinephrine. Hypervascularity in tumors can be demonstrated with computed tomography (CT), magnetic resonance imaging (MRI), ultrasonography (US), optical imaging (OI), and positron emission tomography (PET). Understanding and quantifying enhancement patterns of tumors with imaging studies provides a basis for diagnosis, grading, monitoring, and therapy selection as well as insights into tumor pathophysiology.

A classic enhancement "curve" representing signal (arbitrary units) versus time is shown in Figure 1. In a typical DCE experiment, tumor size enhances briskly after the arrival of the contrast agent, rapidly reaches a peak enhancement, and then gradually washes out. The enhancement is thought to be the result of the contrast agent arriving via the arteries, perfusing the capillaries and venules and diffusing rapidly into the interstitial space (known as the extravascular extracellular space or EES), around these vessels (3). The rate and amplitude of enhancement depends

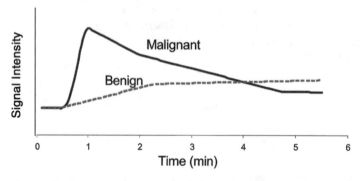

Figure 1 A comparison of typical dynamic enhancement curves in benign and malignant tissue. The "benign" curve slowly enhances over a period of minutes because of well-ordered but high-resistance vessels, which do not leak contrast material. The "malignant" curve typically shows rapid enhancement and washout related to high flow and permeability. Of course, many tumors fall in between these two "classic" curves.

on the density and permeability of the microvasculature and the size of the EES. The contrast agent within the EES eventually leaks back into the venous part of the vascular space, and the contrast media is excreted from the body. Therefore, the degree of enhancement is related to the distribution and the concentration of the contrast agent in the vessels and extracellular interstitial space. The shape of the enhancement curve reflects blood flow, vascular volume, extravascular volume, and vessel permeability. Early observers of DCE studies suggested that such data were amenable to pharmacokinetic (PK) mathematical modeling by which estimates of flow, vascular volume, and permeability could be obtained. The flow, volume fraction, and permeability parameters provide a means of explaining the enhancement patterns in terms of tumor anatomy and physiology thus characterizing tumors and monitoring the response to therapy. PK models are equations that can be used to "fit" the actual data obtained from a raw time–signal curve to a mathematical equation from which fitting "parameters" are derived (e.g., flow, volume, permeability, etc.). The advantages of PK models are its ability (i) to reduce the multitude of data points from time–signal curves to a few concise numerical parameters, whose magnitudes relate to underlying anatomic and physiologic features, (ii) to provide insight into the relationship between the contrast kinetics and the underlying physiology both over time and between regions of the same tumor, (iii) to provide a means of uniformly comparing data from different institutions.

The shape of the time–signal curve gives some diagnostic clues about the nature of the mass (Fig. 1). A highly vascular malignancy would be expected to enhance quickly and then to "de-enhance" as fresh blood washes in and the contrast agents washes out. Benign lesions, with more ordered vessels, more regulated, tight endothelial junctions, and higher vascular resistance, would be expected to enhance and wash out more slowly. Of course, it is not that simple. Nature provides a continuous spectrum of enhancement curves, which leads to families of intermediate curve shapes that combine features of classic "malignant" curves with "normal" curves. Moreover, any single region of interest measurement may encompass both malignant and benign tissues, the relative contribution of each ultimately determines the shape of the contrast enhancement curve.

MRI, CT, nuclear medicine, PET, and US can generate contrast enhancement curves such as shown in Figure 1; however, in practice, MRI is most commonly employed because it lacks ionizing radiation, has good spatial resolution, uses a safe, well-tolerated contrast agent, and is widely available. DCE-MRI studies usually consist of repeated images at several slice locations obtained over time after the injection of an MR contrast agent such as gadolinium-Diethylenetriaminepentaacetate (DTPA). It is not uncommon for such a study to contain 200 to 1000 images. Hence, a central value of PK models is to create relatively compact colorized maps based on well-known physiologic parameters, such as vessel permeability, blood flow, blood volume, and extravascular volume, that reduce the huge data sets to a more manageable size (4,5).

In this chapter, the basic theory and practice of PK modeling of DCE-MRI is presented. Strengths and weaknesses of the PK modeling approach are discussed, and alternative methods of analysis are presented.

GENERAL KINETIC MODEL

The general kinetic model (GKM) is one approach to understand the complex dynamics of contrast enhancement. The GKM simplifies the anatomical regions of

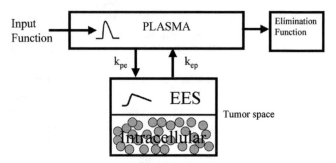

Figure 2 The essential elements of the two compartment pharmacokinetic model. Contrast material enters the plasma (input function) and leaks into the EES at a constant rate. Note that the contrast material remains extracellular so the space given to cells is excluded from the model (although not from real data measurements). The contrast media slowly leaks back from the EES into the plasma and is eventually excreted through the kidneys (elimination function).

the tumor into two functional components, the vascular space and the EES, and one nonfunctional component, the intracellular space (Fig. 2). Most MR contrast agents, specifically the gadolinium chelates, are highly diffusible agents which remain extracellular, and when introduced into the vascular space will leak into the EES at a characteristic rate and then will leak back into the vessel at different rate (3,6,7). The flux from the vascular space into the EES is directly proportional to the concentration (C_p) in the plasma and the permeability–surface (PS) area product, which is a general measure of permeability. The flux from the EES back into the vascular space is the product of the concentration in the EES (C_{EES}) and its PS product. The unit of the PS product is $cm^3 min^{-1} g^{-1}$ or $cm^3 sec^{-1} g^{-1}$ and is not necessarily the same for each direction. Thus the net change of concentration in the tumor, dC_t/dt is

$$dC_t/dt = \frac{(flux_{in} - flux_{out})}{volume} = C_p PS_{in} - C_{EES} PS_{out} \qquad (1)$$

Thus, the rate of change of contrast agent concentration in the tumor, dC_t/dt, equals the flux *into* the EES minus the flux *out of* the EES. When $C_p \gg C_{EES}$ occurs as early after contrast administration, net flux is *into* the tumor, while later, when $C_{EES} > C_p$ net flux is *out of* the EES into the vascular space. Here, let us assume that $PS_{in} = PS_{out} = K^{trans}$ and the contrast agent diffuses only into the EES and not into the intracellular portion of the tumor. Thus,

$$\frac{dC_t}{dt} = K^{trans} C_p - K^{trans} C_{EES} \qquad (2)$$

As $C_{EES} = C_t(V_t/V_{EES})$ where V_t and V_{EES} are the total tumor volume and extravascular volume, respectively, and by definition $V_{EES}/V_t = v_e$ (where v_e is the relative size of the EES compared to the total tumor volume) then Equation (2) can be rewritten as:

$$\frac{dC_t}{dt} = K^{trans} C_p - \left(\frac{K^{trans}}{v_e}\right) C_t \qquad (3)$$

By definition $K^{\text{trans}}/v_e = k_{ep}$, so Equation (2) can be rewritten as:

$$\frac{dC_t}{dt} = K^{\text{trans}}\left[\frac{C_p - C_t}{v_e}\right] = K^{\text{trans}}C_p - k_{ep}C_t \tag{4}$$

This differential equation gives the relationship of the rate of change of tumor concentration at any given time after contrast administration to the plasma and the tumor concentration at that time. The solution of the equation is found in Appendix and is written as:

$$C_t(T) = K^{\text{trans}}\int_0^T C_p(t)e^{-k_{ep}(T-t)}dt \tag{5}$$

This formula is the result of the GKM, and it expresses mathematically the concept that the tumor concentration of the contrast agent at time T, $C_t(T)$ (as opposed to "t" which represents any time point up to time T), is equal to summation of all impulse functions up to time T times the amount of the impulse still remaining at time $T\left(e^{-k_{ep}(T-t)}\right)$. The impulse function [or arterial input function (AIF)] can be viewed as a series of impulses of contrast media. K^{trans} should not be confused with k_{ep}. k_{ep} is usually two to five times the K^{trans}, the transfer constant, as the vascular ratio, v_e is usually 20% to 50% (3,6,7).

If the AIF is divided into a series of individual impulses (Fig. 3), each of which results in a curve with an exponential decay, then the overall tumor curve represents these arterial input response functions (Fig. 3).

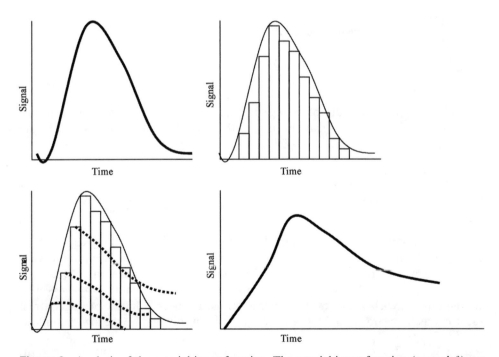

Figure 3 Analysis of the arterial input function. The arterial input function (*upper left*) can actually be thought of as a collection of "mini input functions" (*upper right*) each of which generates their own response curve in the tissue (*lower left*). The summation of these individual response curves is the actual measured response curve. This emphasizes the importance of knowing the arterial input function as it highly influences the shape of the tumor curve.

The basic result of the GKM, summarized in Equation (5), may also be understood in terms of the concept of residence time of contrast agent in the EES where its mean residence time in the EES is $1/k_{ep}$. Tumors with high k_{ep} have short residence times within the EES; the contrast flows in and out rapidly of the tumor space. Residence time is prolonged when k_{ep} is lowered; that is, there is a lower rate of exchange between the vascular space and the EES. Tumors demonstrating high K^{trans} values will tend to have rapid and high amplitude initial rise in signal upon arrival of the contrast agent. High k_{ep} values will be reflected by rapid washout of the contrast media.

The vascular fraction is a measure of biologic interest, particularly, in therapies directed against tumor vasculature. To this point we have ignored the vascular space, assuming that it is a too small component in tumors to influence the signal. To account for the vascular fraction and the vascular space an additional vascular fraction term, v_pC_p can be added to Equation (5):

$$C_t(T) = K^{trans}\int_0^T C_p(t)e^{-k_{ep}(T-t)}dt + v_pC_p(T) \tag{6}$$

The GKM can be used to fit a curve of real data based on the AIF $C_p(t)$ and the tumor curve $C_t(T)$. Changes in K^{trans} and v_e will result in changes in the height and shape of the curve related to the tumor concentration, whereas k_{ep} influences the curve shape. Thus, these parameters can be optimized to fit the actual data.

What does K^{trans} really mean? Until now, we have thought of K^{trans} as a permeability constant. Now, we consider the meaning of K^{trans} in more detail.

If we consider the initial condition just as the contrast arrives in the vessel when $C(T)=0$,

$$\frac{dC_t}{dt} = K^{trans}C_p - k_{ep}C_t \tag{2}$$

then from Equation (2):

$$\frac{dC_t}{dt} = K^{trans}C_p$$

Alternatively, this rate of change in tumor concentrate may be seen as the product of C_p, blood flow (F) and portion of this flow that leaks or is extracted from the vessel, the extraction fraction (E):

$$\frac{dC_t}{dt} = FEC_p \tag{7}$$

Thus by rearrangement:

$$K^{trans} = FE \tag{8}$$

The concept of the extraction fraction (E), introduced by Renkin, helps to clarify the dependence of K^{trans} on tumor flow (F) and permeability surface product (PS) (8). The extraction fraction is defined as the amount of contrast agent removed from the plasma during the first pass divided by the total amount of contrast agent perfusing the tumor (3,9,10). The extraction fraction is the arterial inflow of the contrast agent minus the venous outflow of the contrast agent divided by the arterial inflow:

$$E = \frac{(C_a - C_v)}{C_a} \tag{10}$$

where C_a is the arterial concentration and C_v the venous concentration of the contrast agent (8). The extraction fraction is positive when the net flux is *into* the EES and is negative when net flux is *out of* the EES. However, we are now concerned

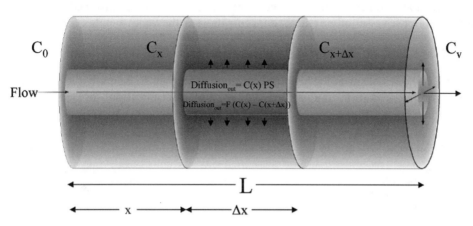

Figure 4 The dual effect of flow and permeability on the leakage rate, K^{trans}. Take a section of a blood vessel with uniform permeability and consider what happens to the concentration (C_x) of the contrast agent as a function of length (L). After the blood has traveled a distance x then the diffusion$_{out}$ is proportional to the concentration of the contrast media at the position x and the permeability surface (PS) area. The net diffusion is also equal to the flow times the concentration at the proximal end minus the flow times the concentration at the distal end ($x + \Delta x$) of the section. Thus, the net diffusion is related to both flow and permeability.

with the first pass or initial extraction fraction before tissue concentrations of the contrast agent build up, that is, early after injection when backflow from EES to the vascular space is zero. Consider a vessel coursing through tissue of length, L (Fig. 4). It has flow, F, and the contrast agent enters the vessel with concentration, C_0. By the time it is downstream a distance, x, it will have a concentration of $C(x)$. For an isolated vessel segment, Δx, the amount leaking out of the vessel is:

$$\text{diffusion}_{out} = F(C(x) - C(x + \Delta x)) \tag{11}$$

where F is the flow. However, when the EES concentration, $C_{EES} = 0$, diffusion also equals:

$$\text{diffusion}_{out} = C(x)\text{PS} \tag{12}$$

where $C(x)$ is the mean concentration for the segment, x, P the permeability, and S the surface area of the vascular segment. For a cylindrical vessel segment, the surface area, S, of the section is $2\pi r\, \Delta x$, where Δx is the length of the section. By rearrangement:

$$\frac{[C(x) - C(x + \Delta x)]}{\Delta x} = \frac{C(x)P2\pi r}{F} \tag{13}$$

Taking the limit as Δx approaches zero produces the differential equation:

$$-\frac{\mathrm{d}C(x)}{\mathrm{d}x} = C(x)\frac{P2\pi r}{F}$$

Solving for $C(x)$ yields:

$$C(x) = C_0 e^{-2\pi r x P/F} \tag{14}$$

where C_0 is the initial upstream concentration. This expression gives the plasma concentration a function of initial concentration, C_0, and the distance along the capillary. For a vessel of length, L, concentration at the venous end, C_v, is:

$$C_v = C_0 e^{-2\pi r x L P/F} = C_0 e^{-PS/F}$$

where S is the vessel surface. The initial extraction fraction, E, is simply the upstream concentration, $C(x)=0$, minus the downstream concentration divided by the upstream concentration:

$$E = \left(C_0 - C_0 e^{-PS/F} \right) C_0 \tag{15}$$

which reduces to:

$$E = 1 - e^{-PS/F} \tag{16}$$

where PS is the permeability–surface area product of the vessel and F the plasma flow. The unit of the PS product is $cm^3 \, min^{-1} \, gm^{-1}$ or $cm^3 \, sec^{-1} \, gm^{-1}$, and the unit of flow is $cm^3 \, gm^{-1} \, min^{-1}$, so that the extraction fraction, E, is unit-less and is dependent on both flow and permeability.

Thus, the GKM yields the following relationship:

$$K^{trans} = F(1 - e^{-PS/F}) \tag{17}$$

This expression simplifies in situations where F or PS dominate. When $F \gg PS$ then $E \approx PS/F$ and $K^{trans} \approx PS$. Thus, in high flow conditions K^{trans} can be thought of as equivalent to permeability. This is called a "permeability limited" condition. When $F \ll PS$, $E \approx 1$, and $K^{trans} = F$. This is known as a "flow limited" condition or Kety condition. Therefore, K^{trans} is not necessarily a pure permeability measure but is also related to flow.

Patlak Approach

Another approach to determine vessel permeability from time concentration curves was proposed by Patlak et al. It uses a graphical method to estimate PS and the fractional vascular space based on the slope and intercept of a derived line. In this method, reflux or flow from the EES to the vascular space is assumed to be negligible, and flow is assumed to be unidirectional. Like the GKM, the Patlak method also includes a vascular term and requires direct measurement of the input function.

To understand this approach consider that the concentration of the contrast agent in the tumor can be expressed as:

$$C_t(T) = PS \int_0^T \frac{C_p(t)}{V_t} \, dt + v_p C_p(T) \tag{18}$$

where v_p is the fractional plasma volume, that is, the plasma volume divided by the total tumor volume, V_t. This method assumes no backflux, therefore, the amount entering the EES at time t is $C_p(t)$ PS. The amount accumulated in the EES equals PS $\int C_p(T) dt$. The contrast agent concentration in the tumor is equal to the summation of the input function over time (i.e., from 0 to T) and the product of the vascular

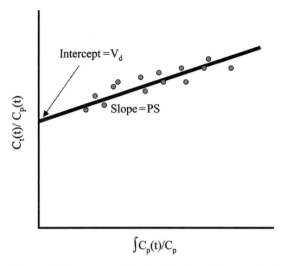

Figure 5 Representative Patlak plot. This graph plots the ratio of the plasma concentration at any given time to the integral of the plasma concentration ($C_p(t)/C_p$) against the ratio of the tumor concentration of contrast to the plasma concentration at the same time. The slope of the line yields the permeability surface (PS) area product, whereas the intercept yields the vascular fraction V_d.

fraction and the concentration in the plasma at any given time, $C_p(t)$. Dividing both sides of the equation by $C_p(t)$ yields:

$$\frac{C_t(T)}{C_p(T)} = \frac{PS}{V_t} \int_0^T \frac{C_p(t)}{C_p} dt + v_p \tag{19}$$

This equation is in the form of the equation of a line ($y = mx + b$). The slope of the line is PS/V_t, whereas the intercept is the vascular fraction, v_p. The horizontal axis is $\int C_p(t)/C_p$, whereas the vertical axis is $C_t(t)/C_p(t)$ (Fig. 5). Thus, the Patlak approach utilizes a simpler approach than do standard PK models. Limitations include the assumption of unidirectional flow from the vascular to the extravascular space and the strength of the fit of the line to the data.

Circumventing the Input Function

The GKM requires the AIF [Eq. (5)]. In reality, the input function cannot be measured directly because it is impossible to resolve the end arteries supplying the tumor. The approach commonly used in applying the GKM is to approximate the input function by measuring the signal from a large artery such as the aorta or left ventricle near the tumor. Other approaches obviate the need for measuring an AIF altogether by making assumptions about the nature/shape of the input function. The problem then reduces to determining the parameters of the input function. This may be accomplished by assuming "normal values" or by including the input function's parameters in the PK model equations for tumor enhancement and then estimating these parameters (and hence the input curve) from the tumor enhancement data alone. The Brix and Tofts methods, both often employed in DCE-MRI analysis, are two such approaches (Fig. 6).

General Kinetic Model

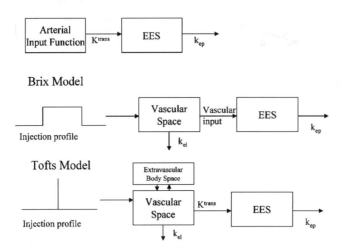

Figure 6 Comparison of several pharmacokinetic models. In the general kinetic model (*top*), the arterial input function is used to calculate the K^{trans} and k_{ep} parameters as the contrast enters and leaves the EES. In the Brix model (*middle*), the injection profile is assumed to be a "step function," that is, a long, slow and steady injection with a relatively stable concentration. This infusion enters the vascular space where it exchanges with the EES. In addition to the parameter k_{ep}, the parameter k_{el} (elimination rate constant) is generated. In the Tofts model (*bottom*), the injection is assumed to be a nearly instantaneous spike which is modulated by the vascular space and the extravascular body space into an input function which then exchanges with the EES. This model yields the parameters K^{trans}, k_{ep}, and k_{el}.

The approach described by Brix is a two-compartment model (plasma and EES) in which the arterial input curve is assumed to be the result of a prolonged constant infusion that takes the shape of a square (i.e., the contrast agent instantly reaches a plateau, remains constant for a while, and then instantly is over), which mixes in the vascular space and is slowly eliminated by renal excretion. The input function is of magnitude K_{in}, its duration is τ, the elimination constant is k_{el}, and the rate constants describing the transfer of contrast agent from the plasma to the tumor space and back are k_{pe} and k_{ep} (11).

If one assumes that the input function is a square wave function of finite duration and amplitude, which undergoes a monoexponential clearance (k_{el}), then the shape of the input function will be predicted thus providing $C_p(T)$ without actually measuring it. The Brix model fits the time–signal curve and derives three fitting parameters, namely, A, k_{ep}, and k_{el}. The former relates to the height of the time–signal curve and is related to K^{trans}, whereas the latter, k_{ep}, relates to the shape of the curve. Sources of error in this model include the assumption of both a square wave injection and a monoexponential decay in plasma concentration of gadolinium. Limitations include the requirement for a slow, steady injection rather than a bolus. In some vascular organs, like the prostate gland and liver, it may be more difficult to discern the lesion against the enhanced background with a slow injection. An advantage of the Brix approach is that scans can be obtained at a slower rate than is required with a rapid bolus of contrast media.

The Tofts model takes a different approach to the AIF, but retains the fundamental assumptions of the GKM (6). In this model, the input function is assumed to be the result of a pulse bolus injected into a two-compartment system. The arterial input is modified by diffusion transfer of contrast material between the vascular space and body's extravascular space; this system of compartments modifies the pulse bolus into a biexponential AIF. The exponential parameter is usually estimated from other "pooled" measurements of the AIF, so it is not measured for each injection. The Tofts model derives two parameters to fit the time–signal curves, K^{trans}, the transfer constant, and v_e. Sources of error in the Tofts model include inaccuracies relating to the input function based on the assumption of an instantaneous bolus.

Lawrence and Lee (12,13) have developed a more complex model, which derives capillary flow, permeability, and transit time. The arterial and tissue concentration must be measured with high temporal resolution (approximately 1–2 seconds) to detect the contrast agent arriving and leaving the capillary bed. Four independent parameters are estimated, namely, F_p (flow), v_b (blood volume), E (extraction fraction), and v_e (extravascular volume). Knowing E and F one can calculate PS. While seemingly ideal, this model is also limited by type and quality of data available during DCE-MRI.

Relation of MR Signal to Concentration

A fundamental problem in DCE-MRI is relating signal intensity to gadolinium concentration. Several solutions have been proposed. These include (a) assuming that the relationship is linear (within the limits of the concentrations employed) or (b) obtaining T1 maps of baseline tissue and calculating estimates of concentration from signal changes after contrast.

PK models require the *concentrations* of contrast agent while DCE-MRI measures *signal*. Are the two the same? While it might be true that signal and concentration are interchangeable for CT and PET, it is not necessarily true for MRI. The relationship between R1(1/T1) and concentration [C] is linear and is related to the baseline $T1_0$ by the equation:

$$\frac{1}{T1} = \frac{1}{T1_0} + \alpha[C]$$

where 1/T1 is the measured R1 after contrast, $1/T1_0$ the baseline R1, and α; is a constant (6,7). If one measures signal intensity and does not convert it to R1(1/T1) then the assumption of linearity may be violated to varying degrees depending on the pulse sequence employed and the concentration of gadolinium chelate. Some models accept the nonlinearity of signal versus gadolinium concentration (as opposed to R1 vs. gadolinium concentration) as a practical compromise for clinical purposes, avoiding the need for generating T1 maps prior to the injection, and then compensating for preinjection T1 of tissue (11). However, the relative signal gain on MRI within a given tissue depends to a large degree on its original R1. Tissues with shorter T1 (e.g., 500 msec) will enhance *much less* than tissues with longer T1s (e.g., 1000 msec) given the same concentration of gadolinium chelate (14). To compensate for this a T1 map is generated prior to obtaining the DCE-MRI. Scans are obtained at multiple TR values or with varying flip angles (typically 2–5 values depending on the required accuracy) with constant TE. T1 and hence R1 are calculated from the Bloch equations. Knowing the R1 (=1/T1) before enhancement allows one to calculate the R1 after injection by applying a multiplier determined empirically.

Another problem complicating the calculation of gadolinium concentration from signal intensity is that MRI does not directly measure gadolinium concentration in the way that CT measures iodine concentration. Rather, MRI measures the effect of gadolinium on the relaxation rate of surrounding water molecules. It is assumed that water is in fast exchange so that the presence of gadolinium is instantly seen as a change in T1. However, Landis et al. (15) have pointed out that not all water compartments are in the fast exchange with each other. This means that significant errors in gadolinium concentration estimation could be made early after injection. This criticism of gadolinium concentration determination is not specific to one model but affects all models. However, the practical significance of this limitation is still unclear.

Limitations of the GKM

As with all models some assumptions are made about the nature of the compartments as illustrated in Figure 2. The vascular space, for example, is assumed to be a perfect mixing chamber in which the contrast media is essentially instantly and evenly diluted. The mixing phase is, in fact, not instantaneous but rather occurs over several minutes following injection (3). Another assumption is that the rate constants of exchange between the compartments are fixed during the time of data collection. This is a reasonable assumption except in instances where the vasculature may be in a state of inhibition or stimulation. Other sources of error include inaccuracies in the T1 map calculation, shape of the AIF, dependency of K^{trans} on both flow and permeability and capillary surface area. The net effect of these assumptions is to reduce the accuracy with which parameters such as K^{trans} can be derived and thereby reduce the confidence with which subtle changes in contrast agent kinetics can be measured.

Empirical Methods

Given the limitations and complexity of application of PK models it is reasonable to consider simpler, more direct approaches to assess the contrast enhancement curves generated during DCE-MRI. Such approaches have also been called heuristic. The term "heuristic" comes from the Greek noun *heuriskein*, which means to discover or find. These methods are purely empiric; their results are descriptors of curves' geometric features without direct physiologic meaning. However, they are simpler and more approachable than PK models.

Time–signal curves can be described by their initial slope, peak value, time to peak, washout slope, and area under the curve. These descriptors are simple to generate and thus widely available. Although they do not attempt to "model" what is known about the underlying biologic system, they may provide equally useful results in monitoring drug therapy within tumors without the complexity of PK models. Of course, these parameters are highly dependent on the method of acquisition. For example, comparison between two studies performed at different injection rates and durations is impossible with heuristic methods. In theory, PK modeling can be adaptable to such differences. Hence, in practice, acquisition of data should be as uniform as possible to avoid experimental error, a problem encountered with all methods. Also, measures such as slope, peak, and washout rates may depend on the MR type, field strength, settings such as gain and scaling, and manufacturer, although these factors also influence pharmocokinetic models. Empiric methods benefit from T1 correction, as "concentration" data are more reproducible than the "signal intensity" data. Thus, empiric methods likely provide similar qualitative information as PK methods. Indeed some investigators take this reductionist approach to the extreme by advocating a three-point method (baseline, peak, and delayed) for characterizing tumor response (16,17).

Methods of Display

Regardless of the actual model or approach employed to analyze time series acquisitions, data display is important. As mentioned, one of the major reasons to employ models or empirical methods is data reduction, the summary of numerous data points of the enhancement curve in terms of a few parameters that reflect curve shape and underlying physiology. The colorized map is superimposed over an anatomic image with relatively high spatial resolution. Thus, the color map reveals lesion size, location, and internal heterogeneity as well as physiologic or functional information (Figs. 7 and 8). And, time–signal curves reflecting the whole tumor as well as specific tumor regions are often displayed. A useful depiction of tumor heterogeneity is an x–y scatter plot of the distribution of parameters within the tumor. Responses to therapy can be visualized as a shift in the distribution of the parameters. Indeed vectors that reflect the magnitude and direction of the shift in the mean and median values can be generated to summarize tumor response to therapy. Histograms of the parameters can also be used to display these complex data sets. Furthermore, superimposition of parameter maps and other kinds of imaging data, such as FDG PET activity, can be used to generate multiparametric analyses of tumors.

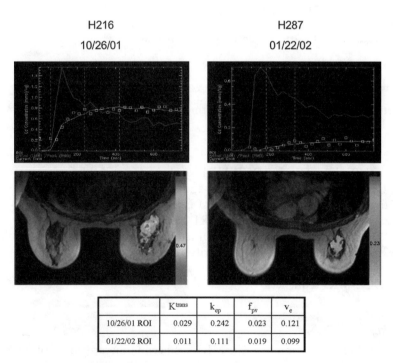

	K^{trans}	k_{ep}	f_{pv}	v_{e}
10/26/01 ROI	0.029	0.242	0.023	0.121
01/22/02 ROI	0.011	0.111	0.019	0.099

Figure 7   Clinical example of a patient with breast cancer undergoing neoadjuvant chemotherapy. At baseline the tumor is large and highly permeable. Several months later the tumor is smaller and the tumor enhancement curve is much lower in amplitude. The K^{trans} and k_{ep} are reduced. The fraction of plasma volume (f_{pv}) and extravascular volume (v_{e}) are also decreased but to a smaller degree. (*See color insert.*)

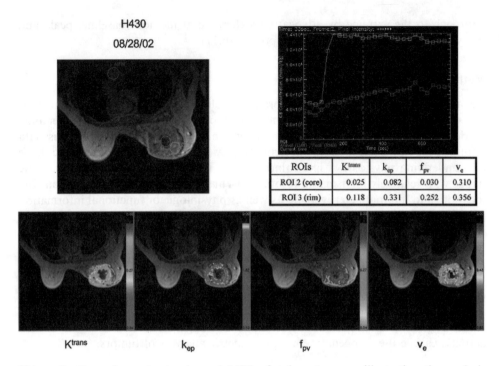

ROIs	K^{trans}	k_{ep}	f_{pv}	v_e
ROI 2 (core)	0.025	0.082	0.030	0.310
ROI 3 (rim)	0.118	0.331	0.252	0.356

K^{trans} k_{ep} f_{pv} v_e

Figure 8 Dynamic contrast enhanced MRI of a breast cancer illustrating the analysis format. The right breast mass contains a necrotic center. The graph reveals region of interest measurements from the rim and the core demonstrating markedly different results. Separate color maps of K^{trans}, k_{ep}, f_{pv}, and v_e can be generated. (*See color insert.*)

Clinical Applications

DCE-MRI is used in diagnosis, staging, and treatment monitoring.

Detection

In women at high risk for breast cancer DCE-MRI is able to detect early cancers and distinguish breast cancers from fibroadenomas and other benign breast lesions. Because it is relatively costly, however, DCE-MRI is not recommended for routine screening for breast cancer. Similarly, DCE-MRI has proven useful in prostate cancer imaging. While abnormalities on T2 weighted scans are nonspecific, when they also demonstrate a high degree of vascularity on DCE-MRI, the likelihood of cancer increases. Biopsies can then be directed to the areas abnormal on both T2 weighted and DCE-MRI sequences.

Therapy Monitoring

Perhaps the most fruitful application of DCE-MRI has been in therapy monitoring. In breast cancer, for example, responses to neo-adjuvant chemotherapy can be detected by decreases in K^{trans} and other parameters after only one to two cycles, well before changes in tumor size. Other examples include bladder, bone sarcomas, cervical, and rectal cancers. Decreases in enhancement, particularly K^{trans} and k_{ep}, have been correlated with improved survival (18).

Challenges

DCE-MRI can be performed at virtually any medical center. However, there are a number of problems that limit its dissemination.

1. Model validation. There are several different types of model validation. *Mathematical validation* assesses how well the model's curves fit the data points. In most cases the current models serve well. *In vitro validation* includes evaluating permeability and estimates of extracellular space within tumors using other indicators of anatomy and physiology and their response to known perturbants. This is inherently difficult as DCE-MRI measures processes within live tumors and as in vitro tests assess fixed tissue. Moreover, it is unclear whether the permeability measured by DCE-MRI is a direct consequence of angiogenesis flow or can occur as a result of other pathways causing leakiness within vessels. Thus, the exact interpretation of these parameters remains controversial. *Clinical validation* is the assessment of DCE-MRI in detecting clinically relevant lesions and determining their histology/prognosis and response to therapy. To date there has been conflicting clinical validation of DCE-MRI with the majority of studies showing that it provides useful clinical information for diagnosis and therapy response.

2. Uniformity of methods. There are multiple variations of the GKM. This has led to a proliferation of names for exchange rate constants making comparisons among studies difficult. Additionally, precontrast T1 maps and AIFs have not been routinely obtained thus further complicating comparisons. The field is in need of a consensus on nomenclature, quantification, performance, and analysis.

3. Macromolecular contrast agents. To date, DCE-MRI has been performed with small molecular weight gadolinium chelates. A new generation of macromolecular agents with larger mean diameters is in the approval process. These agents will have different contrast kinetics, which may not be suitable for modeling with conventional PK approaches because of protein binding and retention in the EES. More sophisticated models may be necessary to adapt to these agents. However, these agents may also provide a purer indication of vessel permeability than existing low molecular weight agents.

CONCLUSION

PK models are used to describe time series data and to provide a biologically meaningful context to analyze and compare these data. It is reflected in enhancement curves that the models are based on knowledge of the microvascular anatomy and physiology. While the exact PK implementation depends on the imaging technique employed, each can be used to fit the data from time–signal series to derive parameters reflecting physiologic/anatomic properties of the tumor. The different models used today are all based on the GKM and differ primarily in their approach to their treatment of the AIF. Empirical methods of analysis of enhancement curves including slope, peak, and washout rates may provide similar data more simply than PK models, although the derived parameters have considerably less physiological meaning. Methods of display include color maps, time–signal curves generated over regions of interest, histograms, and scatter diagrams. Whether empirical or PK methods are used, DCE images provide insight into the vascular nature of tumors and are important methods of analyzing the regional microvascularity of tumors and their response to therapy.

APPENDIX: DERIVATION OF THE GKM

1. We begin with the mass transfer equation:

$$\frac{dC_t(t)}{dt} = K^{trans} C_p(t) - k_{ep} C_t(t)$$

2. By rearrangement:

$$\frac{dC_t(t)}{dt} + k_{ep} C_t(t) = K^{trans} C_p(t)$$

3. To simplify, we will consider $k_{ep} = k$. Multiply both sides by e^{kt}:

$$\frac{dC_t(t)}{dt} e^{kt} + k C_t(t) e^{kt} = K^{trans} C_p(t) e^{kt}$$

4. It is a property of derivatives that:

$$\frac{d(AB)}{dt} = \frac{dA}{dt} B + \frac{dB}{dt} A$$

5. And a property of natural logarithms that:

$$\frac{de^{kt}}{dt} = k e^{kt}$$

6. By rearrangement therefore:

$$\frac{dC_t(t)}{dt} e^{kt} + C_t(t) \frac{de^{kt}}{dt} = K^{trans} C_p(t) e^{kt}$$

7. Which is in a form that could take advantage of step 4:

$$\frac{d\left(C_t(t) e^{kt}\right)}{dt} = K^{trans} C_p(t) e^{kt}$$

8. Integrating both sides:

$$\int_0^T \frac{d\left(C_t(t) e^{kt}\right)}{dt} dt = \int_0^T K^{trans} C_p(t) e^{kt} dt$$

9. Which results in the following simplification:

$$\int_0^T \frac{d\left(C_t(t) e^{kt}\right)}{dt} = K^{trans} \int_0^T C_p(t) e^{kt}$$

10. A property of integrals is:

$$\int_a^b F' dt = F(b) = F(a)$$

11. So that the left part of the equation can be simplified:

$$C_t(T)e^{kT} - C_t(0)e^{kt} = K^{\text{trans}} \int_0^T C_p(t)e^{kt}dt$$

12. Because $C_t(0) = 0$ this term drops out leaving:

$$C_t(T)e^{kT} = K^{\text{trans}} \int_0^T C_p(t)e^{kt}dt$$

13. Multiplying both sides by e^{-kT} eliminates the exponential from the left part of equation.

$$C_t(T)e^{kT}e^{-kT} = K^{\text{trans}} \int_0^T C_p(t)e^{kT}e^{-kt}dt$$

$$C_t(T) = K^{\text{trans}} \int_0^T C_p(t)e^{-k(T-t)}dt$$

which is the GKM.

REFERENCES

1. Folkman J. Tumor angiogenesis: role in regulation of tumor growth. Symp Soc Dev Biol 1974; 30:43–52.
2. McDonald DM, Choyke PL. Imaging of angiogenesis: from microscope to clinic. Nat Med 2003; 9:713–725.
3. Tofts PS. Modeling tracer kinetics in dynamic Gd-DTPA MR imaging. J Magn Reson Imaging 1997; 7:91–101.
4. Choyke PL, Dwyer AJ, Knopp MV. Functional tumor imaging with dynamic contrast-enhanced magnetic resonance imaging. J Magn Reson Imaging 2003; 17:509–520.
5. Knopp MV, Von Tengg-Kobligk H, Choyke PL. Functional magnetic resonance imaging in oncology for diagnosis and therapy monitoring. Mol Cancer Ther 2003; 2:419–426.
6. Tofts PS, Kermode AG. Measurement of the blood-brain barrier permeability and leakage space using dynamic MR imaging. 1. Fundamental concepts. Magn Reson Med 1991; 17:357–367.
7. Tofts PS, Berkowitz B, Schnall MD. Quantitative analysis of dynamic Gd-DTPA enhancement in breast tumors using a permeability model. Magn Reson Med 1995; 33:564–568.
8. Renkin EM. Transport of potassium-42 from blood to tissue in isolated mammalian skeletal muscles. Am J Physiol 1959; 197:1025–1210.
9. Kety SS. The theory and applications of the exchange of inert gas at the lungs and tissue. Pharmacol Rev 1951; 3:1–41.
10. Tofts PS, Brix G, Buckley DL, et al. Estimating kinetic parameters from dynamic contrast-enhanced T(1)-weighted MRI of a diffusible tracer: standardized quantities and symbols. J Magn Reson Imaging 1999; 10:223–232.
11. Brix G, Semmler W, Port R, Schad LR, Layer G, Lorenz WJ. Pharmacokinetic parameters in CNS Gd-DTPA enhanced MR imaging. J Comput Assist Tomogr 1991; 15:621–628.
12. St Lawrence KS, Lee TY. An adiabatic approximation to the tissue homogeneity model for water exchange in the brain: I. Theoretical derivation. J Cereb Blood Flow Metab 1998; 18:1365–1377.

13. St Lawrence KS, Lee TY. An adiabatic approximation to the tissue homogeneity model for water exchange in the brain: II. Experimental validation. J Cereb Blood Flow Metab 1998; 18:1378–1385.

14. Evelhoch JL. Key factors in the acquisition of contrast kinetic data for oncology. J Magn Reson Imaging 1999; 10:254–259.

15. Landis CS, Li X, Telang TW, et al. Determination of the MRI contrast agent concentration time course in vivo following bolus injection: effect of equilibrium transcytolemmal water exchange. Magn Reson Med 2000; 44:563–574.

16. Furman-Haran E, Grobgeld D, Margalit R, Degani H. Response of MCF7 human breast cancer to tamoxifen: evaluation by the three-time-point, contrast-enhanced magnetic resonance imaging method. Clin Cancer Res 1998; 4:2299–2304.

17. Weinstein D, Strano S, Cohen P, Fields S, Gomori JM, Degani H. Breast fibroadenoma: mapping of pathophysiologic features with three-time-point, contrast-enhanced MR imaging – pilot study. Radiology 1999; 210:233–240.

18. Morgan B, Thomas AL, Drevs J, et al. Dynamic contrast enhanced magnetic resonance imaging as a biomarker for the pharmacological response of PTK787/ZK 222584 an inhibitor of the vascular endothelial growth factor receptor tyrosine kinases, in patients with advanced colorectal cancer and liver metastases: results from two Phase I studies. J Clin Oncol 2003; 21:3955–3964.

15

Bioluminescence Reporter Gene Imaging in Small Animal Models of Cancer

Tarik F. Massoud

The Crump Institute for Molecular Imaging, David Geffen School of Medicine, University of California at Los Angeles, Los Angeles, California, U.S.A.; Departments of Radiology and Oncology, University of Cambridge School of Clinical Medicine, Cambridge, U.K.

Sanjiv S. Gambhir

The Crump Institute for Molecular Imaging, Departments of Molecular and Medical Pharmacology and Biomathematics, and UCLA-Johnsson Comprehensive Cancer Center, David Geffen School of Medicine, University of California at Los Angeles, Los Angeles, California, U.S.A.; and Department of Radiology and the Bio-X Program, Stanford University School of Medicine, Stanford, California, U.S.A.

A Note from the Editors

*B*ioluminescence refers to the enzymatic generation of visible light by living organisms and is still exclusively used in animal models. The most commonly used bioluminescence reporter gene has been the luciferase from the North American firefly (Photinus pyralis; Fluc). The sensitivity of bioluminescence imaging is thought to be in the 10^{-15} to 10^{-17} mole/L range, the highest for any available molecular imaging modality. Luciferase does not need external light excitation and self-emits light from green to yellow wavelengths in the presence of D-Luciferin, ATP, magnesium, and oxygen. The relationship between the enzyme concentration and light is linear making quantitation easier. Bioluminescence imaging allows the monitoring of tumor evolution throughout the disease course starting from minimal to late stage disease. Cancer progression, including cell trafficking and development of metastases can be visualized. With continued and rapid technological advancements in this field, bioluminescence imaging has the potential to greatly refine our animal models of cancer and will ultimately contribute to advances in clinical cancer diagnosis, treatment, and prevention.*

INTRODUCTION

Molecular imaging may be defined as the visual representation, characterization, and quantification of biological processes at the cellular and subcellular levels within intact living organisms. It is a novel multidisciplinary field, in which the images produced reflect cellular and molecular pathways and in vivo mechanisms of disease present within the context of physiologically authentic environments. The overall goals of molecular imaging within biomedical research are (i) to develop noninvasive in vivo imaging methods that reflect specific cellular and molecular processes, for example, gene expression, or more complex molecular interactions such as protein–protein interactions; (ii) to monitor multiple molecular events near-simultaneously; (iii) to follow trafficking, differentiation, and targeting of cells; (iv) to optimize drug and gene therapies; (v) to image drug effects at a molecular and cellular levels; (vi) to assess disease progression at a molecular pathological level; (vii) to create the possibility of achieving all of the above goals of imaging in a rapid, reproducible, and quantitative manner, so as to be able to monitor time-dependent experimental, developmental, environmental, and therapeutic influences on gene products in the same animal or patient.

Although the foundations of molecular imaging can be traced to nuclear medicine, the underlying principles of molecular imaging can now be tailored to other imaging modalities such as optical imaging and magnetic resonance imaging (MRI). A relatively recent addition to these techniques is bioluminescence imaging, a noninvasive optical imaging modality, that allows sensitive and quantitative detection of bioluminescence reporter genes in intact small animals. Bioluminescence refers to the enzymatic generation of visible light by living organisms. Bioluminescence imaging is well suited for use with small animal models of cancer, is relatively easily accessible to cancer researchers in their laboratory setting, and offers particular flexibility in experimental cancer investigations (1). Table 1 outlines some of the general advantages and disadvantages of bioluminescence imaging. Bioluminescence imaging probes can now be developed by taking advantage of the rapidly increasing knowledge of available cellular/molecular targets. The merger of molecular biology and imaging is facilitating rapid growth of this new field by providing methods to monitor cellular/molecular events adapted from conventional molecular assays, for example, reporter gene assays (2,3). These developments in bioluminescence imaging of cancer models in animals now enable us to noninvasively track molecular and cellular events contributing to carcinogenesis and cancer progression and to swiftly unveil therapeutic efficacies in preclinical evaluations of novel therapeutic strategies (1).

Principles of Bioluminescence Imaging

The light emission in bioluminescence follows a chemiluminescent reaction that can take place under physiological conditions within living cells in the presence of adenosine triphosphate (ATP), or it can be extracellular (e.g., *Renilla* luciferase) when the reaction is independent of ATP. The most commonly used bioluminescence reporter gene for research purposes has been the luciferase from the North American firefly (*Photinus pyralis*; *Fluc*). Luciferase genes have also been cloned from a variety of other organisms, including corals (*Tenilla*), jellyfish (*Aequorea*), sea pansy (*Renilla, Rluc*), several bacterial species (*Vibrio fischeri* and *V. harveyi*), and dinoflagellates (*Gonyaulax*) (4). Several of these genes, including *Fluc*, have been modified

Table 1 General Advantages and Disadvantages of Bioluminescence Imaging

General advantages

More physiological than conventional in vitro and cell culture assays: Bioluminescence imaging permits both the temporal and the spatial biodistribution of a molecular probe and related biological processes to be determined in a more meaningful manner throughout an intact living subject. Visualization of functions and interactions of a particular gene becomes easier in a more realistic manner that respects the dynamics of complex biological networks and of complete and holistic biological systems in the entire living subject

Whole-body imaging. Surveys many/all tissues simultaneously

Allows repetitive study of the same animal model: Bioluminescence imaging can reveal a dynamic and more meaningful picture of the progressive changes in biological parameters under scrutiny, as well as possible temporal assessment of therapeutic responses, all in the same animal without recourse to its death. The ability to repeat studies means that the same animal can serve as its own control

Quick and convenient: Bioluminescence imaging results may be attainable with less labor, facilitating achievement of a relatively higher-throughput facet to many biological laboratory investigations

Noninvasive, no animal sacrifice, fewer animals used, a more ethical approach than sacrificing many more animals at each follow-up time-point of a study

May be used in phenotype screening of transgenic and gene-targeted animal models

May be used in preclinical trials for drug discovery and validation

General disadvantages

The efficiency of light transmission through an opaque animal can be somewhat limited and depends on tissue type and tissue scattering: Skin and muscle have the highest transmission and are fairly wavelength-dependent, whereas organs with a high vascular content such as liver and spleen have the lowest transmission because of absorption of light by oxyhemoglobin and deoxyhemoglobin

Images obtained from the cooled CCD camera are two-dimensional and lack depth information: It is expected that future bioluminescence image acquisition using rotating CCD cameras or multiple views of the same animal with a single CCD camera may allow volumetric imaging

No equivalent imaging modality applicable for human studies, thus preventing direct translation of developed methods for clinical use

Quantitative comparisons between light signals emanating from different superficial and deeper regions of the body are difficult to make because bioluminescence imaging is a nontomographic modality, and the signals measured are dependent on many factors as discussed in the text

Requires injection of substrate, which represents a relative drawback compared with fluorescence imaging

Source: From Ref. 3.

for optimal expression in mammalian cells and these have been used for many years in bioassays for ATP quantification and to study gene expression in transfected cells in culture. Firefly luciferase (61 kDa) catalyzes the transformation of its substrate D-luciferin [D-(–)-2-(6′-hydroxy-2′-benzothiazolyl)thiazone-4-carboxylic acid] into oxyluciferin in a process dependent on ATP, Mg^{2+}, and O_2, leading to the emission of light, which can be detected using low-light sensing instruments including standard luminometers (Fig. 1). These biochemical assays are typically conducted on cell lysates, although there are several reports of live cell assays that use *Fluc* [reviewed in Edinger et al. (1)].

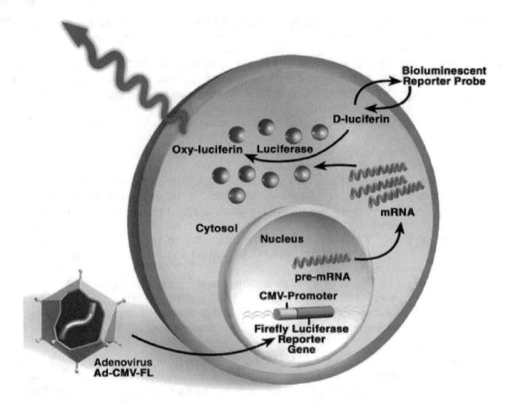

Figure 1 Schematic diagram of the principle of reporter gene imaging using the enzyme firefly luciferase. Once the cell is transduced with a viral vector containing the imaging gene cassette, a promoter of choice drives the transcription of the imaging reporter gene (*Fluc*). If the promoter leads to transcription of *Fluc*, then translation of the imaging reporter gene mRNA leads to a protein product (the enzyme firefly luciferase) that can interact with the imaging reporter probe (D-luciferin). This interaction is a chemiluminescent reaction that catalyses the transformation of the substrate D-luciferin into oxyluciferin in a process dependent on ATP, Mg^{2+}, and O_2, leading to the emission of light, which can be detected using low-light sensing instruments.

Some luciferins require the presence of a cofactor to undergo oxidation, such as $FMNH_2^+$, Ca^{2+}, or ATP. Complexes that contain a luciferase, a luciferin, and generally requiring O_2 are also called photoproteins. Although the most common luciferin–luciferase system used in molecular imaging is that derived from the firefly *Photinus*, the sea pansy *Renilla* luciferase, which uses a different substrate (coelenterazine) is not ATP- or Mg^{2+}-dependent, and has also been validated recently for applications in living subjects (5). *Renilla* luciferase enzyme (36 kDa) is capable of generating a flash of blue light (460–490 nm, peak emission at 482 nm) upon reaction with its substrate. The synthetic *Renilla* luciferase gene (*hRluc*) is a systematically redesigned *Renilla* luciferase gene, encoding the same 311-residue protein as wild-type *Renilla* luciferase, but yielding only codon changes for higher expression in mammalian cells. Both colorimetric (e.g., rhodamine red) and fluorescent (e.g., GFP) reporter proteins require an external source of light for excitation and emit light at a different wavelength for detection, thus making them more susceptible to background noise (autofluorescence). In contrast, the bioluminescence luciferase enzymes and substrate systems described above have several characteristics that make them useful reporter proteins. Firstly, firefly luciferase does not need external light excitation and self-emits light from green to yellow wavelengths (560–610 nm, peak emission at 562 nm) in the presence of D-Luciferin, ATP, magnesium, and oxygen. Secondly, the fast rate of enzyme turnover ($T_{1/2} = 3$ hours) in the presence of substrate D-luciferin allows for real-time measurements, because the enzyme does not accumulate intracellularly to the extent of other reporters. Thirdly, the relationship between the enzyme concentration and amount of emitted light in vitro is linear up to seven to eight orders of magnitude. Therefore, these properties potentially allow for sensitive noninvasive imaging of *Fluc* (and *Rluc*) reporter gene expression in living subjects.

Broadening the use of firefly luciferase as a bioluminescence reporter from biochemical and cell culture assays to living animals was reliant upon the development of low light imaging systems (see below) and two other crucial observations (1). The first observation was the demonstration that D-luciferin would seem to circulate within minutes throughout many body compartments (also readily crossing the blood brain barrier) after intravenous or intraperitoneal (i.p.) administration and rapidly enters many cells (6,7). Studies are underway in our laboratory to accurately quantify the uptake kinetics and biodistribution of the D-luciferin (as well as coelenterazine). The second discovery was that the level and spectrum of emitted light from *Fluc* expressing mammalian cells is adequate to penetrate tissues of small research animals, such as mice and rats, and can be detected externally with low-light imaging cameras (6,7).

Several factors governing interaction of emitted light with tissues deserve particular consideration. The absorption coefficient of light depends on its wavelength (the more the light absorbed, the wavelength is <600 nm), and results from absorbers such as hemoglobin (the main absorber), lipids, and water (8). As the emission spectrum of firefly luciferase is very broad, the lower end of the spectrum is absorbed to a greater extent within tissues, resulting in relatively more red-shifted light emitted from the surface, particularly when the source of light is in a deep location. The blue spectrum emitted from *Renilla* luciferase is absorbed to a greater extent than that of firefly luciferase, but this is counteracted by the much greater initial quantum yield from *Renilla* luciferase. Recently, it has been found that the measurable signal from C6 cells transfected with *hRluc* to be approximately 30- to 40-fold higher than that from C6 cells transfected with *Fluc*, when implanted subcutaneously in the same mouse. The difference in light emission in cell culture is even greater than approximately 120-fold. For deeper tissues (e.g., the lungs), even after absorption, the measurable light when using higher doses of coelenterazine is also higher for cells transfected with *hRluc*. Additional studies are still needed to directly compare firefly luciferase and synthetic *Renilla* luciferase in living subjects.

In mammals, the absorption of light is also affected by the color of skin. Melanin in the skin absorbs light emitted from within the subject. Therefore, the sensitivity of light detection is significantly lower in black mice as compared with white mice (1). Also, hair and fur scatter light, and therefore, albino nude mice yield the highest sensitivity and resolution when used in bioluminescence imaging (9).

The signal intensity of measurable light is further determined to a large extent by attenuation of light owing to the effects of scattering. Scattering results from changes in the refractive index at cell membranes and organelles. The signal intensity from a depth of 1 cm is attenuated by a factor of approximately 10^{-2} for wavelengths at approximately 650 nm (10). This scatter results in the relatively poor spatial resolution of bioluminescence imaging when compared to other modalities that rely on more penetrating electromagnetic radiation to generate images, for example, PET, SPECT, and computed tomography (CT).

TECHNIQUES AND INSTRUMENTATION

Considerable efforts have been directed in recent years toward the development of noninvasive high-resolution imaging technologies for imaging living small animals (3). Optical imaging techniques are well established for in vitro and ex vivo applications in molecular and cellular biology (e.g., fluorescence microscopy and bench-top luminometry using commercial substrate kits for bioluminescence.) An extension of this concept toward noninvasive whole-body imaging with photons represents an interesting avenue for extracting relevant biological information from living subjects. Progress in bioluminescence molecular imaging strategies has come from the recent development of targeted bioluminescence probes, technical advances in detectors for measuring low levels of light emission, and on-going search for more red-shifted bioluminescence proteins or those with varying kinetics of light emission. Bioluminescence imaging allows for a relatively low cost option for studying reporter gene expression in small animal models. Bioluminescence imaging systems are relatively simple in comparison with instrumentation for other molecular or clinical imaging modalities and can be housed in shared resources of basic science laboratories.

A fundamental issue in bioluminescence imaging of living subjects is how to detect light emitted from the subject. In this regard, several technical advances for imaging very low levels of visible light have now emerged, allowing the use of highly sensitive detectors in living subjects and not just restricted to cell cultures and small transparent animals. Charged coupled device (CCD) detectors are made of silicon crystals sliced into thin sheets for fabrication into integrated circuits using similar technologies to those used in making computer silicon chips. For a detailed overview of CCD technology, refer to Spibey et al. (11). One of the properties of silicon-based detectors is their high sensitivity to light, allowing them to detect light in the visible to near-infrared range. When photons at wavelengths between 400 and 1000 nm strike a CCD pixel with energy of just 2–3 eV, the CCD camera can convert these photons into electrons. A CCD contains semiconductors that are connected so that the output of one serves as the input of the next. In this way, an electrical charge pattern, corresponding to the intensity of incoming photons, is read out of the CCD into an output register and amplifier at the edge of the CCD for digitization. Older intensified CCD cameras had much lower sensitivities than newer generation cooled CCD cameras. This is because thermal noise (termed "dark current") from thermal energy within the silicon lattice of a CCD chip resulted in constant release of electrons. Thermal noise is dramatically reduced if the chip is cooled; dark current falls by a factor of 10 for every 20°C decrease in temperature (11). For bioluminescence imaging, CCD cameras are usually mounted in a light-tight specimen chamber and are attached to a cryogenic refrigeration unit (for camera cooling to minus 120–150°C). A camera controller linked to a computer system is used for data acquisition and analysis.

Bioluminescence imaging of neoplastic tissue requires that the gene encoding the bioluminescence reporter protein be transferred to cells or tissues of interest, which can be accomplished using one of three gene transfer methods: ex vivo, in vivo, or as part of a transgenic construct. When cells transfected ex vivo, and transiently or stably expressing the bioluminescence reporter gene, are injected into the research

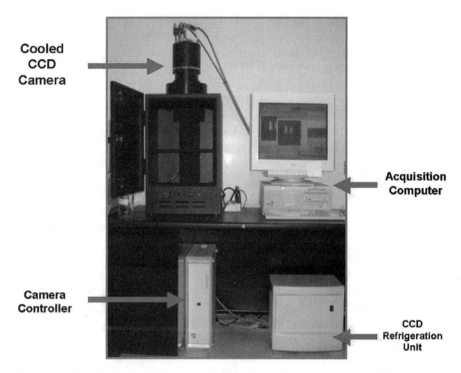

Figure 2 The Xenogen In vivo Imaging System consists of a cooled CCD camera mounted on a light-tight imaging chamber, a cryogenic refrigeration unit, a camera controller, and a computer system for data analysis.

animal, the light emitted from the gene-marked cells can be monitored externally. To generate such an image, the animals are anaesthetized and placed in a light-tight chamber equipped with the CCD camera (Fig. 2). A grayscale reference image (digital photograph) is acquired under weak illumination, and then in complete darkness the photons emitted from within the body of the animal are detected externally using a range of integration times from one second to several minutes. The data are transferred to a computer equipped with image acquisition, overlay, and analysis software for quantification. A bioluminescence image is most often shown as a color image representing light intensity (usually from blue, for least intense, to red, for most intense) that is superimposed on the grayscale photographic image to display the anatomical origin of photon emission. Usually a region of interest is manually selected over an area of signal intensity, and the maximum or average intensity recorded as photons/sec/cm^2/steradian (steradian is a unit of solid angle). Whenever the exposure conditions (including time, f/stop, height of sample shelf, binning ratio, and time after injection with optical substrate) are kept identical, the measurements are highly reproducible (in our laboratory to within 6%).

SENSITIVITY OF BIOLUMINESCENCE IMAGING IN LIVING SUBJECTS

In addition to possession of the general advantageous characteristics outlined in Table 1, bioluminescence imaging stands out specifically because it is quick and easy to perform, and it allows rapid testing of biological hypotheses and proofs-of-principle in living experimental models of cancer. It is also uniquely suited for high-throughput imaging because of its ease of operation, short acquisition, and the possibility of simultaneous measurement of several anesthetized living mice. However, the main advantage of optical bioluminescence imaging is that it can be used to detect very low levels of signal because the light emitted is virtually background-free. Mammalian cells do not possess significant levels of intrinsic bioluminescence (1). Therefore, the presence of an inherently low background of light signifies that photon emission is restricted only to cells expressing bioluminescence reporter genes, and that virtually no signal is detectable from surrounding naive cells or tissues. Moreover, firefly luciferase and its substrate D-luciferin have not been shown to be toxic to mammalian cells, and so far no functional differences have been observed between cells expressing *Fluc* and the parental cell lines, although formal toxicological studies are yet to be conducted (12). Similar observations likely pertain to *Renilla* luciferase and its substrate coelenterazine. However, both absorption and scatter limit the penetration of photons through mammalian tissues (13). Estimates from in vitro studies show that the net reduction of bioluminescence signal is approximately 10-fold for every centimeter of tissue depth, varying with the exact tissue type (6). The sensitivity of detecting internal sources of bioluminescence has been addressed in several studies (13–16). This sensitivity is dependent upon many parameters including the level of reporter gene expression, the emission wavelength spectrum, the depth of gene-marked cells within the body (i.e., the distance that the photons must travel through body tissues), and the sensitivity of the detection system.

In its existing state of advancement, bioluminescence imaging is proving to be one of the most sensitive modalities for the detection of cancer cells in living small research animals. Sensitivity may be regarded as the ability to detect the presence of a molecular probe, relative to the background, measured in mol/L (3). Although not precisely characterized to date, the sensitivity of bioluminescence imaging is thought to be in the order of 10^{-15}–10^{-17} mol/L, the highest of any available molecular imaging modality (3). In syngeneic animal models of leukaemia and lymphoma, A20 and BCL_1 tumor cells could be detected with high sensitivity in internal organs such as the lung, liver, spleen, lymph nodes, and even within the bone marrow of BALB/c mice (1). As few as 1000 cells were detectable after subcutaneous injection; <10,000 cells could be seen in the lungs early after intravenous injection of labeled cells. Tumor infiltration of the spleen was observed earlier with a higher sensitivity than seen by ex vivo flow cytometry after isolation of the splenocytes. Injection of a known number of cells into the peritoneal cavity of living mice has been used to determine the sensitivity and reproducibility of bioluminescence imaging (13,14). As few as 100 cells could be detected above background in these studies. In other gene delivery experiments, Lipshutz et al. (15) used a recombinant adeno-associated virus–based transduction system to deliver *Fluc* into mice in utero. Long-term expression of luciferase in the liver and peritoneum was observed. Limiting dilution polymerase chain reaction performed eight months after the birth of the mice showed that the signal intensity generated from one *Fluc* expressing liver cell among 10^6 nonexpressing liver cells was sufficient to be detected externally. This demonstrated that whole body firefly luciferase imaging was almost as sensitive as luminometry assays on cell lysates, although the liver absorbs light because of its high hemoglobin content (10). Recent experiments using adenoviral-mediated gene transfer to muscle and liver revealed that, in small research animals, bioluminescence imaging is extremely sensitive for detecting transferred genes and may be more sensitive than PET imaging, although formal comparisons are yet to be made (1). Corroboration of this principle was also recently obtained by Ray et al. (2), who developed a fusion reporter gene containing both mutant herpes simplex virus type 1 thymidine kinase (*HSV1-sr39TK*) for PET imaging and *Rluc* for bioluminescence imaging. They found that the higher sensitivity of optical imaging allowed lower levels of reporter gene expression and/or lower numbers of expressing cells to be imaged relative to the PET approach.

Owing to its inherent high sensitivity, bioluminescence imaging has significant potential implications for refining animal models of cancer, for understanding the underlying cancer biology, and for accelerating the preclinical stages of antineoplastic drug development. Typical assays for tumor growth and response to therapy have major limitations in the study of orthotopic, metastatic, and minimal disease animal models, as they are not particularly amenable to frequent measurements of small numbers of cells within deep tissues. Such assays include caliper measurement of gross tumor volume, assessment of weight loss or gain, or demise of the animals. In contrast, bioluminescence imaging now allows tumor cell detection and quantification during the early stages of tumorigenesis, at stages of minimal residual disease, and upon metastasis in living animal models. Moreover, applications of bioluminescence reporter genes in transgenic strategies will make possible the examination in animal models of spontaneous tumor development and of the mechanisms underlying tumor escape after therapy (1).

PRINCIPLES OF REPORTER GENE IMAGING

Intense exploration is taking place in the biological sciences to determine the patterns of gene expression that encode proteins for normal biological processes. There is also a growing belief that diseases result from alterations in normal regulation of gene expression that transform cells to phenotypes of disease, including cancer. These alterations in gene expression can result from interactions with the environment, hereditary deficits, developmental errors, and aging process (17). Imaging of gene expression in living subjects can be directed either at genes externally transferred into cells of organ systems (transgenes) or at endogenous genes. Most current applications of reporter gene imaging are for the former variety. By adopting state-of-the-art molecular biology techniques, it is now possible to better image cellular/molecular events. One can also engineer cells that will accumulate imaging probes of choice, either to act as generic gene "markers" for localizing and tracking these cells or to target a specific biological process or pathway. In the last few years, there has been a veritable explosion in the field of reporter gene imaging, with the aim of determining location, duration, and extent of gene expression within living subjects (18–20).

Reporter genes are used to study promoter/enhancer elements involved in gene expression, inducible promoters to look at the induction of gene expression, and endogenous gene expression through the use of transgenes containing endogenous promoters fused to the reporter (20). In all these cases, transcription of the reporter gene can be tracked and therefore gene expression can be studied. Unlike most conventional reporter gene methods [e.g., chloramphenicol acetyl transferase, lacZ/β-galactosidase, alkaline phosphatase, Bla/β-lactamase, etc.,] molecular imaging techniques offer the possibility of monitoring the location, magnitude, and persistence of reporter gene expression in intact animals or humans

(21). The reporter gene driven by a promoter of choice must be first introduced into the cells of interest (Fig. 1). This is a common feature for all delivery vectors in a reporter gene-imaging paradigm, that is, a complementary DNA expression cassette (an imaging cassette) containing the reporter gene of interest must be used. The promoter can be constitutive or inducible; it can also be cell-specific. If the reporter gene is expressed, an enzyme or receptor product is made, which in turn becomes available to interact with the imaging reporter probe; this may be a substrate for an enzyme (as in the case of bioluminescence imaging) or a ligand for a receptor. The interaction of the reporter protein with the probe leads to an imaging signal, be it from a radioisotope, a photochemical reaction (in bioluminescence imaging), or a magnetic resonance metal cation, depending on the exact nature of the probe itself.

The ideal reporter gene/probe (applicable also to nonbioluminescence imaging systems) would have the following general characteristics (20):

1. to prevent an immune response, the reporter gene should be present in mammalian cells, but not expressed,
2. specific reporter probe should accumulate only where reporter gene is expressed,
3. no reporter probe should accumulate when the reporter gene is not expressed,
4. the product of the reporter gene should also be nonimmunogenic,
5. the reporter probe should be stable in vivo and not be metabolized before reaching its target,
6. the reporter probe should rapidly clear from the circulation and not interfere with detection of specific signal,
7. the reporter probe or its metabolites should not be cytotoxic,
8. the size of the reporter gene and its driving promoter should be small enough to fit into a delivery vehicle (plasmids, viruses), except for transgenic applications,
9. natural biological barriers must not prevent the reporter probe from reaching its destination,
10. the image signal should correlate well with levels of reporter gene mRNA and protein in vivo.

No single reporter gene/reporter probe system currently meets all these criteria. Therefore, the development of multiple systems provides a choice based on the application of interest. The availability of multiple reporter gene/reporter probes also allows monitoring the expression of more than one reporter gene in the same living animal. Ray et al. (18) have previously reviewed the many examples of these imaging reporter systems spanning the several available molecular imaging modalities.

Bioluminescence imaging reporter systems belong to one category where the imaging gene product is intracellular, as opposed to being in/on the cell membrane. Other examples of intracellular reporters include HSV1-TK or its mutant *HSV1-sr39TK*, GFP, cytosine deaminase, and tyrosinase, to name a few. The major advantages of intracellular protein expression are the relatively uncomplicated expression strategy and probable lack of recognition of the expression product by the immune system. The relative theoretical disadvantage is the presence of potentially unfavorable kinetics, requiring the need for the substrate to enter a cell.

However, in practice, there appears to be no hindrance to intracellular penetration by D-luciferin or coelenterazine.

APPLICATIONS OF BIOLUMINESCENCE REPORTER GENE IMAGING IN CANCER MODELS

Four broad categories of applications for bioluminescence reporter gene imaging in animal models of cancer are as follows: gene marking of cells with reporter genes, imaging of gene therapies, imaging of transgenic animals carrying reporter genes, and imaging of molecular interactions such as protein–protein interactions.

Gene Marking of Cancer Cells

Gene marking may be used to track the behavior of almost any tissue (22). It is necessary to stably transfect cells with the imaging marker gene if they and their progeny are to be followed for their entire lifespan within the living subject. However, this assumes that minimal or no promoter attenuation or shutoff takes place. The latter can contribute substantially to decline in transgene expression despite the constitutive nature of the promoter. For example, constitutive CMV promoter attenuation after adenoviral gene transfer may be caused by an inflammatory response, which can lead to the secretion of interferon γ (IFN-γ) and tumor necrosis factor α (TNF-α) by antigen-activated cytotoxic T lymphocytes (23). IFN-γ and TNF-α synergistically inhibit transgene expression from several viral promoters including the CMV promoter–enhancer (24). In practice, transient transfection of cells suffices if these marked cells are to be imaged in a living subject for not more than about 7 to 10 days, depending on the cells in question and other parameters as well (3).

In principle, gene marker studies may be used to follow the behavior of almost any cell type in living subjects. In clinical practice, this has been mostly used with hematopoietic cells (22). However, in molecular imaging research, a variety of cells can be engineered to incorporate reporter genes. Usually, gene marking of cells that are static in one location, for example, subcutaneous tumor xenografts, is used for first assessment and continued validation of reporter genes and their probes or for studying the behavior of the cells themselves within living subjects. This can be accomplished by two ways: ex vivo transfection of the cells in question with a vector containing an imaging cassette followed by placement of these cells in a living subject as a xenograft or an orthotopic transplant. The second approach entails direct in vivo placement, usually via injection, of the vectors carrying the reporter gene as part of the recombinant genome of viruses into the cells of interest within the body.

Evaluation of Reporter Systems in Cancer Cells Grafted in Mice

There are numerous examples of bioluminescence imaging of cells that are mostly destined to remain static in the body after ex vivo gene marking with imaging reporters and subsequent placement in living rodents. A noteworthy advantage in these cancer models is that they create the opportunity for temporal evaluation of cancer biology in a noninvasive manner. Dynamic studies of xenograft growth and regression, either spontaneously or after therapy, can be performed. The enzymatic emission of light by firefly luciferase is ATP-dependent, and therefore, only metabolically active cells contribute to the signal. A decrease in signal intensity occurs as cells die.

For example, growth of *Fluc*-expressing malignant melanoma, B16F10, has been followed over time in severe combined immunodeficiency (SCID) mice (1). Light emission was detected within minutes after subcutaneous injection of 2×10^4 cells, and the signal intensity increased as the tumor progressed and finally formed large, macroscopically visible xenografts. It was also possible to establish in living mice that central tumor necrosis had occurred after three to four weeks, most likely because of insufficient angiogenesis. This observed decrease in signal intensity was likely a reflection on central tumor cell death that was undetected externally using calipers. A potential confounding issue, however, is the fact that as levels of hemo-globin surrounding and within the tumor increases, so does the extent of signal attenuation, without necessarily any cell death. Therefore, future studies will be necessary to examine the relative effects/contributions of these two factors on signal intensity. This notwithstanding, the ability to detect the dynamics of tumor cell death and necrosis in living animals remains a useful feature of *Fluc* bioluminescence imaging, that can be exploited in studies of angiogenesis inhibitors currently being evaluated in preclinical and clinical trials.

Studies where gene-marked xenografts were used in evaluation of biolumines-cence imaging reporters include that of Edinger et al. (13), where a stable line of human cervical carcinoma (HeLa) cells expressing *Fluc* were generated, and proliferation of these cells in irradiated SCID mice was monitored. Tumor cells were introduced into animals through subcutaneous, i.p., and intravenous injections, and whole body images were obtained to reveal tumor location and growth kinetics. Intravenous inoculation resulted in detectable colonies of tumor cells in animals receiving more than 1×10^6 cells. They also demonstrated the ability to detect small numbers of tumor cells in living animals noninvasively suggesting that therapies designed to treat minimal disease states, as occurring early in the disease course and after elimination of the tumor mass, may be monitored using this approach. Similar studies of orthotopic implants of *Fluc*-marked human prostate cells into the prostate glands of mice have been conducted by Honigman et al. (25).

In another study, Bhaumik and Gambhir (5) evaluated *Renilla* luciferase for bioluminescence imaging in living mice. Cells transiently expressing *Rluc* were imaged while located in the peritoneum, subcutaneous layer, as well as in the liver and lungs of living mice tail-vein injected with coelenterazine (Fig. 3). They found that D-luciferin (a substrate for firefly luciferase) did not serve as a substrate for *Renilla* luciferase and coelenterazine (a substrate for *Renilla* luciferase) did not serve as a substrate for firefly luciferase either in cell culture or in living mice (Fig. 4). They also showed that both *Rluc* and *Fluc* expressions could be imaged in the same living mouse and the kinetics of light production were distinct. Unlike the more sustained signal produced upon interaction of D-luciferin and firefly luci-ferase, *Rluc* expression imaging produces a typical pattern of flash kinetics within the first minute of coelenterazine injection (Fig. 5). The approaches they have vali-dated will have direct applications to various studies where two molecular events need to be tracked, including cell trafficking of two cell populations, two gene ther-apy vectors, and indirect monitoring of two endogenous genes through the use of two reporter genes.

Evaluation of Antineoplastic Therapies in Cancer Cells Grafted in Mice

Bioluminescence imaging can also externally monitor the response to chemotherapy. Sweeney et al. (14) evaluated *Fluc*-marked HeLa cells that were engrafted into

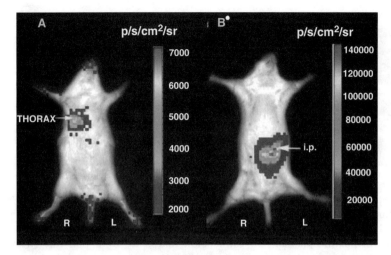

Figure 3 Renilla luciferase bioluminescence from C6-*Rluc* cells present in various tissues in living mice. (**A**) The C6-*Rluc* cells (1.0×10^6) were injected via tail-vein, and coelenterazine was tail-vein injected 90 minutes later. The bioluminescence seen represents the thorax region of the mouse where C6-*Rluc* cells are trapped in the lungs. (**B**) C6-*Rluc* cells (1.0×10^6) were implanted in the peritoneum of a different mouse and coelenterazine was tail-vein injected 90 minutes later. Bioluminescence is seen only from the i.p. region. R and L represent the right and left sides of the mouse resting in a supine position. *Source*: From Ref. 5. (*See color insert.*)

immunodeficient mice. The efficacy of both chemotherapy and immunotherapeutic treatments with ex vivo expanded human T-cell–derived effector cells was studied. In the absence of therapy, animals showed progressive increases in signal intensity over time. Animals treated with cisplatin had significant reductions in tumor signal;

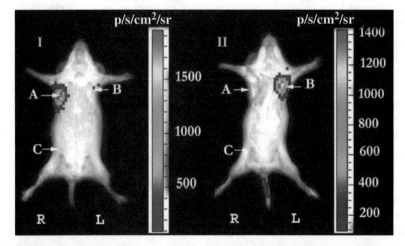

Figure 4 Crossreactivity of *Renilla* luciferase for D-luciferin and firefly luciferase for coelenterazine in living mice. Both C6-*Fluc* (A) and C6-*Rluc* (B) cells were implanted subcutaneously at right axilla and left axilla sites, respectively, in the same mouse with control C6 cell (C) implanted in the right groin region. Injection of D-luciferin via tail-vein in mouse I shows bioluminescence from site A and minimal signal from the B and C sites. Injection of coelenterazine via tail-vein in mouse II produces bioluminescence from site B but minimal signal from the A or C sites. R and L represent the right and left sides of the mouse resting in a supine position. *Source*: From Ref. 5. (*See color insert.*)

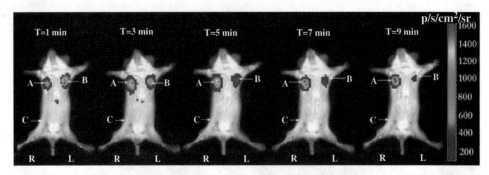

Figure 5 Kinetics of light production from mice carrying subcutaneous C6-*Fluc* and C6-*Rluc* cells after simultaneous tail-vein injection of both D-luciferin and coelenterazine. A mouse was injected subcutaneously with C6-*Fluc* (A), C6-*Rluc* (B), and C6 control cells (C) on right axilla, left axilla, and right groin regions, respectively. Simultaneous injection of both coelenterazine and D-luciferin mixture via tail-vein shows bioluminescence from both the sites simultaneously but with distinct kinetics. A series of images at two minutes intervals is shown from the same mouse. Each image represents a scan time of one minute. The signal from C6-*Rluc* cells (B) peaks early and is near extinguished within 10 minutes. Bioluminescence from C6-*Fluc* cells (A) shows a relatively strong signal beyond 10 minutes. The region of control cells does not show any significant bioluminescence. R and L represent the right and left sides of the mouse resting in a supine position. *Source*: From Ref. 5. (*See color insert.*)

5'-fluorouracil was less effective, and cyclophosphamide was ineffective. Immunotherapy dramatically reduced signals at high effector-to-target cell ratios, and significant decreases were observed with lower ratios. This model system allowed sensitive, quantitative, real-time spatiotemporal analyses of the dynamics of neoplastic cell growth and facilitated rapid optimization of effective treatment regimens. Treatment success and cure of animals could be determined in real-time, whereas relapses were diagnosed long before any clinical signs of disease were detectable or death of the animals occur.

Further evaluations of immunotherapeutic regimens using in vitro stimulated and expanded human CD8$^+$ T cells, which coexpress the natural killer (NK) cell maker CD56 (NKT cells), were performed by Scheffold et al. (26) using bioluminescence imaging. NKT cells have a high cytotoxic activity against a range of tumor cell lines and primary tumor cells, both in vitro and in vivo [reviewed in Edinger et al. (1)]. Adoptive transfer of this cell population into SCID mice cured animals bearing a Her2/neu overexpressing human ovarian cancer (SK-OV-3), if the T cells were redirected to the tumor with a bispecific antibody binding to the CD3 T-cell molecule and Her2/neu. Treatment with a clinically approved anti-Her2/neu antibody (trastuzumab, Herceptin®) also cured the animals in this xenograft tumor model. Although the outcome of the two treatment modalities by traditional read-out systems was identical (long-term survival in both groups), serial imaging revealed that tumor cell clearance occurred rapidly with the T-cell/antibody combination therapy (2–4 days), while trastuzumab treatment led to a gradual tumor regression over a period of weeks, suggesting that different mechanisms were responsible for the therapeutic effect. These observations illustrate that bioluminescence imaging can be used to generate spatial information and also reveals the kinetics of tumor growth, regression, and relapse. The possibility of determining the dynamics of biological processes in a living subject is a powerful tool for many research areas. Although most malignant diseases in humans are not treated with a single chemotherapeutic agent but with combination chemotherapy, the evaluation of cytostatic drugs in preclinical trials is usually done in single agent experiments. Bioluminescence imaging allows for the examination of combination chemotherapy regimens in the living animal, where timing, dosage, and specific combinations of drugs can be investigated to determine the ideal time intervals between treatments in animal models, which can provide useful insights for clinical trials (1).

Orthotopic mouse brain implants of rat 9L gliosarcoma cells gene-marked with *Fluc* have also been attempted by Rehemtulla et al. (27). Intracerebral tumor burden was monitored over time by quantification of light emission and tumor volume using bioluminescence imaging and MRI, respectively. There was excellent correlation ($r = 0.91$) between detected photons and tumor volume. A quantitative comparison of tumor cell kill determined from serial MRI volume measurements and bioluminescence imaging photon counts following 1,3-*bis*(2-chloroethyl)-1-nitrosourea (BCNU) treatment revealed that both imaging modalities yielded statistically similar cell kill values ($p = 0.951$). These results provide direct validation of bioluminescence imaging as a powerful and quantitative tool for the assessment of antineoplastic therapies in living animals.

Evaluation of Metastatic Trafficking of Gene-Marked Cancer Cells in Mice

In vivo imaging of cell trafficking is currently performed in clinical practice (e.g., using ^{111}In-Oxine for SPECT imaging of infection and inflammation) and is the objective of many immunological and oncological studies (28).

Marrow micrometastases elude radiographic detection and, therefore, more sensitive methods are needed for their direct identification. Recently, cancer cells marked with *Fluc* and injected into the left ventricle have helped in the study of micrometastatic spread to bone marrow (29). Whole-body bioluminescence imaging detected microscopic bone marrow metastases of approximately $0.5\,mm^3$ volume, a size below the limit in which tumors need to induce angiogenesis for further growth. This sensitivity translates into early detection of intramedullary tumor growth, preceding the appearance of a radiologically evident osteolysis by approximately two weeks. Bioluminescence imaging also enables continuous monitoring in the same animal of growth kinetics for each metastatic site and guides end-point analyses (e.g., histopathology) specifically to the bones affected by metastatic growth. This model could accelerate the understanding of the molecular events in metastasis and the evaluation of novel therapies aimed at repressing the initial stages of metastatic growth.

El Hilali et al. (30) analyzed quantitative aspects of noninvasive bioluminescence imaging of *Fluc*-marked tumors by comparing the efficiency of noninvasive whole-body light detection with in vitro quantification of firefly luciferase activity in cell lysates derived from the same tumors. Three *Fluc*-marked human prostate cell lines were grafted in nude mice. Repeated imaging after intervening growth periods allowed monitoring of tumor and metastases development. The cytostatic effects of paclitaxel in these different human prostate tumors and their metastases were also evaluated.

Noninvasive imaging and transcriptional targeting can improve the safety of therapeutic approaches in cancer. Adams et al. (31) have also demonstrated the ability to identify metastases in a human-prostate cancer model, employing a prostate-specific adenovirus vector (AdPSE-BC-luc) and bioluminescence imaging. AdPSE-BC-luc, which expresses *Fluc* from an enhanced prostate-specific antigen promoter, restricted expression in the liver but produced robust signals in prostate tumors. Expression was found to be higher in advanced, androgen-independent tumors than in androgen-dependent lesions. Repetitive imaging over a three-week period after AdPSE-BC-luc injection into tumor-bearing mice revealed that the virus could locate and illuminate metastases in the lung and the spine. Systemic injection of low doses of AdPSE-BC-luc illuminated lung metastasis. Their results demonstrated the potential use of bioluminescence imaging in therapeutic and diagnostic strategies to manage prostate cancer.

Edinger et al. (32) recently gene-marked two murine lymphoma cell lines with *Fluc* and monitored radiation and chemotherapy as well as immune-based strategies that employ the tumorcidal activity of ex vivo–expanded CD8(+) natural killer (NK)-T cells. Using bioluminescence imaging they were able to visualize the entire course of malignant disease including engraftment, expansion, metastasis, response to therapy, and unique patterns of relapse. They also gene-marked the effector NK-T cells and monitored their homing to the sites of tumor growth followed by tumor eradication. These studies revealed the efficacy of immune cell therapies and the dynamics of NK-T cell trafficking in living mice.

Imaging of Cancer Gene Therapies in Living Mice

Although various methods of gene therapy have met with limited success, it is probable that eventually many diseases, including cancer, will be successfully treated with the delivery of one or more transgenes to target tissue(s). A concern in applying gene therapy is achievement of controlled and effective delivery of genes to target cells and avoidance of ectopic expression. Molecular imaging of reporters on particular therapeutic genes could be critical in optimizing gene therapy. The aim of these approaches is to quantitatively image reporter gene expression, and to infer from this the levels, location, and duration of therapeutic gene expression (20). There are several strategies to achieve linkage of expression of the therapeutic transgene and the imaging reporter gene (18,19). A fusion approach can be used where two or more different genes are joined in such a way that their coding sequences are in the same reading frame, and thus a single protein with properties of both the original proteins is produced. Another approach is to insert an internal ribosomal entry site (IRES) sequence between the two genes so that they are transcribed into a single mRNA from the same promoter but translated into two separate proteins. A third approach uses two different genes expressed from distinct promoters within a single vector. A fourth approach entails co-administering both genes cloned in two different vectors but driven by the same promoter type. These various techniques can be adopted with bioluminescence imaging reporter genes.

There are only a few examples where bioluminescence imaging has been used in experimental gene therapy protocols for quantification of transgene expression. Rehemtulla et al. (33) developed an adenoviral vector containing both the therapeutic transgene for yeast cytosine deaminase (yCD) along with *Fluc*. Following intra-tumoral injection of the vector into orthotopic 9L gliomas in rats, anatomical and diffusion-weighted MRI images were obtained over time to provide for quantitative assessment of overall therapeutic efficacy and spatial heterogeneity of cell kill, respectively. In addition, bioluminescence images assessed the duration and magnitude of gene expression. MR images revealed significant reduction in tumor growth rates associated with yCD/5-fluorocytosine (5FC) gene therapy. Significant increases in mean tumor diffusion values were also observed during treatment with 5FC. Moreover, spatial heterogeneity in tumor diffusion changes were also observed revealing that diffusion MRI could detect regional therapeutic effects because of the nonuniform delivery and/or expression of the therapeutic yCD transgene within the tumor mass. In addition, bioluminescence imaging in the living mice detected *Fluc* expression, which was found to decrease over time during administration of the prodrug providing a noninvasive surrogate marker for monitoring gene expression. These results demonstrated the efficacy of the yCD/5FC strategy for the treatment of brain tumors and revealed the feasibility of using multimodality molecular and functional imaging for assessment of gene expression and therapeutic efficacy.

Imaging of Transgenic Models of Spontaneous Cancer in Mice

The strong merits of noninvasive imaging in the assessment of transgenic animals can be readily appreciated from the above discussion of the overall advantages of molecular imaging in living subjects. To date, several research groups have employed bioluminescence imaging in their assessment of transgenic mice. Transgenic models of spontaneous cancer in which tumor formation is dependent on defined genetic alterations provide a powerful test system for evaluating the therapeutic efficacy of pathway-specific antineoplastics. Vooijs et al. (34) have generated a conditional mouse model for retinoblastoma-dependent sporadic cancer that permits non-invasive monitoring of pituitary tumor development in living mice by bioluminescence imaging of *Fluc* expression. Bioluminescence imaging of pituitary cancer development with co-expression of the *Fluc* gene enabled longitudinal monitoring of tumor onset, progression, and response to therapy and may be used effectively for testing cancer prevention and treatment strategies based on therapeutics that specifically target the retinoblastoma pathway.

Imaging of Molecular Interactions in Living Mice

Some interesting variations of standard reporter gene assays described earlier have also been adapted recently for imaging of molecular interactions in living subjects. A two-step transcriptional amplification (TSTA) method for imaging gene expression using weak promoters (i.e., many tissue-specific ones) has been described by Iyer et al. (35) and in a follow-up study by Zhang et al. (36). The TSTA system was used to amplify expression of *Fluc* and *HSV1-sr39tk* in a prostate cancer cell line using a duplicated variant of the prostate-specific antigen gene enhancer to express GAL4 derivatives fused to one, two, or four VP16 activation domains. The resulting activators were targeted to cells with reporter templates bearing one, two, or five GAL4 binding sites upstream of the reporter gene. It was found, for example, that the expression of *Fluc* could be varied over an 800-fold range. It has been recently shown that these approaches can be adapted for amplifying endogenous promoters in transgenic models of cancer and the use of the TSTA system would seem to have no undesirable toxicity in living mice.

To image protein–protein interactions in living mice, Ray et al. (37) have used the well-studied yeast two-hybrid system adapted for mammalian cells and modified it to be inducible. They employed the NF-κB promoter to drive expression of two fusion proteins (VP16-MyoD and GAL4-Id) and modulated the NF-κB promoter through TNFα. *Fluc* reporter gene expression was driven by the interaction of MyoD and Id through a transcriptional activation strategy. They demonstrated the ability to detect this induced protein–protein interaction in cell culture and to image it in living mice by using transiently transfected cancer cells (Fig. 6). More recently,

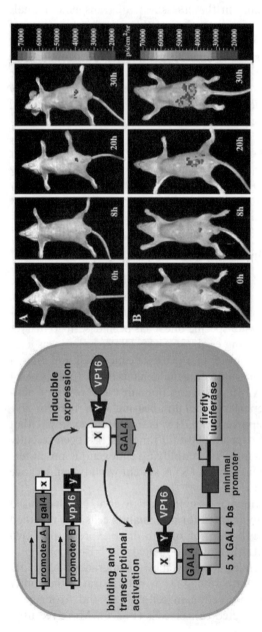

Figure 6 Imaging protein–protein interaction in living mice. Schematic diagram of the system for imaging the interaction of proteins X and Y. The first step involves the vectors pA-gal4-x and pB-vp16-y, which are used to drive transcription of *gal4-x* and *vp16-y* through use of promoters A and B. In the second step, the two fusion proteins GAL4-X and VP16-Y interact because of the specificity of protein X for protein Y. Subsequently, GAL4-X-Y-VP16 binds to GAL4-binding sites (bs) (five GAL4-bs are available) on a reporter template. This leads to VP16-mediated transactivation of firefly luciferase reporter gene expression under the control of GAL4 response elements in a minimal promoter. Transcription of the firefly luciferase reporter gene leads to firefly luciferase protein, which, in turn, leads to a detectable visible light signal in the presence of the appropriate substrate (D-luciferin), ATP, Mg^{2+}, and oxygen. The NF-κB promoter was used for either pA or pB and TNF-α–mediated induction. In vivo optical CCD imaging of mice carrying transiently transfected 293T cells for induction of the yeast two-hybrid system. All images shown are the visible light image superimposed on the optical CCD bioluminescence image with a scale in photons/sec/cm^2/steridian (sr). Mice in top row were imaged after injection of D-luciferin but with no TNF-α–mediated induction. Mice in bottom row were imaged after injection of D-luciferin after TNF-α–mediated induction, showing marked gain in signal from the peritoneum over 30 hours. *Source:* From Ref. 2. (*See color insert.*)

Paulmurugan and Gambhir (38) have also validated the use of split reporter technology to show that both complementation and intein-mediated reconstitution of firefly luciferase can also be used to image protein–protein interactions in cancer cells in living mice (Fig. 7). This approach has the advantage of potentially imaging the interactions anywhere in the cell, whereas the yeast two-hybrid approaches are limited to interactions in the nucleus. In a separate study, Paulmurugan et al. (39) have also developed an inducible synthetic *Renilla* luciferase protein-fragment–assisted complementation-based bioluminescence assay to quantitatively measure real-time protein–protein interactions in mammalian cells. They identified suitable sites to generate fragments of N-terminal and C-terminal portions of the protein that yielded significant recovered activity through complementation. Again, they validated complementation-based activation of split synthetic *Renilla* luciferase protein driven by the interaction of two strongly interacting proteins, MyoD and Id, in five different cell lines using transient transfection studies. The expression level of the system was also modulated by TNF-α through NF-κB-promoter/enhancer elements used to drive expression of the N-terminal portion of *hRluc* reporter gene. A further technique recently evaluated in our laboratory for imaging of protein–protein interactions (and potentially for other intracellular events such as, protein phosphorylation, caspase induction, and ion influx) is that of bioluminescence resonance energy transfer (BRET). BRET occurs when the emission wavelength of a bioluminescence light excites an adjacent (within 50–100 Å) fluorescent protein and causes it to emit light. BRET partners which may be attached to interacting proteins include *Renilla* luciferase and yellow fluorescent protein or synthetic *Renilla* luciferase and GFP. Advantages of BRET over conventional FRET imaging include the avoidance of autofluorescence, light scattering, photobleaching and/or photoisomerization of the donor moiety, or photodamage to cells. Initial experimental results of BRET imaging in living mouse tumor models are encouraging.

These above systems described should above help to study protein–protein interactions, and when used in various combinations should help to monitor different components of intracellular pathways and networks, including their application to logical circuitry analysis within cells to provide protein- and transcription-based biological "computation," with potential for future extrapolation to imaging in living subjects (40). Imaging interacting protein partners in living subjects could pave the way to functional proteomics in whole animals, the assessment of dysfunctional signaling networks in cancer cells, and provide a tool for evaluation of new pharmaceuticals targeted to modulate protein–protein interactions.

Wang and El-Deiry (41) have recently detected noninvasively the real-time p53 activity in tumor cells both in cell culture and in living mice using bioluminescence imaging. HCT116 colon cancer cells were stably transduced with PG13-luc, a p53 reporter with *Fluc* under the control of 13 p53 response elements, together with *Rluc* under an MMLV long terminal repeat promoter. Basic conditions for both in vivo and in vitro imaging were explored. Signals from as few as 3000 cells in a 96-well plate were detected following addition of D-luciferin at a concentration of 100 µg/mL. Bioluminescence from 15×10^3 cells with PG13-luc inoculated subcutaneously was detected following intravenous injection of D-luciferin at a dose of 100 mg/kg. The maximal luminescence intensity after i.p. injection was 4 to 10 times lower than that from intravenous injection. Bioluminescence from *Renilla* luciferase constitutively expressed in tumor cells was also imaged both in vitro and in vivo and served as an internal control to monitor the physiological state of the cells or tumor volume. Infection of the cells with adenovirus carrying p53 increased the

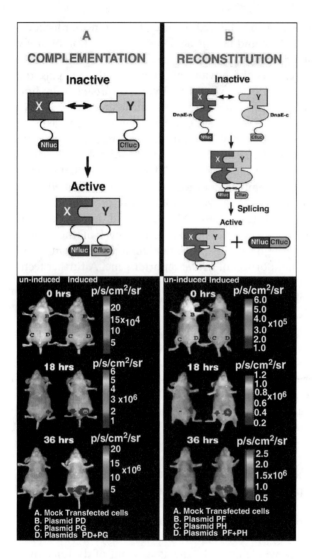

Figure 7   (*Caption on facing page*)

bioluminescence intensity both in vitro and in vivo. This study demonstrated that noninvasive imaging of p53 transcriptional activity could provide a practical way to monitor the p53 response in cell culture and in animal models.

Objective and quantitative noninvasive imaging of apoptosis would be a significant advancement for rapid and dynamic screening as well as validation of experimental therapeutic agents. Laxman et al. (42) reported the development of a recombinant firefly luciferase reporter molecule, which when expressed in mammalian cells, has attenuated levels of reporter activity. In cells undergoing apoptosis, a caspase-3–specific cleavage of the recombinant product occurs, resulting in the restoration of firefly luciferase activity that can be detected in living animals with bioluminescence imaging. The ability to image apoptosis noninvasively and dynamically over time provides an opportunity for high-throughput screening of pro- and antiapoptotic compounds and for target validation in vivo in both cell lines and transgenic animals.

MULTIPLEX AND MULTIMODALITY BIOLUMINESCENCE IMAGING IN LIVING MICE

A notable theoretical advantage of bioluminescence and other optical imaging techniques is the fact that multiple probes with different spectral characteristics could potentially be used for multichannel imaging, similar to in vivo karyotyping. For example, the different kinetics of light emission when using firefly luciferase and *Renilla* luciferase (wild-type or synthetic) provide us with the ability to perform simultaneous imaging of multiple molecular events in one population of cancer cells in living subjects. This may be attainable by combining two or more of the above described strategies for gene marking and imaging the trafficking of cells with those entailing linked expression of an imaging gene to an endogenous promoter or to an exogenous therapeutic gene. As such, in these experiments it is foreseeable that one reporter may reveal the spatial distribution of cells and whether they have reached a specific target, and another reporter may indicate whether a certain gene becomes upregulated at this site or if a more complex interaction occurs. Efforts are underway in our laboratories to demonstrate the feasibility of this concept of simultaneous multiplexing of molecular imaging strategies, with a view to a better understanding of the complexities of molecular pathways and networks.

Figure 7 (*Facing page*) Schematic diagram of two strategies for using split reporters to monitor protein–protein interactions. (**A**) Complementation-mediated restoration of firefly luciferase activity. N-terminal half of firefly luciferase is attached to protein X through a short peptide FFAGYC, and the C-terminal half of firefly luciferase is connected to protein Y through the peptide CLKS. Interaction of protein X and Y recovers *Fluc* activity through protein complementation. (**B**) Split Intein (DnaE)–mediated protein splicing leads to firefly luciferase reconstitution. The N-terminal half of firefly luciferase is connected to the DnaE-n with peptide FFAGYC. The N-terminal half of DnaE in turn is connected to protein X. Similarly, the C-terminal half of firefly luciferase is connected to the DnaE-c with peptide CLKS, and the C-terminal half of intein is in turn connected to protein Y. The interaction of proteins X and Y mediates reconstitution through splicing of the N and C halves of DnaE. In vivo optical CCD imaging of mice carrying transiently transfected 293T cells for induction of the complementation-based (**A**) and intein-mediated reconstitution (**B**) of split luciferase system. All images shown are the visible light image superimposed on the optical CCD bioluminescence image with a scale in photons/sec/cm^2/steridian (sr). Mice were imaged in a supine position after i.p. injection of D-luciferin. (**A**) Set of nude mice were repetitively imaged after subcutaneous implantation of 293T cells transiently transfected with various plasmids as described in Ref. (39). One group of mice was induced with TNF-α and the other group was not induced. Images are from one representative mouse from each group immediately after implanting cells (0 hour) and 18 and 36 hour after TNF-α induction. The induced mouse showed higher *Fluc* signal at site D (where interacting proteins result in reporter complementation) when compared with the mouse not receiving TNF-α. The *Fluc* signal significantly increases after receiving TNF-α. (**B**) Set of nude mice were repetitively imaged after subcutaneous implantation of 293T cells transiently transfected with various plasmids as described in Ref. (39) to test the reconstitution-based split-luciferase system. One group of mice was induced with TNF-α and the other group was not induced. Images are from one representative mouse from each group immediately after implanting cells (0 hour), 18 and 36 hour after TNF-α induction. The induced mouse showed significantly higher *Fluc* signal at site D (where interacting proteins result in intein-mediated reconstitution of the reporter) when compared to the mouse not receiving TNF-α. *Abbreviations*: DnaE-n, N-terminal half of DnaE; DnaE-c, C-terminal half of DnaE. *Source*: From Ref. 39. (*See color insert.*)

Noninvasive imaging of the expression of multiple fused reporter genes using multiple imaging modalities is likely to play an increasingly important role in defining molecular events in the field of cancer biology, cell biology, and gene therapy. In a recent study, Ray et al. (2) have constructed a novel reporter vector encoding a fusion protein that comprises mutant herpes simplex virus type 1 thymidine kinase (*HSV1-sr39tk*), a PET reporter gene, and *Rluc*, a bioluminescence optical reporter gene joined by a 20 amino acid long spacer sequence. They validated the activity of the two enzymes encoded by the fusion gene in cell culture. Tumors stably expressing this fusion gene were imaged both by microPET and a CCD camera in xenograft-bearing living mice. Further extension of this useful concept has resulted in development of a triple fusion reporter construct combining synthetic *Renilla* luciferase for bioluminescence imaging, a monomeric red fluorescence protein for fluorescence imaging/microscopy/cell sorting, and HSV1-sr39TK for PET imaging. The use of a single fusion reporter (PET/bioluminescence/fluorescence) gene should accelerate the validation of reporter gene approaches developed in cell culture for translation into preclinical and clinical cancer models.

COMBINED IN VITRO, EX VIVO, AND LIVING SUBJECT BIOLUMINESCENCE IMAGING

Fluc activity has been used to assess gene expression in in vitro assays for many years. This has provided us with extensive knowledge of the molecular and biochemical properties of the firefly luciferase enzyme. This knowledge has facilitated applications in living subjects and has therefore helped to link the study of biological events by in vitro and living-subject assays employing a single reporter gene (1). Scheffold et al. (26) used luminometric data from *Fluc*-transfected human ovarian tumor cell line, SK-OV-3, to establish a nonradioactive cell killing assay in vitro. The addition of activated and expanded (CD3[+], CD8[+], CD56[+]) NKT cells to the cancer cells in a 96-well plate led to a dose-dependent reduction of light emission in a four hours cytotoxicity assay, which was further enhanced by crosslinking tumor and effector cells with a bispecific antibody against CD3 and Her2/neu. This measured tumor cell killing correlated with results generated by standard chromium-release cytotoxicity assay and predicted the outcome of experiments in living subjects.

Bioluminescence imaging allows the monitoring of tumor evolution throughout the disease course starting from minimal to late stage disease. Cancer progression, including cell trafficking and development of metastases can be visualized, which is otherwise difficult to study by other means because very few cells are present at any number of tissue sites (1). This allows for defining the location and measurement of tumor growth at metastatic sites of disease before sacrificing the experimental animal. Therefore, more labor-intensive assays, for example, histopathology, which may also be prone to missing sites of disease can be directed to key target tissues. Of note, because the bioluminescence reporter genes are present in the tumor cells, it is also possible to confirm that the lesion was recovered because the gene marked cells will continue to emit light after biopsy or at postmortem examination. In this manner, imaging in living subjects can facilitate and direct ex vivo assays. A good example of the utility of this approach can be found in studies where cancer tissue may be recovered for examining gene expression patterns in metastatic lesions using DNA microarray technologies. The value of these studies may be further enhanced by the use of dual optical reporter genes. Several groups have recently constructed fusion bioluminescence (firefly or *Renilla* luciferase) and fluorescence (GFP or its variants) proteins (43) [also refer Ray et al. (2)]. These fusion genes effectively couple the powerful in vivo capabilities of bioluminescence imaging with the subset-discriminating capabilities of fluorescence-activated cell sorting. Unfortunately, the latter is necessary because subcellular spatial resolution is sacrificed with the bioluminescence approach. Although bioluminescence microscopy of single cells has been attempted before, the inherent low levels of light emission at the single cell level precludes microscopic and cell-sorting applications as for fluorescence-based approaches (44). Thus, bioluminescence imaging of a tumor can be made in living subjects, and examination of the biopsied tissues can be evaluated by fluorescence microscopy, and reisolation of labeled cells by flow cytometry is made possible.

FUTURE OUTLOOK

We can expect progress to be made in many aspects of bioluminescence imaging so that it can further integrate with on-going cancer functional genomic and proteomic endeavors. The initial methodological and technological descriptions and validations are being made in bioluminescence imaging, and soon it is anticipated that the second generation of experiments will face the interesting task of applying these techniques to help answer specific hypothesis-driven questions in many areas of cancer biological study.

Many developments in bioluminescence imaging are anticipated over the next decade. The developing trend of housing CCD cameras in core facilities of basic science laboratories will likely expand significantly in the future as more research groups acquire these technologies. Adoption of molecular imaging approaches and establishment of a molecular imaging facility within a basic biological research setup is likely to be cost-effective in the long-term. Although some start-up expenses are necessary to lay the foundation for this research methodology, it is anticipated that the cost of small-animal imaging instrumentation and the required core facilities will continue to fall with continued future developments and demands.

Improved instrumentation will make use of advances in detector technology and better image reconstruction techniques. This should help to produce newer generations of cameras, likely with better resolution, sensitivity, and even higher-throughput time, which will aid substantially in the screening of mice (45). There are also on-going developments for construction of tomographic three-dimensional imaging systems that can accurately quantify bioluminescence in deep heterogeneous media in living subjects. Although progress is being made, these attempts are hindered currently by the complex data that has to be acquired and analyzed as a series of two-dimensional images from multiple viewing angles. This data is then used to model surface radiance of photons emitted from deep within tissues by mathematical techniques dependent on diffusion equations and partial-current boundary condition models.

Linked to the development of better instrumentation is the search for better bioluminescence reporters. The luciferases comprise a whole family of photoproteins that use different substrates and emit light of varying wavelengths. Unfortunately, substrates for many of luciferases from different organisms are not readily available, which precludes their use in biomedical research applications. Current searches are underway for naturally occurring reporters (with available substrates) that may emit more red-shifted light, and therefore, would likely result in improved light transmission through deeper body structures. Moreover, an increasing number of bioluminescence reporter genes may undergo site-directed mutagenesis for the purpose of yielding reporter proteins that are also more red-shifted and/or with codon changes for higher expression in mammalian cells. Improving the thermo-stability of firefly luciferase has already been investigated using mutagenesis directed at amino acid position 354 (46). An intriguing future possibility might entail the genetic engineering of cells or creation of transgenic animals that could make their own substrates (e.g., D-luciferin and/or coelenterazine) without having to provide these substrates (by injection in the case of imaging in living subjects).

A new class of molecular imaging probes is being developed in our laboratory for imaging of cancer cells that have available cell surface targets for specific protein binding. Bifunctional chimeric proteins, each containing a cell surface targeting protein fused to a bioluminescence reporter protein can be used to image cancer cells without recourse to prior expression of the reporter protein via the delivery of imaging transgenes, as in conventional reporter gene imaging. To date, this novel approach has been attempted with a *Renilla* luciferase and epidermal growth factor fusion protein to image A431 human epidermoid carcinoma cells and an anti-CEA diabody and synthetic *Renilla* luciferase fusion protein to image CEA-expressing xenografts in mice.

Ongoing experiments will determine the feasibility of these novel approaches for cancer imaging prior to potential future clinical applications.

Given the inherent advantages of optical imaging, these approaches are likely to be used increasingly in bridging imaging studies from small animals to larger ones and humans. For limited applications, for example, in endoscopic or breast imaging, optical imaging may even have the potential to be directly translated to human investigations in the future, assuming mass amounts of substrate that have to be given to patients are proven to be safe. In addition, newer multimodality imaging systems for small animals will provide anatomical and functional image registration. Several microPET/CT scanners are in current development, as are attempts at building instruments that combine MRI or optical imaging with PET.

Stem cells are cells that have the ability to perpetuate themselves through self-renewal and to generate into mature cells of a particular tissue through differentiation. Striking parallels can be found between stem cells and cancer cells through their property of self-renewal (47). As such, a great deal of interest is emerging in overlapping aspects of stem cell and cancer biology. As cancer can be considered as a disease of unregulated self-renewal, it is anticipated that the above-described full repertoire of reporter gene imaging may be applied to stem cells to help understand the regulation of normal stem cell self-renewal and its balance with differentiation. Also, these imaging techniques in living subjects could be adapted to investigate tumors that might originate from transformation of normal stem cells through inappropriate activation of signaling pathways [e.g., the sonic hedgehog-Gli pathway (48)] or differentiation of "cancer stem cells," that is, rare cells with indefinite potential for self-replication that drive tumorigensis (47,48). Reporter gene imaging may also be adapted to future strategies using hematopoietic stem cells for the treatment of solid tumors. This would entail imaging the effects of treatment on the cancer cells and/or the fate of the hematopoetic stem cells themselves used for treatment in both "autologous" or "allogeneic" approaches (49).

Bioluminescence imaging in living rodents is already revealing interesting new insights in cancer research. Further integration of bioluminescence imaging reporters into the constructs of transgenic and knockout animals should considerably enhance studies of carcinogenesis, as spatial and temporal information on abnormal molecular events will be generated in real time, allowing for insights into disease development in the preclinical stage. With continued and rapid technological advancements in this field, bioluminescence imaging has the potential to greatly refine our animal models of cancer and will ultimately contribute to better understanding of integrative cancer biology, and the discovery, validation, and fine-tuning of new and improved clinical cancer diagnosis, treatment, and prevention regimens.

REFERENCES

1. Edinger M, Cao YA, Hornig YS, et al. Advancing animal models of neoplasia through in vivo bioluminescence imaging. Eur J Cancer 2002; 38:2128–2136.
2. Ray P, Wu AM, Gambhir SS. Optical bioluminescence and positron emission tomography imaging of a novel fusion reporter gene in tumor xenografts of living mice. Cancer Res 2003; 63:1160–1165.
3. Massoud TF, Gambhir SS. Molecular imaging in living subjects: seeing fundamental biological processes in a new light. Genes Dev 2003; 1:545–580.
4. Hastings JW. Chemistries and colors of bioluminescent reactions: a review. Gene 1996; 173:5–11.
5. Bhaumik S, Gambhir SS. Optical imaging of Renilla luciferase reporter gene expression in living mice. Proc Natl Acad Sci USA 2002; 99:377–382.
6. Contag CH, Contag PR, Mullins JI, Spilman SD, Stevenson DK, Benaron DA. Photonic detection of bacterial pathogens in living hosts. Mol Microbiol 1995; 18:593–603.
7. Contag CH, Spilman SD, Contag PR, et al. Visualizing gene expression in living mammals using a bioluminescent reporter. Photochem Photobiol 1997; 66:523–531.
8. Weissleder R, Ntziachristos V. Shedding light onto live molecular targets. Nat Med 2003; 9:123–128.
9. Rocchetta HL, Boylan CJ, Foley JW, et al. Validation of a noninvasive, real-time imaging technology using bioluminescent *Escherichia coli* in the neutropenic mouse thigh model of infection. Antimicrob Agents Chemother 2001; 45:129–137.
10. Rice BW, Cable MD, Nelson MB. In vivo imaging of light-emitting probes. J Biomed Opt 2001; 6:432–440.
11. Spibey CA, Jackson P, Herick K. A unique charge-coupled device/xenon arc lamp based imaging system for the accurate detection and quantitation of multicolour fluorescence. Electrophoresis 2001; 22:829–836.
12. Tuchin VV. Laser light scattering in biomedical diagnostics and therapy. J Laser Appl 1993; 5:43–60.
13. Edinger M, Sweeney TJ, Tucker AA, Olomu AB, Negrin RS, Contag CH. Noninvasive assessment of tumor cell proliferation in animal models. Neoplasia 1999; 1:303–310.
14. Sweeney TJ, Mailander V, Tucker AA, et al. Visualizing the kinetics of tumor-cell clearance in living animals. Proc Natl Acad Sci USA 1999; 96:12044–12049.
15. Lipshutz GS, Gruber CA, Cao Y, Hardy J, Contag CH, Gaensler KM. In utero delivery of adeno-associated viral vectors: intraperitoneal gene transfer produces long-term expression. Mol Ther 2001; 3:284–292.
16. Wu JC, Sundaresan G, Iyer M, Gambhir SS. Noninvasive optical imaging of firefly luciferase reporter gene expression in skeletal muscles of living mice. Mol Ther 2001; 4: 297–306.
17. Phelps M. Inaugural article: positron emission tomography provides molecular imaging of biological processes. Proc Natl Acad Sci USA 2000; 97:9226–9233.
18. Ray P, Bauer E, Iyer M, et al. Monitoring gene therapy with reporter gene imaging. Semin Nucl Med 2001; 31:312–320.
19. Sundaresan G, Gambhir SS. Radionuclide imaging of reporter gene expression. In: Toga AW, Mazziotta JC, eds. Brain Mapping: The Methods. San Diego, CA: Academic Press, 2002:799–818.

20. Gambhir SS. Imaging gene expression: concepts and future outlook. In: Schiepers C, ed. Diagnostic Nuclear Medicine. Berlin: Springer-Verlag, 2000:253–272.

21. Spergel DJ, Kruth U, Shimshek DR, Sprengel R, Seeburg PH. Using reporter genes to label selected neuronal populations in transgenic mice for gene promoter, anatomical, and physiological studies. Prog Neurobiol 2001; 63:673–686.

22. Brenner M. Gene marking. Hum Gene Ther 1996; 7:1927–1936.

23. De Geest B, Van Linthout S, Lox M, Collen D, Holvoet P. Sustained expression of human apolipoprotein A-I after adenoviral gene transfer in C57BL/6 mice: role of apolipoprotein A-I promoter, apolipoprotein A-I introns, and human apolipoprotein E enhancer. Hum Gene Ther 2000; 11:101–112.

24. Qin L, Ding Y, Pahud DR, Chang E, Imperiale MJ, Bromberg JS. Promoter attenuation in gene therapy: interferon-gamma and tumor necrosis factor-alpha inhibit transgene expression. Hum Gene Ther 1997; 8:2019–2029.

25. Honigman A, Zeira E, Ohana P, et al. Imaging transgene expression in live animals. Mol Ther 2001; 4:239–249.

26. Scheffold C, Kornacker M, Scheffold YC, Contag CH, Negrin RS. Visualization of effective tumor targeting by CD8+ natural killer T cells redirected with bispecific antibody F(ab′)(2)HER2xCD3. Cancer Res 2002; 62:5785–5791.

27. Rehemtulla A, Stegman LD, Cardozo SJ, et al. Rapid and quantitative assessment of cancer treatment response using in vivo bioluminescence imaging. Neoplasia 2000; 2:491–495.

28. Becker W, Meller J. The role of nuclear medicine in infection and inflammation. Lancet Infect Dis 2001; 1:326–333.

29. Wetterwald A, van der Pluijm G, Que I, et al. Optical imaging of cancer metastasis to bone marrow: a mouse model of minimal residual disease. Am J Pathol 2002; 160:1143–1153.

30. El Hilali N, Rubio N, Martinez-Villacampa M, Blanco J. Combined noninvasive imaging and luminometric quantification of luciferase-labeled human prostate tumors and metastases. Lab Invest 2002; 82:1563–1571.

31. Adams JY, Johnson M, Sato M, et al. Visualization of advanced human prostate cancer lesions in living mice by a targeted gene transfer vector and optical imaging. Nat Med 2002; 8:891–897.

32. Edinger M, Cao YA, Verneris MR, Bachmann MH, Contag CH, Negrin RS. Revealing lymphoma growth and the efficacy of immune cell therapies using in vivo bioluminescence imaging. Blood 2003; 101:640–648.

33. Rehemtulla A, Hall DE, Stegman LD, et al. Molecular imaging of gene expression and efficacy following adenoviral-mediated brain tumor gene therapy. Mol Imaging 2002; 1:43–55.

34. Vooijs M, Jonkers J, Lyons S, Berns A. Noninvasive imaging of spontaneous retinoblastoma pathway-dependent tumors in mice. Cancer Res 2002; 62:1862–1867.

35. Iyer M, Wu L, Carey M, Wang Y, Smallwood A, Gambhir SS. Two-step transcriptional amplification as a method for imaging reporter gene expression using weak promoters. Proc Natl Acad Sci USA 2001; 98:14595–14600.

36. Zhang L, Adams JY, Billick E, et al. Molecular engineering of a two-step transcription amplification (TSTA) system for transgene delivery in prostate cancer. Mol Ther 2002; 5:223–232.

37. Ray P, Pimenta H, Paulmurugan R. Non invasive quantitative imaging of protein-protein interactions in living subjects. Proc Natl Acad Sci USA 2002; 99:3105–3110.

38. Paulmurugan R, Gambhir SS. Monitoring protein-protein interactions using split synthetic renilla luciferase protein-fragment-assisted complementation. Anal Chem 2003; 75:1584–1589.

39. Paulmurugan R, Umezawa Y, Gambhir SS. Noninvasive imaging of protein–protein interactions in living subjects by using reporter protein complementation and reconstitution strategies. Proc Natl Acad Sci USA 2002; 99:15608–15613.

40. Xu CW, Mendelsohn AR, Brent R. Cells that register logical relationships among proteins. Proc Natl Acad Sci USA 1997; 94:12473–12478.

41. Wang W, El-Deiry WS. Bioluminescent Molecular Imaging of Endogenous and Exogenous p53-Mediated Transcription In Vitro and In Vivo Using an HCT116 Human Colon Carcinoma Xenograft Model. Cancer Biol Ther 2003; 2:196–202.

42. Laxman B, Hall DE, Bhojani MS, et al. Noninvasive real-time imaging of apoptosis. Proc Natl Acad Sci USA 2002; 99:16551–16555.

43. Wang Y, Yu YA, Shabahang S, Wang G, Szalay AA. Renilla luciferase – Aequorea GFP (Ruc-GFP) fusion protein, a novel dual reporter for real-time imaging of gene expression in cell cultures and in live animals. Mol Genet Genomics 2002; 268:160–168.

44. Hooper CE, Ansorge RE, Browne HM, Tomkins P. CCD imaging of luciferase gene expression in single mammalian cells. J Biolumin Chemilumin 1990; 5:123–130.

45. Kudo T, Fukuchi K, Annala AJ, et al. Noninvasive measurement of myocardial activity concentrations and perfusion defect sizes in rats with a new small-animal positron emission tomograph. Circulation 2002; 106:118–123.

46. White PJ, Squirrell DJ, Arnaud P, Lowe CR, Murray JA. Improved 47 thermostability of the North American firefly luciferase: saturation mutagenesis at position 354. Biochem J 1996; 319(Pt 2):343–350.

47. Reya T, Morrison SJ, Clarke MF, Weissman IL. Stem cells, cancer, and cancer stem cells. Nature 2001; 414:105–111.

48. Ruizi Altaba A, Sanchez P, Dahmane N. Gli and hedgehog in cancer: tumours, embryos and stem cells. Nat Rev Cancer 2002; 2:361–372.

49. Perillo A, Pierelli L, Scambia G, Leone G, Mancuso S. The role of hematopoietic stem cells in the treatment of ovarian cancer. Panminerva Med 2002; 44:197–204.

16

Diffusion MR Imaging in Tumors

Andrzej Dzik-Jurasz
CR UK Clinical Magnetic Resonance Research Group, Institute of Cancer Research and Royal Marsden NHS Trust, Sutton, U.K.

Simon Doran
University of Surrey, Guildford, Surrey, U.K.

A Note from the Editors

*D*iffusion magnetic resonance imaging (MRI) interrogates the restricted random Brownian motion of tissue water. The structured environment of biological tissues restricts random water motion. Structural influences include macromolecules including proteins, proteoglycans, collagen fibres, cell membranes, and white matter tracts. Thus, diffusion MRI allows the non-invasive investigation of the average structure of tissues. Diffusion measurements in tissues are also affected by tissue perfusion and temperature. Anisotropy refers to restriction of water diffusion that is greater in some directions than others, a situation found in the white matter of the brain and spinal cord. Tumor diffusion is usually considered and has been shown to be isotropic. The apparent diffusion coefficient (ADC) is a quantitative variable that indicates the restrictions present in a tissue sample. Diffusion weighted images can formulate such that they are more or less sensitive to perfusion effects (low and high b values). Potential clinical roles of diffusion imaging include diagnosis and grading of tumors, predicting and assessing response to anticancer treatments and for therapy planning. Several studies have shown strong correlations between ADC and tumor cellularity of gliomas. Studies of diffusion in extracranial malignancy are limited but studies of the liver, pancreas, and pelvic malignancy are emerging where lesion detection (prostate) and characterization have been explored (liver, pancreas, ovary). Early studies also suggest that the success of treatment can be assessed early after starting therapy before structural changes are seen, perhaps indicating the onset of apoptosis.

INTRODUCTION

The application of diffusion weighted-magnetic resonance imaging (DW-MRI) studies to biologic processes in vivo is a recent development given that it is 50 years since the first description of the effects of diffusion on the nuclear magnetic resonance (NMR) signal. Although considerable effort has gone into explaining the biology underlying the diffusion effects monitored via NMR, these often remain unappreciated by clinicians and life scientists. The purpose of this chapter is to provide an introduction to the physical principles governing the study of diffusion processes in biology and their application in vivo.

PHYSICAL PRINCIPLES AND TECHNICAL CONSIDERATIONS

What Is Diffusion?

The term *"diffusion"* describes the process by which fluids and, to a much lesser extent, solids mix with each other when placed in contact. This occurs via random motion of particles at a molecular scale. Complete mixing between different species eventually occurs unless there are perturbing effects such as gravity, which is significant where one set of particles is much more massive than another and sedimentation occurs, or active transport of molecules, as in cellular homeostasis.

Tracer Diffusion

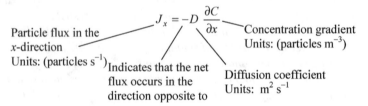

Diffusion is perhaps most familiarly encountered in medicine in the form of "tracer" diffusion—the spreading out of an exogenous agent within the body. With this example in mind, it is useful to distinguish between straightforward mixing, which occurs because of differences in macroscopic flow rates, such as might occur with an injected bolus of magnetic resonance (MR) contrast agent, and genuine diffusion, seen, for example in the dissolution of a tablet of drug and its subsequent spread.

Illustrated in Figure 1, tracer diffusion is traditionally described in terms of a *concentration gradient*, i.e., the change per unit distance of the concentration of the particles of interest. Fick's first law of diffusion states that the concentration gradient is directly proportional to the net flux of particles (i.e., the number of particles crossing a unit area per unit time). The *diffusion coefficient* is simply the constant of proportionality in this relation.

As indicated in the equation above, the SI unit of the diffusion coefficient is $m^2 s^{-1}$. In practice, this unit is very large, with typical values met in MRI of the order of $10^{-9} m^2 s^{-1}$, and the unit $mm^2 s^{-1}$ is often more appropriate.

It is often of interest to consider a given concentration of tracer and to find how far it gets in a given time. The lines on the graph in Figure 2A represent concentration profiles at successively later stages following introduction of a small initial quantity of

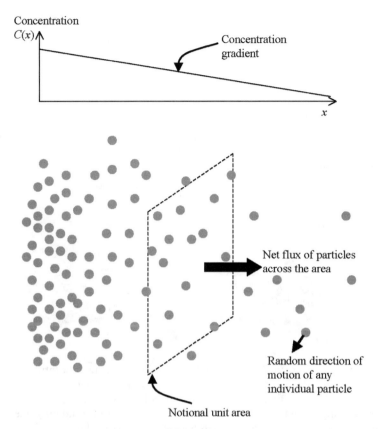

Concentration
$C(x)$

Concentration gradient

x

Net flux of particles across the area

Random direction of motion of any individual particle

Notional unit area

Figure 1 Explanation of tracer diffusion. A concentration gradient leads to a net flux of particles across a given area. Diffusion is a stochastic process and the individual particles are in fact moving randomly in all directions. The large arrow indicates the net effect of adding up contributions from all the particles, with appropriate weightings for particles moving at an angle to the plane.

tracer (the central rectangular region). Figure 2B shows how the "diffusion front" $C = C_0$ moves outward in proportion to $\sqrt{t}$. At a molecular level, the so-called "random walk model," illustrated in Figure 2C, explains how this arises. It can be shown mathematically that, while it is impossible to predict where any given particle will end up, the distance traveled will *on average* be $\sqrt{6Dt}$, where D is the diffusion coefficient described earlier. This is the well-known Einstein relation.

For further information on the general physics of diffusion, the reader is referred to the monograph by Crank (1).

Self Diffusion

In MRI, where we look at tissue water, we are not primarily interested in tracers but in *self diffusion*. In a solvent such as water, individual molecules are moving randomly as in Figure 2C, but in what sense is this diffusion as defined above? It does not appear to have a mixing of different species. Nevertheless, self diffusion is not something different from the foregoing; rather it is simply the special case where the two fluids mixing are identical. How then are we to interpret the term "concentration gradient" and apply the above analysis?

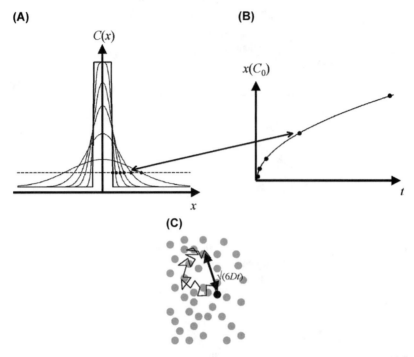

Figure 2 Tracer diffusion portrayed in three different ways. **(A)** Changing concentration profiles with time—the substance starts off as a discrete bolus with uniform density and the bolus edges gradually blur, **(B)** changing position with time of the concentration front $C = C_0$, and **(C)** the path of an individual molecule, which changes direction randomly due to collisions with its neighbors, and, on average, travels a distance $(\sqrt{6Dt})$ in time t.

It is at this point that the unique abilities of NMR come to the fore. By applying appropriate radiofrequency pulses, we can "magnetically label" the nuclear spins in part of the sample. Now we have a detectably different set of water molecules, whose concentration we can measure as they diffuse through the sample. Figure 3 shows such an example: Water molecules within a narrow strip of the sample were labeled by exciting magnetization from the longitudinal axis to the transverse plane, using a delays alternating with nutation for tailored excitation (DANTE) pulse

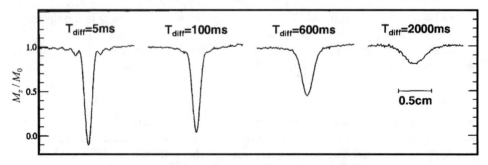

Figure 3 Experimental data showing how water, "labeled magnetically" via a DANTE NMR pulse sequence, behaves in exactly the way described in the text for tracer diffusion and shown schematically in Figure 2. *Abbreviations*: DANTE, delays alternating with nutation for tailored excitation pulse sequence; NMR, nuclear magnetic resonance. *Source*: From Refs. 2, 3.

sequence. The longitudinal magnetization was then sampled at subsequent times to "watch the labeled spins move." This magnetic labeling does not affect *how* the molecules move, unlike radioactive labeling, which leads to a minor perturbation, because it changes the mass. Hence, using MRI, we are able to make "tracer" measurements of one set of particles moving through another set that is in all physical ways identical, save for the spin states of the nuclei.

Diffusion and MRI

Whilst the measurements of Figure 3 make it easy to visualize pictorially the process of self diffusion, they are not the most efficient or accurate way of measuring the diffusion coefficient. Early in the development of NMR, Hahn (4) noted that the amplitudes of spin echoes were attenuated because of self-diffusion of the sample molecules. Subsequently, Carr and Purcell (5) gave a full explanation of this phenomenon and Stejskal and Tanner (6) applied the theory to make measurements of D. Consider the simple pulse sequence in Figure 4, with reference to a spin initially at position x_1. During the first gradient lobe, the spin acquires a phase $\varphi_1 = \omega(x_1)\delta$ $= -\gamma x_1 G_x \delta$. After the 180° pulse, a refocusing lobe causes the spin to acquire a further phase $\varphi_2 = \omega(x_2)\delta = +\gamma x_2 G_x \delta$, where x_2 is the position of the spin at the time of application of the second gradient pulse. (The sign of this second contribution is opposite because of the presence of the 180° pulse). Clearly, if the spin has not moved, then $x_2 = x_1$ and the two phases φ_1 and φ_2 cancel exactly. However, in general, the spin has a residual phase $\Delta\varphi = \varphi_1 + \varphi_2 = \gamma G \delta(x_2 - x_1)$. If one considers many different spins undergoing random diffusion, then there will be a large number of different values of $(x_2 - x_1)$ and, hence, many different spin phases. When we sum up all these different spins to get our net magnetization, they add up partially (but

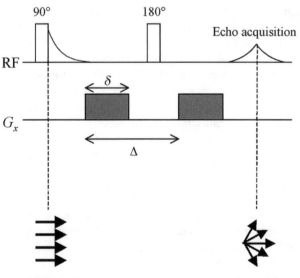

Spins all in phase
Net magnetisation M_0

Spins dephased due to motion in G_x
Net magnetisation $< M_0$

Figure 4 Basic PGSE pulse sequence. *Abbreviations*: PGSE, pulsed-field gradient spin-echo. *Source*: From Ref. 6.

not completely) out of phase (Fig. 4). This leads to an attenuation of the amplitude of the spin echo, which is given by the following formula:

$$S(b) = S(0) \exp(-bD)$$

where $S(0)$ is the echo amplitude with no diffusion gradient present, $S(b)$ is the value measured with a diffusion gradient on, D is the self-diffusion coefficient of the sample and b is the so-called "diffusion b-value," which is dependent on the pulse sequence parameters. For the basic Stejskal-Tanner sequence of Figure 4 (often also called the pulsed field-gradient (PFG) or pulsed-gradient spin-echo (PGSE) sequence),

$$b = (\gamma G)^2 \delta^2 (\Delta - \delta/3)$$

This formula shows that increased sensitivity to diffusion effects (i.e., a larger b-value) can be obtained (i) by increasing the strength of the diffusion gradient G, (ii) by increasing its duration δ (the most efficient way), and (iii) by increasing the gap Δ between the two gradient lobes.

Why Is Diffusion a Useful "Probe" in Medical Imaging?

If all the samples imaged by MRI were simple liquids, then the ability to measure diffusion coefficients would be, perhaps, no more than a curiosity: for a given temperature, every liquid has a well-defined self-diffusion coefficient. In fact, the human body provides a wide range of *structured environments*, through which water molecules diffuse. Measuring quantitatively the way in which an environment modifies the self-diffusion coefficient of water gives us a unique probe for investigating tissue structure noninvasively. Clearly, an exact determination of the 3-D microstructure of a tissue would require an imaging resolution far superior to anything available clinically. It would also entail the acquisition of much unnecessary information—we are not interested in the exact location of every twist and turn of every tumor microvessel. Instead, measurement of the self-diffusion coefficient with the resolution of a typical MRI clinical scan allows one to infer *average* properties of the tissue inside the voxel. This can provide metrics that may be diagnostically useful. In the following paragraphs, we provide a brief overview of the physical basis of five ways in which diffusion measurements can enhance our knowledge of tissues. Later in the Chapter, the clinical and research uses of diffusion imaging are described in detail.

Restricted Diffusion and the ADC

The immediate consequence of the cellular structure of tissue is that cell walls *restrict* the diffusion of water molecules. Consider a molecule that is initially within a given cell—the argument is very similar for a molecule that starts outside. Initially, the molecule is diffusing freely: It moves randomly, jostled by the other particles present, but experiences no restriction in its direction of movement. Its distance from the starting point increases with $\sqrt{t}$, as described above by the Einstein relation. However, after a certain time, the molecule comes into contact with the cell walls and its motion is impeded. It remains within the cell and the distance from its initial position stops increasing. Suppose we measure the self-diffusion coefficient of this molecule with the NMR sequence of Figure 4. If Δ, the diffusion time, is less than the time taken to cross the cell, i.e., $\sqrt{6D\Delta}$ is less than the cell radius, then the NMR experiment measures a value of D that is the "free diffusion coefficient," i.e., it is determined by the fluid composition in the cell. However, if Δ is longer than this, which is very often the case in DW-MRI, then the diffusion coefficient measured is *lower* than the free diffusion coefficient. We term this as the *apparent diffusion coefficient* (ADC) and it gives us an indication of the restrictions present in the sample. In principle, measurement of ADC as a function of diffusion time Δ could yield a measurement of cell size. However, the mathematics involved in extracting this is in practice very complicated (7).

Anisotropic Diffusion and the Diffusion Tensor

In the previous example, we implicitly assumed that the cell in which our molecule was diffusing was approximately spherical and that the restrictions would be the same in all directions. The human body contains a number of diffusion environments in which this is not the case, for example, muscle fibres or cerebral white-matter tracts. In these cases, diffusion is said to be *anisotropic*: particle movement occurs with fewer restrictions in some directions than others. This effect can be very marked: in white-matter tracts with a regular, parallel-fibre arrangement, water ADC is almost ten times greater along the fibre (1.4–1.8×10^{-3} mm^2 s^{-1}) than the average value in the perpendicular direction (0.15–0.3×10^{-3} mm^2 s^{-1}) (8).

This immediately suggests an interesting MR experiment. In the basic Stejskal-Tanner sequence of Figure 4, the physical *axis* (i.e., x, y, z, or some combination thereof) chosen for the diffusion gradient is arbitrary. If one is able to apply the gradients parallel and perpendicular to the fibre of interest, then one should measure *different ADCs*. The difficulty arising is that not one configuration of the gradients will be correctly aligned with all the fibres, since they all have different orientations. At this point, some useful mathematics known as *tensor diagonalisation* comes to our aid. It can be shown that provided diffusion data with a certain minimum number of gradient orientations—this can be as little as four diffusion-weighted images, plus an unweighted image—are acquired, then we can calculate not only the values of the ADC parallel and perpendicular to the fibre, but also the direction of the fibre. This has led, in recent years, to the growth of a whole new field of research, *fibre tracking* or *tractography*. The reader is referred to the special "diffusion tensor" edition of *NMR in Biomedicine* [15 (7,8): NOV-DEC 2002], which contains an impressive set of review articles on this subject.

Multicomponent Diffusion

Compared with the length scales relevant to tissue microstructure, voxels in standard clinical imaging are very large. This raises the possibility that more than one diffusion environment may be present in any given voxel. In such cases, the diffusion behaviour is characterised by a *number of different ADC values*. Our previous equation for the decay of the spin echo amplitude is now changed to

$$S(b) = \sum_i S_i(0) \exp(-bD_i)$$

where $S_i(0)$ represents the fractional signal from the ith diffusion "compartment," characterised by diffusion coefficient D_i. (In practice, restriction, discussed above, means that D_i will become ADC$_i$.) Analysis of multicomponent diffusion is

(A)   **(B)**

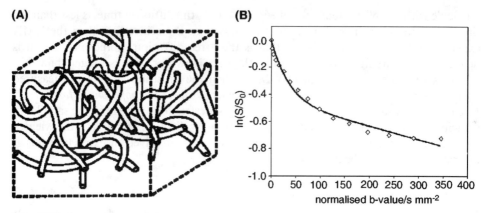

Figure 5 (**A**) Principle of IVIM. A single voxel contains many separate segments of blood capillary, all pointing in different directions. Perfusive flow in this network of capillaries is analogous to the random diffusive motion that is measured by NMR, but leads to effects approximately 1–2 orders of magnitude greater, (**B**) IVIM effects give rise to a multiexponential signal decay in a PGSE experiment. Averaged data from a tumour ROI in a rectal carcinoma patient show a steep initial slope corresponding to IVIM decay, which becomes shallower. The solid line is a bi-exponential fit to the data. *Abbreviations*: IVIM, intravoxel incoherent motion; PGSE, basic pulsed-field gradient spin-echo; ROI, region of interest. *Source*: From Ref. 11.

problematic, because many different distributions of exponentials lead to almost identical results for $S(b)$. Distinguishing between them requires extremely high signal-to-noise ratios in the diffusion images. However, in recent years, this approach has started to yield interesting results (9).

Intravoxel Incoherent Motion (IVIM) and Perfusion

As early as 1986, Le Bihan et al. (10) suggested that tissue *perfusion* could be measured using a DW-MRI experiment. The basic premise is that a single imaging voxel contains a very large number of tumor microvessels, all at different orientations, (Fig. 5A). If standard Stejskal-Tanner diffusion gradients are applied, then water molecules in the blood flowing along these vessels will exhibit a random distribution of phases, just like the randomly diffusing spins described earlier. The difference here is that the *pseudo-diffusion* coefficient corresponding to perfusive flow is between one and two orders of magnitude larger than that for normal diffusion and is thus easy to separate using multicomponent analysis. This is illustrated in Figure 5B, which shows diffusion data obtained from a rectal carcinoma.

Temperature Measurements

As a final illustration of the potential utility of measurements of diffusion coefficient, we note that increasing the temperature of the sample results in faster molecular motion of the water and hence to an increased diffusion coefficient. This effect can easily be observed via MRI and, although the alternative method of proton resonance frequency measurement has emerged as being the method of choice, DW-MRI has successfully been used in temperature mapping for clinical hyperthermia studies (12,13).

Measurement of Diffusion in an Imaging Context

A standard spin-echo imaging sequence may be turned into a diffusion-weighted sequence by the simple addition of two diffusion gradient lobes on either side of the 180° pulse. Figure 6A may thus be seen simply as the imaging version of the basic Stejskal-Tanner sequence of Figure 4. Each different amplitude of the diffusion gradient G_{diff} leads to an image with a different diffusion weighting. However, there are

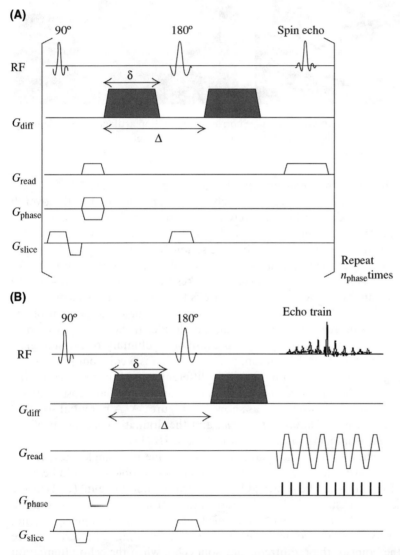

Figure 6 (**A**) Pulsed-gradient spin-echo diffusion imaging sequence—addition of standard Fourier imaging gradients to the Stejskal-Tanner sequence. In order to obtain the required b-values, it is often necessary to make the diffusion gradients significantly larger and longer than the imaging gradients. Note that the diffusion gradients act as crushers round the 180° pulse, (**B**) EPI single-shot diffusion imaging sequence. The central echo in the train (corresponding to the zero phase-encode line, which is largely responsible for the image contrast) is weighted by the same attenuation factor as in the spin-echo case above. *Abbreviation*: EPI, echo-planar imaging.

(A)   **(B)**

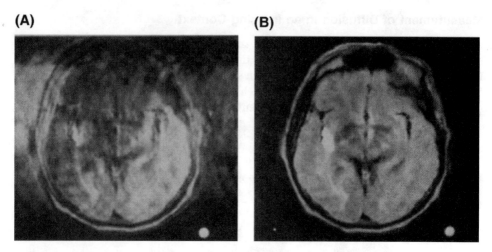

Figure 7   (**A**) Diffusion-weighted brain image corrupted by motion artifacts; (**B**) same image after correction using the navigator-echo method. *Source*: From Ref. 14.

two major drawbacks of this sequence. Firstly, a full spin-echo image, lasting perhaps a couple of minutes, is required for each b-value and this makes the overall acquisition time for the dataset prohibitively long for routine clinical practice. Secondly, motion causes a number of *artifacts*. Motion between the different b-value images leads to misregistration, but, much more seriously, motion during the acquisition of each phase-encoding step causes the individual images to be corrupted. The presence of the diffusion gradients (necessarily) makes the data acquisition sensitive to motion of the spins. What we wish to measure is the random diffusive motion of the water molecules, which, as described earlier, leads to a phase dispersion of the spins and hence to a decrease in the spin echo amplitude. If, however, all or part of the sample moves en masse, for example because of involuntary or physiological motion, then superimposed on the random phase variation is a coherent phase shift, the same for all of the spins. This phase shift is different at each phase-encode step and its influence on the final reconstructed image can destroy all possibility of obtaining useful diffusion information, as shown in, Figure 7A. A potential solution to this problem is the use of a *navigator echo*, and the dramatic restoration of the image using navigator information is shown in Figure 7B (14).

If one was able to obtain the image for each b-value in a single shot, rather than over multiple phase-encoding steps, then both of these problems would be overcome. In many cases, this can be achieved by using echo-planar imaging (EPI) as the imaging module (15). As shown in Figure 6B, diffusion information is encoded using our standard Stejskal-Tanner gradients, but this time, instead of a single spin echo, multiple gradient echoes are acquired with EPI spatial encoding. The zero k-space line occurs at the point of the radiofrequency spin echo, when the echo attenuation due to diffusion is exactly as described earlier.

DW-EPI is probably the most commonly used method of DW-MRI at the present time. However, it does have limitations: (i) A relatively long sample T_2 is required to allow both diffusion gradients and the echo-planar readout. A compromise must normally be made between the image resolution and the attainable b-value. (ii) Variations in magnetic susceptibility lead to image artifacts, particularly extracranially. These problems have tended to restrict DW-EPI to intracranial applications, although some work has been done on diffusion imaging of the spinal cord and in the abdomen (16–18).

Most rapid imaging sequences can be made sensitive to diffusion and, in recent years, competitors to EPI have begun to emerge. These include versions of the standard clinical sequences fast low angle shot (FLASH) and half-fourier single-shot turbo spin echo (HASTE) incorporating Stejskal-Tanner gradients, but also more unusual sequences such as line-scan and Burst imaging (19–22). In all of these cases, diffusion attenuation is described by the formulae above. By contrast, the PSIF (time reversed fast imaging with steady state precession) sequence, currently under active investigation because of the high image quality and signal-to-noise obtainable, requires a knowledge of T_1, T_2, and the spin flip angle to extract accurate diffusion information from the measured data.

Biological and Clinical Perspectives

Given the outline of the physical principles governing the assessment of diffusion in the previous section, this section will review the current role and likely future directions of DW-MRI in oncological imaging. The role of DW-MRI in oncological imaging is presented under three themes: (i) The diagnosis, grading, and physiological significance of diffusion measurements in cancer, (ii) The prediction and assessment of anticancer treatment, and (iii) The role of DW-MRI in treatment planning. In order to provide structure to the discussion, each theme will be discussed on a systems (organ) basis.

DIAGNOSIS, GRADING, AND PHYSIOLOGICAL SIGNIFICANCE OF DW-MRI IN CANCER

Intracranial Malignancy: DW-MRI is most commonly applied to the study of intracranial malignancies and is a reflection of the technical issues of physiological motion, susceptibility, and lipid-induced chemical shift artifact commonly encountered extracranially. DW-MRI has made a significant impact on the assessment of stroke (23,24). Early studies in neuro-oncology have shown its potential to improve tumor diagnosis and grading of brain tumors. Most DW-MRI studies have a complementary role in diagnosis and are almost always reported together with pre- and post-contrast T1W, T2W, and fast low angle inversion recovery (FLAIR) images. Given these brief comments, diagnostic benefit was found in differentiating purulent brain processes from cystic or necrotic brain tumors giving a positive predictive value of 93% and a negative predictive value of 91% (25,26). The high signal intensity (SI) seen in abscesses on DW-MRI are being taken to represent the viscous nature of abscess contents. DW-MRI also provides better conspicuity of intracranial epidermoids over fast-FLAIR with the intense high SI of epidermoids being attributed to "T2 shine-through," a phenomenon typically observed with sequences incorporating low b-values (27).

Several studies have now histologically verified the strong correlation between the measured ADC of gliomas and tumor cellularity (23). Low-grade gliomas typically return significantly higher ADC values than high-grade or intracranial lymphoma in keeping with the hypothesis that higher cellularity contributes to a more restricted diffusion (24,28). In addition, ADC values have been found to correlate with the total nuclear area (a measure of the area taken up by a cell nucleus in a high power view) and histology in several paediatric tumors (29). In addition, that same study demonstrated near zero values for all measures of anisotropy using diffusion tensor imaging. This is an important point since isotropic diffusion is often assumed but rarely assessed in tumors. The assessment of anisotropy should be encouraged particularly in view of the ordered structure reported in some meningiomas (30). Nevertheless, a clearly defined role remains to be established in the differential diagnosis and grading of intracranial tumors because of limitations of DW-MRI in clearly defining tumor boundaries and grade (31,32). Although these latter two studies might be criticized on aspects of methodology including sample number, they highlight the continuing need to assess the clinical impact and cost of these emerging technologies.

Abdominal and Pelvic Malignancies: The technical issues surrounding respiratory motion compounded by issues of susceptibility and chemical shift artefacts have led to a limited literature on extracranial DW-MRI. Recent advances particularly in motion compensation strategies such as navigator echoes and spatially selective fat suppression pulses have promoted studies into abdominal and pelvic malignancy (14).

The pancreas is a deep-seated abdominal organ that continues to pose diagnostic-imaging problems particularly if nonspecific abnormalities such as cysts are detected. The differentiation of benign from malignant cystic lesions of the pancreas is facilitated by echo-planar generated images and ADC maps (33). The greater viscosity of mucin producing tumors caused these lesions to have a low ADC and high SI that convincingly differentiated them from benign cysts on DW-MRI. In a similar fashion, hepatic abscesses were demonstrated to have a significantly lower ADC than cystic or necrotic tumor, mirroring findings in the brain (see above) (34). In the liver, diagnostic specificity was still partly dependent on the appearance of the postgadolinium rim enhancement despite the ADC of abscesses being half that of cysts. In an attempt to exploit the high perfusion in abdominal organs, an alternative DW-MRI approach was taken using intravoxel incoherent motion imaging (see previous section). In this approach, a double exponential characterizes the ADC of flowing spins (D^*) and the true diffusion coefficient (D) of the tissues. An additional value in the expression represents the fractional volume (f) occupied in the voxel by flowing spins. D and f values were useful in the characterization of hepatic lesions using either EPI or turbo FLASH (35,36). Unsurprisingly, hepatic carcinoma had the lowest D with the highest values recorded in cysts. Some variation was seen in D^* and f values particularly for cysts where inertial motion in the fluid is likely to have contributed to the recorded values.

Currently, only a limited number of studies have reported the use of DW-MRI in pelvic malignancy. These have assessed the potential of the ADC to discriminate benign from malignant ovarian tumor and to differentiate endometrial from other pelvic cysts (37,38). Both studies concluded that although malignant lesions tended to have a lower ADC, no diagnostic advantage could be found over conventional use of T1 and T2 weighted imaging. Some value was detected in adding ADC to the conventional MR protocol when differentiating endometrial from other pelvic cysts but not to the extent of excluding other sequences in favor of DW-MRI. Surprisingly, DW-MRI studies of prostate cancer are only beginning to be reported despite it being a common male malignancy. The feasibility of performing DW-MRI in the normal and malignant prostate has been reported though formal studies assessing the diagnostic and predictive value of DW-MRI in the prostate remain to be performed (39). Some hope that DW-MRI might provide increased lesion conspicuity over conventional T2 imaging has recently been reported as a result of an animal study in which a twofold difference in ADC between benign and malignant tissue was reported (40). The prostate also offers considerable opportunity for the integration of functional studies in addition to that of DW-MRI (41).

Musculoskeletal and Soft Tissues: DW-MRI of head and neck lesions and soft-tissue tumors have seldom but nevertheless been reported (42,43). In several head and neck malignancies, setting a threshold ADC to less than $1.22 \times 10\text{--}3$ mm^2 s^{-1} was predictive for malignancy with an accuracy of 86% and a sensitivity and specificity of 84% and 91% respectively. As in tumors at other sites, soft-tissue malignancies tended to have a lower ADC than benign lesions.

In the realm of musculoskeletal imaging, DW-MRI has most commonly been applied to the differentiation of benign from malignant vertebral fractures. Metastatic vertebral disease occurs in 5% to10% of all malignancy and most commonly involves the thoracic spine. Histologically verified studies have demonstrated a positive correlation between ADC and bone marrow cellularity which, in the case of leukemia was used to segment abnormal from uninvolved marrow (44,45). The typically lower ADC of malignant hypercellularity was therefore useful in the differentiation of osteoporotic from malignant vertebral fracture though technical features such as the use of low b-values might explain the absence of diagnostic sensitivity in some reports (46–50). It is however becoming apparent that DW-MRI does not always image all bony malignancy advantageously. In bony lymphoma, for example, DW-MRI conferred no diagnostic advantage over T1 weighted spin-echo and STIR imaging (51).

Breast Tumors: Spurred partly by the limited sensitivity (70–90%) of X ray mammography in the detection and differentiation of breast lesions, several studies have assessed the feasibility and role of DW-MRI in breast malignancy. In keeping with other malignancies, breast carcinomas are characterized by a lower ADC than benign lesions and there is a strong association between mean ADC and tumor cellularity (52,53). Interestingly, despite low tumor detectability, diffusion weighted HASTE demonstrated a lower mean ADC in invasive ductal carcinoma when compared to fibroadenoma with the added advantage of limited susceptibility and chemical shift artifact inherent in the sequence (54). In keeping with other pathologies, DW-MRI remains promising but not essential to diagnosis.

PREDICTION AND ASSESSMENT OF THE RESPONSE TO ANTICANCER TREATMENT

The ability to noninvasively predict or assess response at an earlier stage than is currently possible would have considerable clinical advantages. Such an assessment could ultimately lead to individualized patient treatment. Currently tumor response is assessed on size criteria that rarely reflect underlying tumor biology (55). Such poor sensitivity is partly due to organism survival being more dependent on cell kill and repopulation kinetics than the fraction of tumor cells killed (56). Human studies have reported changes in the appearance of diffusion-weighted images following successful treatment in, for example, metastatic vertebral disease but such changes were noted only following the end of conventional treatment (57). It was first pointed out several years ago that a dose dependent increase in ADC preceded morphological change in a murine model bearing a RIF-1 tumor treated with cyclophosphamide (58). Since then, several workers have reported that an increase in ADC indicates early response in animal tumor models treated by conventional or gene therapy and similar behaviour has been reported in a limited number of human brain tumors (59–66). The exact mechanisms underlying the detected ADC changes remain to be fully established though it is generally accepted that the ADC rises as a result of cell

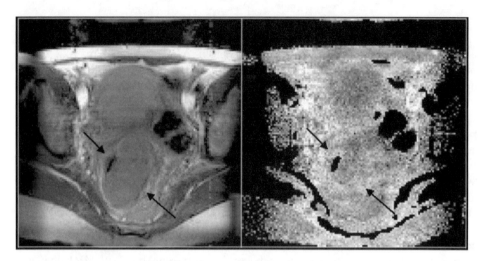

Figure 8 ADC map of a locally advanced rectal cancer. This large mid-rectal cancer invading the mesorectum is clearly outlined (*arrows*) on this axial T2-weighted image (**A**). The image on the right (**B**) is the ADC map. Note the different distribution of contrast and the low signal intensity crescentic region due to luminal air.

loss and an increase in the size of the extracellular volume often in parallel with treatment-induced apoptosis (67,68). This explanation is necessarily an oversimplification since the biophysical characteristics of tissues including the extracellular space are complex (69). Nevertheless, DW-MRI is being increasingly used preclinically as an early measure of therapeutic response including in studies of drug delivery and action (70,71).

Where assessment of early response is desirable, response prediction is invaluable. In a recent study of locally advanced rectal cancer, (Fig. 8) the mean pretreatment ADC of tumors was found to be strongly correlated, (Fig. 9) with response following chemotherapy and chemoradiotherapy (72). With the exception of one report this has not been noted in other animal studies and may reflect the common use of xenotransplanted tumors (61). Given that the ADC is known to correlate with necrotic fraction, it was postulated that in locally advanced rectal tumors the ADC was acting as a surrogate marker of necrosis. Consequently, the ADC was reflecting the recognized poor outcome of necrotic tumors to therapy. Furthermore those rectal tumors demonstrating a drop in ADC following initial therapy subsequently showed the best response, contrary to findings in other tumors (see above). The preferential sloughing of necrotic tumor over viable tissue might explain the resulting low ADC. This hypothesis remains to be verified since those measurements were taken several weeks following initial treatment whilst the rise in ADC detected in other publications occurred only days following initiation of treatment. Nevertheless, an important issue is raised and highlights the fact that although cell density and necrotic fraction of grafted tumors often correlates with ADC this is not always the case for all cell lines (74,75). This may also be the case in human tumors. In a preliminary report no correlation was found between the pretreatment ADC in low-grade glioma and mean tumor ADC (Fig. 10) (76). Although this might be the result of sampling error, it might equally be a manifestation of the underlying tumor biology. By definition low-grade gliomas are not necrotic. If ADC is primarily a surrogate marker of necrosis, then the absence of a correlation with ADC in this instance is understandable.

(A)

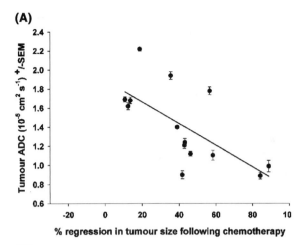

% regression in tumour size following chemotherapy

(B)

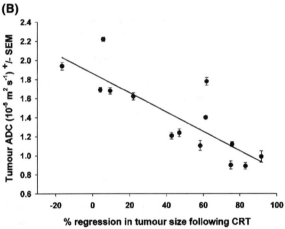

% regression in tumour size following CRT

Figure 9 Association between pretreatment rectal tumor ADC and tumor regression following **(A)** chemotherapy and **(B)** chemoradiation. Note the strong negative correlation in both instances: **(A)** $r = -0.66$ $p = 0.011$; **(B)** $r = -0.78$ $p = 0.001$. Although histological validation is awaited, the mean ADC in this instance is likely to be a surrogate marker of necrosis. *Source*: From Ref. 73.

DW-MRI IN TREATMENT PLANNING

Here treatment planning is taken to include medical and surgical approaches including experimental therapies such as thermal tumor ablation (77).

White matter tractography is a particularly elegant application of diffusion tensor imaging that has been used to delineate uninvolved from infiltrated white matter tracts prior to resection or radiotherapy. In tractography, the anisotropy inherent in white matter tracts is exploited to generate detailed color maps of their disposition. The technique is now established in animals (78,79) and humans (76,80–83). These studies have firmly established that tensor DW-MRI can distinguish involved from noninvolved tracts and can accurately delineate the paths of white matter tracts in disease. It remains to be established what impact this will have on patient morbidity though with the advent of precise radiation dose delivery via

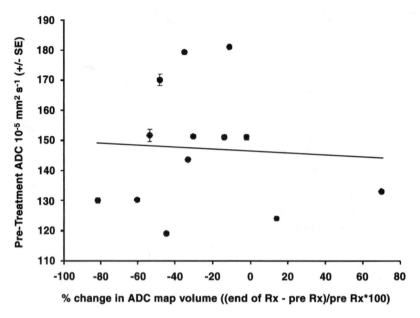

Figure 10 Absence of an association (r = 0.05, p = 0.81) between pretreatment ADC and response to treatment with the anticancer agent temozolomide in low-grade glioma. Although the absence of an association may be a sampling issue, it may represent the absence of necrosis in low-grade glioma.

IMRT (Intensity Modulated Radiotherapy) tensor imaging has the potential to play a central role in radiotherapy planning.

An interesting application of DW-MRI has been the assessment of events related to the administration of dexamethasone. Dexamethasone is recognised to have a dramatic effect on the symptoms of raised intracranial pressure. Although it is generally assumed that the effects relate to reductions in tumor or peritumoral water content, the effects remain incompletely understood. As part of a multifunctional imaging approach, DW-MRI was used to assess changes in the degree of oedema (84). In that study, dexamethasone was found to cause a dramatic and rapid decrease in blood-brain barrier permeability and regional cerebral blood volume but without significant change in cerebral blood flow or degree of oedema as assessed by diffusion tensor imaging. Clearly the issues are not straightforward since other studies have detected significant changes in the ADC of tumoral and peritumoral areas (85). As the mechanisms underlying these changes become established, it may be that DW-MRI will have a role to play in planned treatment based on the response to dexamethasone.

Despite the evident strengths of DW-MRI in reporting on the structural features of tissues in vivo, it is unlikely that the modality will alone have a significant impact on patient management. Several recent studies incorporating DW-MRI, perfusion and permeability imaging, and ^{1}H-MR spectroscopy have been reported. Their role has been to provide additional insight into human tumor biology. In a study of gliomas incorporating histological verification, a significant inverse correlation was found between tumor ADC and cell density (86). The spectroscopically determined choline signal was also linearly correlated with cell density suggesting a combined approach delineating dense cellular lesions from necrotic regions could influence patient management. Additional functional findings that might bear on future targeting of tumors include an inverse correlation between the percentage enhancement in pediatric brain tumors and ADC, and an inverse correlation between relative cerebral blood volume and ADC, and a similar correlation with the choline/creatine ratio (87,88). The increasing understanding of the biological significance of such imaging/spectroscopic findings has the potential to improve targeted therapies in the future.

CONCLUSIONS

We have seen how diffusion describes the random manner in which particles progress down a concentration gradient. Such molecular behaviour can be observed by DW-MRI by the appropriate choreography of nuclear species. Much of current development is targeted towards resolving physiological issues of organ motion and tissue content. In oncology, DW-MRI is proving to be a useful but not unique adjunct to diagnosis whilst its role in treatment planning is being assessed. The early assessment and prediction of response however appears to be a real advantage of DW-MRI.

ACKNOWLEDGMENTS

Cancer Research UK C1060/A808/G7643 and EPSRC (GR/M60613) generously funded part of the research work described in this chapter.

REFERENCES

1. Crank J. The Mathematics of Diffusion. Oxford, 1975.
2. Morris GA, Freeman R. Selective excitation in Fourier transform nuclear magnetic resonance. J Magn Reson 1978; 29:433–462.
3. Doran SJ, Jakob P, Decorps M. Rapid repetition of the "Burst" sequence: The role of diffusion and consequences for imaging. Magnetic Resonance in Medicine 1996; 35(4): 547–553
4. Hahn EL. Spin echoes. Phys Rev 1950; 80(1):580–594.
5. Carr HY, Purcell EM. Effects of diffusion on free precession in nuclear magnetic resonance experiments. Phys Rev 1956; 94(3):630–638.
6. Stejskal EO, Tanner JE. Spin diffusion measurements: spin echoes in the presence of a time-dependent field gradient. J Chem Phys 1965; 42(1):288–292.
7. Mitra PP, Sen PN. Effects of microgeometry and surface relaxation on NMR pulsed-field-gradient experiments: simple pore geometries. Phys Rev B 1992; 45(1):143–156.
8. Pierpaoli C, Basser PJ. Toward a quantitative assessment of diffusion anisotropy. Magn Reson Med 1996; 36:893–906.
9. Assaf Y, Ben-Bashat D, et al. High b-value q-space analyzed diffusion-weighted MRI: application to multiple sclerosis. Magn Reson Med 2002; 47:115–126.
10. Le Bihan D, Breton E, et al. MR imaging of intravoxel incoherent motions: application to diffusion and perfusion in neurologic disorders. Radiology 1986; 161:401–407.
11. Le Bihan D, Breton E, Lallemand D. Separation of diffusion and perfusion in intravoxel incoherent motion MR imaging. Radiology 1988; 168:497–505.
12. Le Bihan D, Delannoy J, Levin RL. Temperature mapping with MR imaging of molecular diffusion: application to hyperthermia. Radiol 1989; 171(3):853–857.
13. Zhang Y, Samulski TV, Joines WT, Mattiello J, Levin RL, LeBihan D. On the accuracy of noninvasive thermometry using molecular diffusion magnetic resonance imaging. Int J Hyperthermia 1992; 8(2):263–274.

14. Anderson AW, Gore JC. Analysis and correction of motion artifacts in diffusion weighted imaging. Magn Reson Med 1994; 32:379–387.
15. Turner R, Le Bihan D. Single-shot diffusion imaging at 2.0 Tesla. J Magn Reson 1990; 86(3):445–452.
16. Clark CA, Werring DJ. Diffusion tensor imaging in spinal cord: methods and applications – a review. NMR Biomed 2002; 15(7–8):578–586.
17. Issa B. In vivo measurement of the apparent diffusion coefficient in normal and malignant prostatic tissues using echo-planar imaging. J Magn Reson Imaging 2002; 16(2):196–200.
18. Ries M, Jones RA, Basseau F, Moonen CTW, Grenier N. Diffusion tensor MRI of the human kidney. J Magn Reson Imaging 2001; 14(1):42–49.
19. Thomas DL, Pell GS, Lythgoe MF, Gadian DG, Ordidge RJ. A quantitative method for fast diffusion imaging using magnetization-prepared TurboFLASH. Magn Reson Med 1998; 39(6):950–960.
20. Schick F. SPLICE: Sub-second diffusion-sensitive MR imaging using a modified fast spin-echo acquisition made. Magn Reson Med 1997; 38(4):638–644.
21. Gudbjartson H, Maier SE, Jolesz FA. Double line scan diffusion imaging. Magn Reson Med 1997; 38:101–109.
22. Wheeler-Kingshott CA, Thomas DL, Lythgoe MF, Guilfoyle D, Williams SR, Doran SJ. Burst excitation for quantitative diffusion imaging with multiple b-values. Magn Reson Med 2001; 44(5):737–745.
23. Sugahara T, Korogi Y, et al. Usefulness of diffusion-weighted MRI with echo-planar technique in the evaluation of cellularity in gliomas. J Magn Reson Imaging 1999; 9(1):53–60.
24. Kono K, Inoue Y, et al. The role of diffusion-weighted imaging in patients with brain tumors. Am J Neuroradiol 2001; 22(6):1081–1088.
25. Guzman R, Barth A, Lovblad KO, El-Koussy M, Weis J, Schroth G, Seiler RW. Use of diffusion-weighted magnetic resonance imaging in differentiating purulent brain processes from cystic brain tumors. J Neurosurg 2002; 97(5):1101–1107.
26. Chang SC, Lai PH, Chen WL, Weng HH, Ho JT, Wang JS, Chang CY, Pan HB, Yang CF. Diffusion-weighted MRI features of brain abscess and cystic or necrotic brain tumors: comparison with conventional MRI. Clin Imaging 2002; 26(4):227–236.
27. Chen S, Ikawa F, Kurisu K, Arita K, Takaba J, Kanou Y. Quantitative MR evaluation of intracranial epidermoid tumors by fast fluid-attenuated inversion recovery imaging and echo-planar diffusion-weighted imaging. Am J Neuroradiol 2001; 22(6):1089–1096.
28. Guo AC, Cummings TJ, Dash RC, Provenzale JM. Lymphomas and high-grade astrocytomas: comparison of water diffusibility and histologic characteristics. Radiology 2002; 224(1):177–183.
29. Gauvain KM, McKinstry RC, et al. Evaluating pediatric brain tumor cellularity with diffusion-tensor imaging. Am J Roentgenol 2001; 177(2):449–454.
30. Filippi CG, Edgar MA, Ulug AM, Prowda JC, Heier LA, Zimmerman RD. Appearance of meningiomas on diffusion-weighted images: correlating diffusion constants with histopathologic findings. Am J Neuroradiol 2001; 22(1):65–72.
31. Stadnik TW, Chaskis C, Michotte A, Shabana WM, van Rompaey K, Luypaert R, Budinsky L, Jellus V, Osteaux M. Diffusion-weighted MR imaging of intracerebral masses: comparison with conventional MR imaging and histologic findings. Am J Neuroradiol 2001; 22(5):969–976.
32. Lam WW, Poon WS, Metreweli C. Diffusion MR imaging in glioma: does it have any role in the pre-operation determination of grading of glioma? Clin Radiol 2002; 57(3):219–225
33. Yamashita Y, Namimoto T, et al. Mucin-producing tumor of the pancreas: diagnostic value of diffusion-weighted echo-planar MR imaging. Radiology 1998; 208(3):605–609.
34. Chan JH, Tsui EY, Luk SH, Fung AS, Yuen MK, Szeto ML, Cheung YK, Wong KP. Diffusion-weighted MR imaging of the liver: distinguishing hepatic abscess from cystic or necrotic tumor. Abdom Imaging 2001; 26(2):161–165.

35. Yamada I, Aung W, Himeno Y, Nakagawa T, Shibuya H. Diffusion coefficients in abdominal organs and hepatic lesions: evaluation with intravoxel incoherent motion echo-planar MR imaging. Radiology 1999; 210(3):617–623.

36. Moteki T, Horikoshi H, Oya N, Aoki J, Endo K. Evaluation of hepatic lesions and hepatic parenchyma using diffusion-weighted reordered turboFLASH magnetic resonance images. J Magn Reson Imaging 2002; 15(5):564–572.

37. Katayama M, Masui T, Kobayashi S, Ito T, Sakahara H, Nozaki A, Kabasawa H. Diffusion-weighted echo planar imaging of ovarian tumors: is it useful to measure apparent diffusion coefficients? J Comput Assist Tomogr 2002; 26(2):250–256.

38. Moteki T, Horikoshi H, Endo K. Relationship between apparent diffusion coefficient and signal intensity in endometrial and other pelvic cysts. Magn Reson Imaging 2002; 20(6):463–470.

39. Gibbs P, Tozer DJ, Liney GP, Turnbull LW. Comparison of quantitative T2 mapping and diffusion-weighted imaging in the normal and pathologic prostate. Magn Reson Med 2001; 46(6):1054–1058.

40. Song SK, Qu Z, Garabedian EM, Gordon JI, Milbrandt J, Ackerman JJ. Improved magnetic resonance imaging detection of prostate cancer in a transgenic mouse model. Cancer Res 2002; 62(5):1555–1558.

41. Kurhanewicz J, Swanson MG, Nelson SJ, Vigneron DB. Combined magnetic resonance imaging and spectroscopic imaging approach to molecular imaging of prostate cancer. J Magn Reson Imaging 2002; 16(4):451–463.

42. Wang J, Takashima S, et al. Head and neck lesions: characterization with diffusion-weighted echo-planar MR imaging. Radiology 2001; 220(3):621–630.

43. van Rijswijk CS, Kunz P, Hogendoorn PC, Taminiau AH, Doornbos J, Bloem JL. Diffusion-weighted MRI in the characterization of soft-tissue tumors. J Magn Reson Imaging 2002; 15(3):302–307.

44. Nonomura Y, Yasumoto M, Yoshimura R, Haraguchi K, Ito S, Akashi T, Ohashi I. Relationship between bone marrow cellularity and apparent diffusion coefficient. J Magn Reson Imaging 2001; 13(5):757–760.

45. Ballon D, Dyke J, Schwartz LH, Lis E, Schneider E, Lauto A, Jakubowski AA. Bone marrow segmentation in leukemia using diffusion and T (2) weighted echo planar magnetic resonance imaging. NMR Biomed 2000; 13(6):321–328.

46. Chan JH, Peh WC, Tsui EY, Chau LF, Cheung KK, Chan KB, Yuen MK, Wong ET, Wong KP. Acute vertebral body compression fractures: discrimination between benign and malignant causes using apparent diffusion coefficients. Br J Radiol 2002; 75: 207–214.

47. Spuentrup E, Buecker A, Adam G, van Vaals JJ, Guenther RW. Diffusion-weighted MR imaging for differentiation of benign fracture edema and tumor infiltration of the vertebral body. Am J Roentgenol 2001; 176(2):351–358.

48. Zhou XJ, Leeds NE, McKinnon GC, Kumar AJ. Characterization of benign and metastatic vertebral compression fractures with quantitative diffusion MR imaging. Am J Neuroradiol 2002; 23(1):165–170.

49. Castillo M, Arbelaez A, Smith JK, Fisher LL. Diffusion-weighted MR imaging offers no advantage over routine noncontrast MR imaging in the detection of vertebral metastases. Am J Neuroradiol 2000; 21(5):948–953.

50. Baur A, Stabler A, et al. Diffusion-weighted MR imaging of bone marrow: differentiation of benign versus pathologic compression fractures. Radiology 1998; 207(2):349–356.

51. Yasumoto M, Nonomura Y, Yoshimura R, Haraguchi K, Ito S, Ohashi I, Shibuya H. MR detection of iliac bone marrow involvement by malignant lymphoma with various MR sequences including diffusion-weighted echo-planar imaging. Skeletal Radiol 2002; 31(5):263–269.

52. Guo Y, Cai YQ, Cai ZL, Gao YG, An NY, Ma L, Mahankali S, Gao JH. Differentiation of clinically benign and malignant breast lesions using diffusion-weighted imaging. J Magn Reson Imaging 2002; 16(2):172–178.

53. Sinha S, Lucas-Quesada FA, Sinha U, DeBruhl N, Bassett LW. In vivo diffusion-weighted MRI of the breast: potential for lesion characterization. J Magn Reson Imaging 2002; 15(6):693–704.

54. Kinoshita T, Yashiro N, Ihara N, Funatu H, Fukuma E, Narita M. Diffusion-weighted half-Fourier single-shot turbo spin echo imaging in breast tumors: differentiation of invasive ductal carcinoma from fibroadenoma. J Comput Assist Tomogr 2002; 26(6):1042–1046.

55. Husband JE, Gwyther SJ, Rankin S. Monitoring tumor response. Abdom Imaging 1999; 24(6):618–621.

56. Ross BD, Zhao YJ, Neal ER, Stegman LD, Ercolani M, Ben-Yoseph O, Chenevert TL. Contributions of cell kill and posttreatment tumor growth rates to the repopulation of intracerebral 9L tumors after chemotherapy: an MRI study. Proc Natl Acad Sci USA 1998; 95(12):7012–7017.

57. Byun WM, Shin SO, Chang Y, Lee SJ, Finsterbusch J, Frahm J. Diffusion-weighted MR imaging of metastatic disease of the spine: assessment of response to therapy. Am J Neuroradiol 2002; 23(6):906–912.

58. Zhao M, Pipe JG, Bonnett J, Evelhoch JL. Early detection of treatment response by diffusion-weighted 1H-NMR spectroscopy in a murine tumor in vivo. Br J Cancer 1996; 73(1):61–64.

59. Galons JP, Altbach MI, Paine-Murrieta GD, Taylor CW, Gillies RJ. Early increases in breast tumor xenograft water mobility in response to paclitaxel therapy detected by non-invasive diffusion magnetic resonance imaging. Neoplasia 1999; 1(2):113–117.

60. Chinnaiyan AM, Prasad U, Shankar S, Hamstra DA, Shanaiah M, Chenevert TL, Ross BD, Rehemtulla A. Combined effect of tumor necrosis factor-related apoptosis-inducing ligand and ionizing radiation in breast cancer therapy. Proc Natl Acad Sci USA 2000; 97:1754–1759.

61. Lemaire L, Howe FA, Rodrigues LM, Griffiths JR. Assessment of induced rat mammary tumor response to chemotherapy using the apparent diffusion coefficient of tissue water as determined by diffusion-weighted 1H-NMR spectroscopy in vivo. Magma 1999; 8(1): 20–26.

62. Jennings D, Hatton BN, Guo J, Galons JP, Trouard TP, Raghunand N, Marshall J, Gillies RJ. Early response of prostate carcinoma xenografts to docetaxel chemotherapy monitored with diffusion MRI. Neoplasia 2002; 4(3):255–262.

63. Stegman LD, Rehemtulla A, Hamstra DA, Rice DJ, Jonas SJ, Stout KL, Chenevert TL, Ross BD. Diffusion MRI detects early events in the response of a glioma model to the yeast cytosine deaminase gene therapy strategy. Gene Ther 2000; 7(12):1005–1010.

64. Poptani H, Puumalainen AM, et al. Monitoring thymidine kinase and ganciclovir-induced changes in rat malignant glioma in vivo by nuclear magnetic resonance imaging. Cancer Gene Ther 1998; 5(2):101–109.

65. Chenevert TL, Stegman LD, Taylor JM, Robertson PL, Greenberg HS, Rehemtulla A, Ross BD. Diffusion magnetic resonance imaging: an early surrogate marker of therapeutic efficacy in brain tumors. J Natl Cancer Inst 2000; 92(24):2029–2036.

66. Mardor Y, Roth Y, et al. Monitoring response to convection-enhanced taxol delivery in brain tumor patients using diffusion-weighted magnetic resonance imaging. Cancer Res 2001; 61(13):4971–4973.

67. Kauppinen RA. Monitoring cytotoxic tumor treatment response by diffusion magnetic resonance imaging and proton spectroscopy. NMR Biomed 2002; 15(1):6–17.

68. Hakumaki JM, Poptani H, et al. Quantitative 1H nuclear magnetic resonance diffusion spectroscopy of BT4C rat glioma during thymidine kinase-mediated gene therapy in vivo: identification of apoptotic response. Cancer Res 1998; 58(17):3791–3799.

69. Rusakov DA, Kullmann DM. Geometric and viscous components of the tortuosity of the extracellular space in the brain. Proc Natl Acad Sci USA 1998; 95(15):8975–8980.

70. Dev SB, Caban JB, Nanda GS, Bleecher SD, Rabussay DP, Moerland TS, Gibbs SJ, Locke BR. Magnetic resonance studies of laryngeal tumors implanted in nude mice: effect of treatment with bleomycin and electroporation. Magn Reson Imaging 2002; 20(5):389–394.

71. Beauregard DA, Thelwall PE, Chaplin DJ, Hill SA, Adams GE, Brindle KM. Magnetic resonance imaging and spectroscopy of combretastatin A4 prodrug-induced disruption of tumor perfusion and energetic status. Br J Cancer 1998; 77(11):1761–1767.

72. Dzik-Jurasz A, Domenig C, George M, Wolber J, Padhani A, Brown G, Doran S. Diffusion MRI for prediction of response of rectal cancer to chemoradiation. Lancet 2002; 360(9329):307–308.

73. Dzik-Jurasz A, Domenig C, George M, Wolber J, Padhani A, Brown G, Doran S. Diffusion MRI for prediction of response of rectal cancer to chemoradiation.The Lancet 2002; 360:307.

74. Maier SE, Bogner P, et al. Normal brain and brain tumor: multicomponent apparent diffusion coefficient line scan imaging. Radiology 2001; 219(3):842–849.

75. Lyng H, Haraldseth O, Rofstad EK. Measurement of cell density and necrotic fraction in human melanoma xenografts by diffusion weighted magnetic resonance imaging. Magn Reson Med 2000; 43(6):828–836.

76. Krings T, Reinges MH, Thiex R, Gilsbach JM, Thron A. Functional and diffusion-weighted magnetic resonance images of space-occupying lesions affecting the motor system: imaging the motor cortex and pyramidal tracts. J Neurosurg 2001; 95(5):816–824.

77. Germain D, Chevallier P, Laurent A, Saint-Jalmes H. MR monitoring of tumor thermal therapy. Magma 2001; 13(1):47–59.

78. Melhem ER, Mori S, Mukundan G, Kraut MA, Pomper MG, van Zijl PC. Diffusion tensor MR imaging of the brain and white matter tractography. Am J Roentgenol 2002; 178(1):3–16.

79. Clark CA, Hedehus M, Moseley ME. Diffusion time dependence of the apparent diffusion tensor in healthy human brain and white matter disease. Magn Reson Med 2001; 45(6):1126–1129.

80. Inglis BA, Neubauer D, Yang L Plant D, Mareci TH, Muir D. Diffusion tensor MR imaging and comparative histology of glioma engrafted in the rat spinal cord. Am J Neuroradiol 1999; 20(4):713–716.

81. Wieshmann UC, Symms MR, et al. Diffusion tensor imaging demonstrates deviation of fibres in normal appearing white matter adjacent to a brain tumor. J Neurol Neurosurg Psychiatry 2000; 68(4):501–503.

82. Witwer BP, Moftakhar R, et al. Diffusion-tensor imaging of white matter tracts in patients with cerebral neoplasm. J Neurosurg 2002; 97(3):568–575.

83. Mori S, Frederiksen K, van Zijl PC, Stieltjes B, Kraut MA, Solaiyappan M, Pomper MG. Brain white matter anatomy of tumor patients evaluated with diffusion tensor imaging. Ann Neurol 2002; 51(3):377–380..

84. Ostergaard L, Hochberg FH, Rabinov JD, Sorensen AG, Lev M, Kim L, Weisskoff RM, Gonzalez RG, Gyldensted C, Rosen BR. Early changes measured by magnetic resonance imaging in cerebral blood flow, blood volume, and blood-brain barrier permeability following dexamethasone treatment in patients with brain tumors. J Neurosurg 1999; 90(2):300–305.

85. Bastin ME, Delgado M, Whittle IR, Cannon J, Wardlaw JM. The use of diffusion tensor imaging in quantifying the effect of dexamethasone on brain tumors. Neuroreport 1999; 10(7):1385–1391.

86. Gupta RK, Cloughesy TF, Sinha U, Garakian J, Lazareff J, Rubino G, Rubino L, Becker DP, Vinters HV, Alger JR. Relationships between choline magnetic resonance spectroscopy, apparent diffusion coefficient and quantitative histopathology in human glioma. J Neurooncol 2000; 50(3):215–226.

87. Tzika AA, Zarifi MK, et al. Neuroimaging in pediatric brain tumors: Gd-DTPA-enhanced, hemodynamic, and diffusion MR imaging compared with MR spectroscopic imaging. Am J Neuroradiol 2002; 23(2):322–333.

88. Yang D, Korogi Y, Sugahara T, Kitajima M, Shigematsu Y, Liang L, Ushio Y, Takahashi M. Cerebral gliomas: prospective comparison of multivoxel 2D chemical-shift imaging proton MR spectroscopy, echoplanar perfusion and diffusion-weighted MRI. Neuroradiology 2002; 44(8):656–666.

17

Noninvasive Determination of Tissue Oxygen Concentration by Overhauser Enhanced Magnetic Resonance Imaging

Sean J. English, Koen Reijnders, Kenichi Yamada, Nallathamby Devasahayam, John A. Cook, James B. Mitchell, Sankaran Subramanian, and Murali C. Krishna
Radiation Biology Branch, Center for Cancer Research, National Cancer Institute, Bethesda, Maryland, U.S.A.

A Note from the Editors

*H**ypoxia is an important attribute of tumors, one that influences tumor response to radiation and systemic therapy. In vivo non-invasive measurement of oxygenation, however, remains an elusive goal. Electron paramagnetic resonance (EPR) is a technique that induces resonance in the unpaired electrons of paramagnetic atoms rather than protons as occurs in magnetic resonance imaging (MRI). Since paramagnetics are in low abundance, they must be introduced as contrast agents. The characteristic line width of the signal arising from paramagnetic species is directly dependent on oxygen concentration and thus becomes a non-invasive method to determine tissue oxygenation. The Overhauser effect can be utilized to generate MRIs based on EPR effects. While several technical hurdles need to be overcome before EPR is useful clinically, it represents a highly promising technology for measuring oxygenation within tumors.*

INTRODUCTION

Thomlinson and Gray originally proposed the concept of tumor hypoxia in the 1950s (1). They based this notion on examinations of histological sections of human lung tumors, which revealed a constant distance in the range of 100 to 150 μm between blood vessels and the edge of necrotic zones (1). This hypothesis was verified in other human tumors by measuring pO_2 values by inserting polarographic electrodes in accessible sites such as head and neck tumors (2). These measurements revealed significant levels of hypoxia (10 mmHg), which was correlated with treatment failure in fractionated radiotherapy. It is estimated that approximately one half of solid human tumors have median oxygen levels <10 mmHg, prior to therapy (3,4). Subsequent studies, using oxygen electrodes inserted into various of human tumors, have demonstrated that significant levels of hypoxia are associated with compromised response to radiation treatment for breast cancer, head and neck cancer, sarcomas, cervix cancer, and for prostate cancer (5–9). The radiobiological basis for the failure of fractionated radiation treatment of hypoxic tumors is well documented and is attributed to its efficient chemical repair of radiation-induced lesions on DNA (10). More recent clinical studies have noted that patients with tumors with low pO_2 levels exhibited higher incidence of loco-regional failures (with or without distant metastases), irrespective of whether surgery or radiotherapy was performed (8). Not only did the presence of hypoxic cells in the tumor compromise therapy, but also their presence denoted a more aggressive disease.

Collectively, the studies cited suggest that the ability to measure and track changes in the oxygenation of a tumor is necessary to select the most appropriate and effective treatment(s). The use of oxygen electrodes is both invasive and inaccurate. This is particularly the case as pO_2 levels fall below 20 mmHg when the electrode consumes the oxygen in a region of the tissue during the process of measurement. Likewise, it is often not practical or even possible to obtain oxygen measurements for deep-seated tumors. Therefore, a noninvasive means of making pO_2 measurements with sensitivity ≤20 mmHg range would be desirable.

Magnetic resonance imaging (MRI) is a widely used imaging technique, that uses nuclear magnetic resonance (NMR), a spectroscopic technique that detects protons among other magnetic nuclei. Water protons ubiquitous in soft tissue are detected and imaged giving high-resolution images with anatomic detail that have become extremely useful in diagnosis. Additional contrast, specific to local regions, is achieved from these imaging techniques using appropriate exogenous contrast agents, to obtain tissue/organ or tumor-specific information. Techniques such as dynamic contrast enhanced (DCE) MRI or blood oxygen level dependent (BOLD) MRI, provide information pertaining to tissue perfusion, microvessel density, tumor oxygenation, and vessel leakiness. These techniques have been employed recently in monitoring treatment response of tumors.

Electron paramagnetic resonance (EPR) is a spectroscopic technique similar to NMR spectroscopy. While NMR detects nuclei such as $^1H, ^{13}C, ^{19}F, ^{31}P$, etc., which possess magnetic moments, EPR spectroscopy probes paramagnetic species that are atoms or molecules containing unpaired electrons. Examples of paramagnetic species are transition metal complexes (Fe^{3+}, Cu^{2+}, Mn^{2+}, etc.) and free radicals (organic and inorganic). NMR and EPR have both similarities and differences. While both are resonance absorption techniques requiring externally applied magnetic fields to create the energy levels, the magnitude of the magnetic field at a given radiofrequency (RF) of operation is quite different. At a given magnetic field, the frequency of RF for EPR is approximately 660 times greater than for proton NMR because of the fact that the electron magnetic moment is 660 times stronger than that of protons. Although both NMR and EPR were discovered almost simultaneously in the mid 1940s, NMR evolved into clinically useful MRI because of the abundance of tissue water protons that can be detected and imaged. EPR could not be implemented as a medical imaging technique becuaseof the lack of detectable levels of endogenous, paramagnetic species and the lack of exogenous probes compatible for in vivo use. The experiences that have accumulated from using MRI suggest that the paramagnetic species suitable for in vivo EPR imaging (EPRI) should have the following characteristics: (i) water-soluble, (ii) chemically stable, (iii) exhibit simple EPR spectra, preferably a single line, (iv) nontoxic at concentrations needed for in vivo imaging, and (v) have in vivo lifetime longer than imaging time. With the recent availability of paramagnetic species exhibiting these characteristics, in vivo EPRI is now feasible (11). Extensively derivatized symmetric trityl radicals exhibit single line EPR spectra and are useful for in vivo EPRI. One unique advantage of EPRI is that unlike protons NMR spectra that are not sensitive to the presence of dissolved oxygen, paramagnetic species such as trityl radicals exhibit an oxygen concentration–dependent linewidth. Imaging strategies that can use this property and extract pixel- or voxel-dependent EPR spectral linewidths will therefore provide spatially resolved pO_2 information or pO_2 "maps."

OVERHAUSER ENHANCED MRI: COMBINATION OF MRI AND EPRI

Overhauser enhanced MRI (OMRI) is a double resonance imaging technique, that uses paramagnetic spin probes to enhance the image intensity of a typical magnetic resonance (MR) image (12–14). The difference between images obtained using standard MRI scans and OMRI scans is that while the intensity of images in MRI scans primarily depend on tissue water, the image intensity of images from OMRI is governed by factors such as perfusion, oxygenation, vessel density, etc. When such information is coregistered with anatomic images, functional/physiologic images are obtained.

The resonator coils are tuned simultaneously to the NMR and EPR frequency. The operating magnetic fields are typically in the range of 6–15 mT; at least 500 times lower than that of standard clinical scanners. The loss in image resolution at such low magnetic fields employed in OMRI is overcome by utilizing trityl radicals. The properties of the contrast agent are suited to interact with relaxation processes of tissue protons and enhance their signals. The hardware of the OMRI scanner differs from conventional MRI scanners in that it includes an EPR transmit chain. The MRI scan sequence is initiated after irradiation of the object by a strong RF pulse (EPR) corresponding to the resonance frequency of the paramagnetic contrast agent present in the object (Fig. 1). The reason for including high-frequency irradiation prior to the MRI sequence is to elicit enhanced signal from protons, at very low magnetic fields, by the "Overhauser effect" also known as "dynamic nuclear polarization" (15). In this process, the poor signal from protons obtained using these low magnetic fields are enhanced in the presence of suitable paramagnetic contrast agents via the Overhauser effect. Andrew (16) first pointed out the use of OMRI for medical imaging and it was first implemented for in vivo imaging by Lurie et al. (12). The details of the scanner are described in an earlier report (14). Experimentally, the object under examination is placed in a specially designed coil assembly. The coil assembly comprises an EPR coil

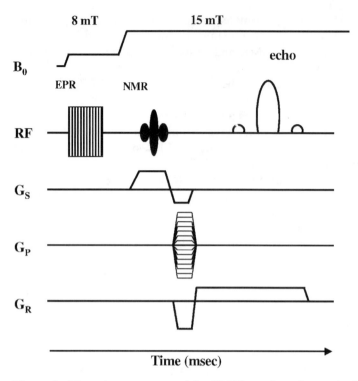

Figure 1 The pulse sequence used for OMRI consists of a standard spin warp gradient echo MRI sequence, with each phase-encoding step preceded by an EPR saturation pulse to elicit Overhauser enhancement. The pulse sequence begins with an 8 mT B_0 field for EPR irradiation. An EPR RF pulse (226 MHz) is applied for 300 msec; whereby B_0 field is then ramped to 13 mT before the NMR RF pulse and the associated field gradients are turned on. For pO_2 imaging, OMRI images are collected with interleaving pulse sequences in which the EPR irradiation is applied at two different power levels (45 W and 3 W), before each phase-encoding gradient step. A conventional MRI, without EPR pulsing, is independently collected for calculating enhancement factors.

that at a magnetic field of 8 mT is tuned to a frequency in the range of 200–300 MHz. Within the EPR coil, a standard MRI coil is incorporated to accommodate the object and tuned to the proton resonance frequency. The proton resonance frequency is approximately 650 times lower than that of the EPR frequency and is in the range of 300–500 kHz. For imaging experiments, the paramagnetic trityl radical is introduced in a system containing protons and irradiated by an RF radiation corresponding to its resonance frequency and the proton MRI signals are detected. Figure 1 shows the timing sequence of the OMRI experiment. After the EPR irradiation, the MR signals are recovered using standard gradient echo sequences.

The enhancement of the intensity is given by:

$$E = -(\gamma_e/\gamma_p)fkS$$

where E is the enhancement, γ_e and γ_p are the electron and proton magnetic moments, respectively. Factor "f" is called the leakage factor, "k" is the coupling factor, and "S" is the saturation factor. The contributions of the leakage factor "f," the coupling factor "k," and the saturation factor "S" to the enhancement E and the underlying reasons are discussed in detail in Ref. 14 and can be simplified in terms of:

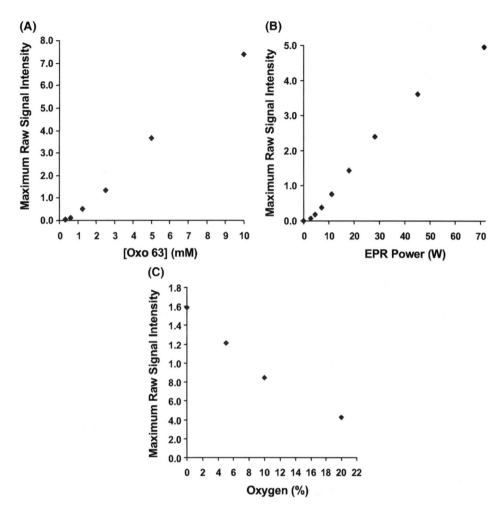

Figure 2 The maximum proton signal intensity for a one-dimensional projection of an Oxo63 phantom is plotted as a function of the EPR irradiation power (**A**), the concentration of Oxo63 constituting the phantom (**B**), and the concentration of dissolved oxygen in the phantom (**C**). A 5 mM, in 5 mL Oxo63 phantom was used for plots A and C, while the EPR irradiation power was held constant at 45 W for plots B and C.

(a) concentration of the paramagnetic contrast agent, (b) inverse of oxygen concentration, and (c) strength of the RF power at the EPR frequency. The maximum enhancement achievable is 329. However, practically achievable enhancement value ranges between 5 and 100 depending on the tissue concentration of the contrast agent, tissue oxygenation, and strength of the EPR irradiation. While the concentration of the contrast agent and oxygen are tissue/organ-specific and are to be determined, the strength of the RF irradiation is under the experimenter's control and can be varied.

To demonstrate the enhancement of proton MR image intensities, experiments were carried out on phantom objects of aqueous solutions containing the trityl radical Oxo63 at a concentration of 5 mM and the results obtained are summarized in Figure 2. The enhancement of the image intensity as a function of the concentration of the paramagnetic probe is shown in Figure 2A. This experiment was done in air-saturated solutions of Oxo63 at different concentrations from 0 to 10 mM irradiated at a constant power at the EPR frequency. The signal enhancement shows a linear increase as a function of Oxo63 concentration and is consistent with the enhancement equation where a linear increase is predicted based on the linear dependence with the leakage factor f. When the experiment is performed at a fixed concentration of Oxo63 in air-saturated solutions at different EPR powers, again a linear response was observed, consistent with the involvement of the saturation factor S in the enhancement equation (Fig. 2B). However, when the experiment was performed at fixed RF power and Oxo63 concentration, but at different oxygen levels, an inverse dependence was observed (Fig. 2C). This behavior can be explained in terms of inefficient saturation of the EPR transition in the presence of increasing oxygen at a given EPR power and Oxo63 concentration. In defined phantoms, where oxygen levels and Oxo63 concentrations are known, it is straightforward to understand the signal enhancement. However, for in vivo experiments, the concentration of the paramagnetic agent and oxygen level are to be determined. EPR power is the only variable in the hands of the experimenter that can be varied to obtain images with characteristic enhancement profiles. When a set of two images are collected at two different powers of EPR, it is possible to estimate the concentration of the spin probe and the concentration of oxygen by solving for the enhancement equations, knowing certain scanner conditions and the relaxation properties of the paramagnetic probe. The details of these calculations have been discussed earlier (13,14).

The capabilities of OMRI to obtain anatomically coregistered pO_2 images were tested in tumor-bearing mice. Figure 3 shows the MR images from an anesthetized mouse placed in the coil. The abdominal region and lower extremities were in the active volume of the coil, infused with a bolus of Oxo63 (2.5 mmol/kg) delivered through a tail vein cannula. The image shown in Figure 3A was collected without EPR irradiation, whereas the image shown in Figure 3B was collected with EPR irradiation. The poor resolution of the image shown in Figure 3A is consistent with the low field of operation (15 mT) for MRI signal recovery. However, the image shown in Figure 3B, while collected at the same magnetic field, shows improved reso-

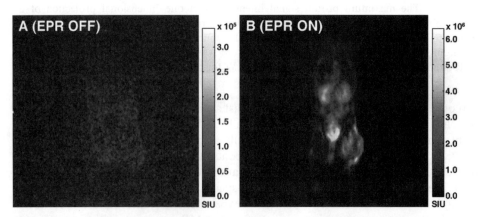

Figure 3 (**A**) A conventional MR image of a mouse collected at 13 mT, without an EPR saturation pulse, demonstrates the lack of anatomical resolution associated with MRI at such a low B_0 field. (**B**) An OMR image of a mouse that received a loading dose (1.5 mmol/kg) of Oxo63, followed by continuous infusion (0.15 mmol/kg/min) of Oxo63, collected with an EPR saturation pulse (45 W), demonstrates the increased anatomical resolution resulting from the Overhauser energy transfer.

lution. The improvement in image quality can be attributed to the presence of Oxo63 as well as irradiation at its resonance prior to MR image sequence.

MAPPING pO_2 WITH OMRI

As discussed earlier, the image enhancement is related to the concentration of the contrast agent, degree of hypoxia, and the strength of the EPR irradiation. While the contrast agent concentration distribution in vivo after bolus administration and oxygenation are the factors to be determined, the strength of the EPR irradiation is a variable that can be set by the experimenter. Spatially resolved pO_2 distribution and contrast agent concentration can be determined using the procedure described subsequently. By collecting two sets of images at two different RF powers, two images are obtained. From the enhancement profile in each pixel at these two powers of irradiation, tissue oxygen and concentration of the contrast agent can be determined. Figures 4A and 4B show OMRI images collected from a mouse after intravenous administration of Oxo63 when the strength of the EPR irradiation was 3 W and 45 W, respectively. As expected, the image intensity was higher with higher EPR power. Using the methods described earlier, images shown in Figures 4A and 4B are parametric images representing the contrast agent concentration. From these images, the pO_2 distribution can be calculated. Experiments were carried out to monitor the changes in concentration and pO_2 in response to changes in oxygen content in the breathing gas. The tumor-bearing mouse was anesthetized and infused with Oxo63 and low-power and high-power images were collected, when the animal was first breathing air and then followed by carbogen (95% oxygen, 5% CO_2). Parametric images of concentration of the contrast agent and pO_2 were obtained using the procedures described earlier (13,14). Figure 5 shows the changes in the contrast agent concentration (A and C) and pO_2 (B and D) when the tumor-bearing mouse was breathing air (A and B) and carbogen (C and D), respectively. As can be seen, the concentration of the contrast agent was high in the kidneys and the tumor but not significant in muscle and liver. The differences in concentration of the contrast agent, when the mouse was breathing air (Fig. 5A) and when the mouse was breathing carbogen

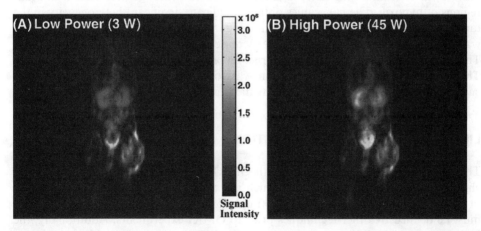

Figure 4 OMRI images of a mouse that received a loading dose (1.5 mmol/kg) of Oxo63, followed by continuous infusion (0.15 mmol/kg/min) of Oxo63 were collected with EPR saturation pulses at **(A)** 3 W and **(B)** 45 W.

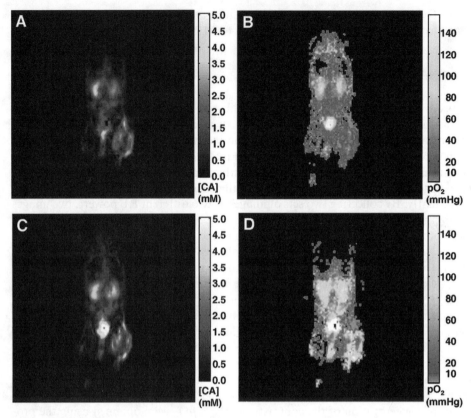

Figure 5 Parametric maps of the pixelwise concentration of Oxo63 (CA) when breathing air (**A**) or carbogen (**C**) and concentration of oxygen when breathing air (**B**) or carbogen (**D**). These images were computed from two successive images obtained from the same animal while breathing air (**A, B**) or carbogen (**C, D**). (*See color insert.*)

(Fig. 5C), were not significant except for increasing accumulation in the bladder. The tumor, while accumulating fairly high levels of the contrast agent, showed significant regions of hypoxia. The pO_2 values obtained indicate significant heterogeneity in the tumor while the mouse was breathing air (Fig. 5B). However, when the inspired gas was changed to carbogen, a significant increase in tumor pO_2 was noted (Fig. 5D). This observation is in agreement with earlier reports using similar experimental models. The spatially resolved pO_2 information was found to be in good agreement with currently used standard methods such as the Clark electrode pO_2 histogram (14).

LIMITATIONS AND FUTURE DIRECTIONS

There are certain issues associated with OMRI, which need to be resolved before clinical use. Unlike standard MRI, which is a multislice imaging modality, the use of OMRI for multislice imaging is not straightforward. Therefore, the slice of interest must be defined by other techniques prior to OMRI experiments. Additionally, the high-frequency irradiation associated with the EPR frequency to achieve the image enhancement may in some cases exceed the specific absorption rate (SAR) limits and cause undesired heating as a result of the nonresonant absorption of the incident

RF. These are some of the factors, which impose certain limitations on this technique when it is scaled up for human use. The future of this modality depends on developments in technology associated with magnetic field ramping, coil design, and contrast agent properties. With respect to magnetic field ramping, the current system operates at 8 mT for the EPR saturation to keep the SAR low, and the field is ramped to 15 mT to increase the sensitivity of detection. However, if the magnetic field can be ramped from 8 mT to even higher fields such as 0.5 T, the sensitivity improvement, which is linear with magnetic field, will be significant. The coils currently used are in a configuration where the EPR irradiation is performed using linearly polarized RF. As a result, 50% of the incident RF is not used in realizing the desired enhancement while still causing the undesired heating. If circularly polarized RF irradiation is employed using quadrature coils, the RF is better utilized while keeping the heating lower. Additional improvements in signal to noise ratio can be realized using cooled NMR coils. Contrast agents with narrower EPR spectra, when they become available, can provide improved enhancement at low RF powers and therefore improve the image quality. Improvements in the above mentioned three aspects are necessary for the further development and human use of OMRI.

A distinct advantage in using the OMRI scanner is the possibility of detecting and imaging the paramagnetic probes directly by EPR. From EPR images, it is then possible to extract spatially resolved spectroscopic information of the probe such as the oxygen-dependent EPR linewidth (17). Although image resolution in EPRI may be poor because of the larger linewidths of paramagnetic probes, recent implementation of phase-encoded imaging strategies have made it possible to recover image resolution significantly (18). Efficient data acquisition strategies have made it possible to collect three-dimensional image data in less than three minutes with spatial resolution less than 1 mm. Coregistering the functional information (oxygen-dependent linewidth) with anatomic images obtained from OMRI will give pO_2 maps. One distinct advantage of using EPRI is that it is possible to collect three-dimensional images using the same scanner at voxel sizes of $\sim$ mm from which pO_2 information can be obtained using T_2^* weighted image processing (19). As the RF power required for EPRI is well below the SAR limits, undesired tissue heating can also be minimized.

SUMMARY

It is possible to obtain spatially resolved pO_2 information from living objects using paramagnetic spin probes as reporter molecules and imaging modalities such as OMRI or EPRI. The physical interaction between molecular oxygen and the paramagnetic probe provides the capability to obtain useful functional information of tissue pO_2 levels.

REFERENCES

1. Thomlinson RH, Gray LH. The histological structure of some human lung cancers and the possible implications for radiotherapy. Br J Cancer 1955; 9:539–549.
2. Gatenby RA, Kessler HB, Rosenblum JS, et al. Oxygen distribution in squamous cell carcinoma metastases and its relationship to outcome of radiation therapy. Int J Radiat Oncol Biol Phys 1988; 14:831–838.

3. Hockel M, Vaupel P. Tumor hypoxia: definitions and current clinical, biologic, and molecular aspects. J Natl Cancer Inst 2001; 93:266–276.

4. Brown JM. Tumor microenvironment and the response to anticancer therapy. Cancer Biol Ther 2002; 1:453–458.

5. Vaupel P, Schlenger K, Knoop C, Hockel M. Oxygenation of human tumors: evaluation of tissue oxygen distribution in breast cancers by computerized O_2 tension measurements. Cancer Res 1991; 51:3316–3322.

6. Brizel DM, Dodge RK, Clough RW, Dewhirst MW. Oxygenation of head and neck cancer: changes during radiotherapy and impact on treatment outcome. Radiother Oncol 1999; 53:113–117.

7. Brizel DM, Scully SP, Harrelson JM, et al. Tumor oxygenation predicts for the likelihood of distant metastases in human soft tissue sarcoma. Cancer Res 1996; 56:941–943.

8. Hockel M, Schlenger K, Aral B, Mitze M, Schaffer U, Vaupel P. Association between tumor hypoxia and malignant progression in advanced cancer of the uterine cervix. Cancer Res 1996; 56:4509–4515.

9. Movsas B, Chapman JD, Hanlon AL, et al. Hypoxic prostate/muscle pO_2 ratio predicts for biochemical failure in patients with prostate cancer: preliminary findings. Urology 2002; 60:634–639.

10. von Sonntag C. The Chemical Basis of Radiation Biology. London: Taylor & Francis, 1987.

11. Golman K, Leunbach I, Ardenkjaer-Larsen JH, et al. Overhauser-enhanced MR imaging (OMRI). Acta Radiol 1998; 39:10–17.

12. Lurie DJ, Bussell DM, Bell LH, Mallard JR. Proton–electron double magnetic resonance imaging of free radical solutions. J Magn Reson 1988; 76:366–370.

13. Golman K, Petersson JS, Ardenkjaer-Larsen JH, et al. Dynamic in vivo oxymetry using overhauser enhanced MR imaging. J Magn Reson Imaging 2000; 12:929–938.

14. Krishna MC, English S, Yamada K, et al. Overhauser enhanced magnetic resonance imaging for tumor oximetry: coregistration of tumor anatomy and tissue oxygen concentration. Proc Natl Acad Sci 2002; 99:2216–2221.

15. Overhauser AW. Polarization of nuclei in metals. Phys Rev 1953; 92:411–415.

16. Andrew ER. NMR imaging of intact biological systems. Philos Trans R Soc Lond B Biol Sci 1980; 289:471–481.

17. Afeworki M, Van Dam GM, Devasahayam N, et al. Three-dimensional whole body imaging of spin probes in mice by time-domain radiofrequency electron paramagnetic resonance. Magn Reson Med 2000; 43:375–382.

18. Subramanian S, Devasahayam N, Murugesan R, et al. Single-point (constant-time) imaging in radiofrequency Fourier transform electron paramagnetic resonance. Magn Reson Med 2002; 48:370–379.

19. Subramanian S, Yamada K, Irie A, et al. Noninvasive in vivo oximetric imaging by radiofrequency FT EPR. Magn Reson Med 2002; 47:1001–1008.

18
Advances in Optical Imaging of Cancer

Alexander M. Gorbach
Department of Diagnostic Radiology, National Institutes of Health, Bethesda, Maryland, U.S.A.

Vasilis Ntziachristos
Massachusetts General Hospital, Harvard Medical School, Boston, Massachusetts, U.S.A.

Lev T. Perelman
Beth Israel Deaconess Medical Center, Harvard Medical School, Boston, Massachusetts, U.S.A.

A Note from the Editors

*O*ptical methods represent an exciting new branch of imaging technology for cancer. Optical imaging is divided into intrinsic and extrinsic contrast mechanisms. Intrinsic optical imaging includes infrared (thermal), near infrared (oxygen saturation of hemoglobin), and light scattering. The latter can be used to detect early dysplastic and neoplastic tissue during endoscopy. Intrinsic optical imaging does not require the injection of a contrast agent but relies on the optical properties of tumors to differentiate them from normal tissue. Extrinsic optical imaging is provided by specially designed optical contrast agents. A class of these agents, termed "activatible," are engineered fluorochromes that are non fluorescing in their native state but fluoresce only in the presence of a specific molecular target. These agents, often designed for the near-infrared spectrum, may provide highly specific information about the characteristics of human tumors in the future.

In the recent decades, substantial progress has been made in medical diagnostic technologies that target functional and anatomic changes related to cancer. Techniques such as magnetic resonance imaging (MRI) and spectroscopy, X-ray computed tomography, and ultrasound (US) made it possible to "see through the human body." At the same time, there is clearly a need for the development of clinical techniques that would combine better sensitivity and specificity to cancer with cost-effectiveness and simplicity of operation.

In comparison with the mature technologies for cancer imaging, optical imaging promises to be highly accurate for cancer identification, relatively inexpensive, and readily implemented. Studies in physiology and pathology of tumors have revealed multiple cancer "signatures," which can be utilized for optical imaging as internal (natural) and external (artificial) optical contrasts.

This chapter describes how intrinsic optical properties of malignant tumors can be used in clinical imaging. Additionally, in an attempt to improve the sensitivity and specificity of optical imaging, multiple-extrinsic optical contrasts agents will be described. Although, compared with internal contrast agents, clinical use of external contrast agents is currently limited, they are already very useful in basic cancer research and represent the "next generation" in optical technology.

OPTICAL IMAGING BASED ON INTERNAL CONTRASTS TO IDENTIFY CANCER

Intraoperative Infrared Imaging During Tumor Resection in the Human Brain

Temperature as a source of internal contrast has been thought of as useful for human diagnostics for more than 2000 years (1). The temperature of the surface of the skin overlying a tumor has been measured and visualized by a medical imaging technique known as thermography. An understanding of the energy of infrared (IR) photons in the 3 to 5 μm wavelength range, emitted from deeper body structures is dramatically attenuated by surface tissues, made it highly unlikely that an IR camera capable of imaging deep within the human body could be developed (2). However, clinical applications have been found for tissues that are more superficial especially during surgical exposure of structures otherwise unavailable to imaging. To show that brain tumors have distinctive temperature signatures we used IR imaging of the cortical surface intraoperatively. The focal plane array detector of the camera used in this study was sensitive to IR photons emitted from the exposed brain surface because of natural IR radiation (3,4). With the brain exposed during surgery, arterial blood, which is at core-body temperature, is warmer than the surface of the exposed brain, which has been cooled by evaporation and by the room air (5). The evaporation would increase the rate of heat dissipation, enhancing discrimination of local thermal gradients and thus enhancing the capacity to localize superficial capillary blood flow (6,7). Therefore, local microvascular cerebral blood flow (CBF) can be used as an internal, natural thermal contrast agent for IR monitoring and precise imaging of tumor blood flow in time and space can be performed during cranial surgery (8).

Surface cortical IR images were obtained in 34 patients undergoing surgery for brain lesions. This study included 21 patients with intrinsic brain tumors (eight high and low grade *oligodendroglioma*, two *mixed anaplastic oligodendroglioma/ astrocytoma,* one *astrocytoma,* and 10 *glioblastoma*), 10 patients with brain metastases (five *melanoma*, three *adenocarcinoma*, two *carcinoma*), and one each with a falx *meningioma*, a *cavernous angioma*, and *radiation necrosis/astrocytosis*. Local anesthesia with intravenous sedation (fentanyl, midazolam, and propofol) was chosen for 18 patients. The other sixteen patients received surgery under general anesthesia.

An advanced digital IR camera (Infrared Focal Plane Array camera, Lockheed Martin IR Imaging Systems, Inc., Goleta, California, U.S.) was used to image local thermal gradients across the cerebral cortex by passively detecting IR emission. As IR emission at the measured wavelength (3–5 μm) is directly proportional to temperature, the camera was calibrated in units of temperature. It has a sensitivity of 0.02°C. One hundred images (256×256 pixels) were obtained at intervals of 0.01 to 120 seconds and digitized at 14 bits per pixel. The camera was placed 10 to 30 cm above the exposed brain surface to achieve a field-of-view that fits the exposed area of the cortex (35×35 mm to 100×100 mm), which produced a spatial resolution for individual pixels of 100×100 μm to 350×350 μm.

Sequential digital images were taken with the plane of the IR camera's lens positioned parallel to the plane of the exposed brain. Imaging was performed on all 34 patients by passive acquisition of spontaneous IR emission for one minute. In four cases, IR images were acquired during tumor resection, which allowed real time visualization of temperature changes during surgical manipulations. When cortical incision was indicated, as for temporal lobectomy, a small (approximately 0.5 mm diameter) surface artery was temporarily occluded at the cortical incision site for one minute with a temporary aneurysm clip. IR imaging was started 30 seconds before the occlusion, continued during the occlusion period, and terminated 60 seconds after the occlusion was relieved by removal of the clip.

To analyze the data *on-line*, a representative image was selected and was color-coded to visualize cortical thermal gradients during surgery. To analyze the data *off-line*, the temperature difference between the tumor and the surroundings was quantified for each patient by extracting a temperature profile from a representative IR image. The line of the region of interest (ROI), a one-pixel-wide line across an IR image, was placed on both pre- and postresection IR images so as to retrace the same areas of normal cortex, cortex adjacent to the tumor, and central mass of the tumor area or a projection of it on the cortical surface.

For each case, IR images before and after tumor resection, digital photographs of the cortical surface before and after tumor resection, and a three-dimensional (3D) MRI representation of the exposed cortical area were placed in separate layers, scaled, rotated, coregistered, and superimposed using anatomical landmarks (Adobe PhotoShop 5.01). The area with tumor-induced thermal gradients on the IR image was colocalized with the area identified as tumor by preoperative MRI imaging (T1-weighted 3D MRI; SPGR sequences), intraoperative US images, and the pathology report.

IR images revealed temperature heterogeneity between 27°C and 34°C on the exposed cortical surface in all cases. The images consisted of multiple thermal compartments (warm and cool patches) with irregular form and distinctive vascular patterns. In general, the arteries appeared bright (highest temperature), the cortical surfaces appeared dark (low temperature), and the veins appeared light (intermediate temperature). The difference between arteries and veins was 1.5°C to 2.0°C, and between veins and brain parenchyma was 0.2°C to 1.0°C.

Temporary occlusion of a small cortical artery (four patients) reduced the IR signal within the vessel immediately (Fig. 1C, J, and I) and transiently reduced the temperature from the cortical regions perfused by it (Fig. 1D and G). Temperature

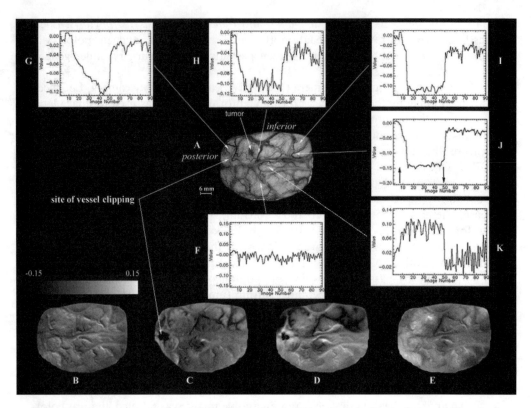

Figure 1 Cortical temperature during occlusion and reperfusion of a single vessel. Vessel of 0.9 mm diameter at the area of a cortical tumor was chosen for temporary (14.7 seconds) occlusion (visible light image, **A**). Two small arrows on **J** mark the start and the end of occlusion. Four IR images (results of subtracting the baseline image from each collected IR image) were chosen from a series of 90 images (350 msec/image) to represent the changes in differential temperature from 0.35 seconds before clipping (**B**), 1.4 seconds after clipping (**C**), 0.35 seconds before reperfusion (**D**), to 12.9 seconds after reperfusion (**E**). Notice that temperature profiles (temperature changes in relative value vs. image number) from ROI (4 × 4 pixels) close to clipping site (**G**, **H**) and at distances of 40 mm (**K**) and 70 mm (**I**, **J**) show remarkable differences from the temperature in an unrelated cortical site (**F**). Notice an inverse temperature change between **K** and **J**. Notice a different rate of temperature change between **G** and **J** during occlusion, but not reperfusion. Notice a difference between temperature before occlusion and after reperfusion on **H** and **I**, also reflected on the **B** and **E** images.

elevation was observed in some areas remote from the occluded vessel (Fig. 1D and K). After the occlusion was relieved, the IR signal rapidly returned to normal in some areas (Fig. 1J and G). However, in other areas it took more than 35 seconds for the tissue to regain the preocclusion temperature level (Fig. 1E, H, and I). These experiments revealed high specificity of IR signal to the flow of preheated blood (8).

Certain vascular patterns on the IR image appeared different from visible light photographs. Some vessels (mostly at the tumor site) showed no temperature gradients with the surrounding brain and, therefore, were not visible on the IR image. This happens if the vessels have no blood flow, have a leak of blood, or are collapsed.

Noticeable thermal gradients were observed in all cases in the region where MRI and intraoperative US localized the surgically verified tumors (Fig. 2A, D).

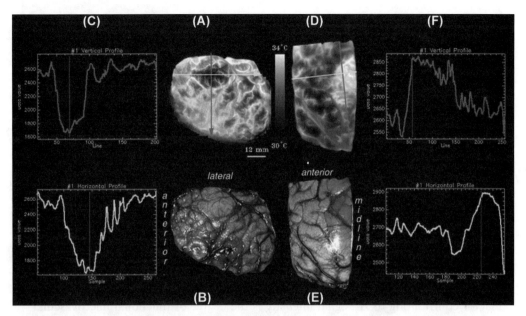

Figure 2 IR image of the cortex with *oligodendroglioma* (**A**) reveals a steep local decrease in temperature (hypothermia) at the site of the tumor (dark area with central mass of the tumor at the intersection of yellow and blue arrows). IR image of the cortex with *astrocytoma* (**D**) shows a local increase in temperature (hyperthermia) at the site of the tumor (bright area with central mass of the tumor at the intersection of yellow and blue arrows). Vertical (*blue*) and horizontal (*yellow*) temperature profiles (**C** and **F**) show pixel's values along blue and yellow arrows on **A** and **D**. Visible light images of the cortex with *oligodendroma* (**B**) and *astrosytoma* (**E**) show orientation. (*See color insert.*)

In general, a 0.5°C to 2.0°C temperature difference between the cortex overlying the tumors and surrounding areas was visualized on IR images (Fig. 2C, F). As observed on histological sections and cortical digital photographs, vessel-rich regions corresponded to the warmest areas within the tumor region. Areas that are surrounded by bulk tumor and comprised of the mixed necrotic regions with a reduced number of blood vessels correspond to the coolest areas on IR images. Although the region of tumor involvement could be distinguished from the adjacent brain, temperature heterogeneity occurred within individual parts of the lesion. Regions of signal intensity change were evident over central areas of focal necrosis and also over viable tumor surrounding these areas.

In 18 cases, the cortex over the tumor colocalized with the coolest area on IR images and was hypothermic relative to the surrounding, normal, regions of the brain. In 14 cases, the cortex overlying the tumor was warmer than surrounding tissue and, therefore, was relatively hyperthermic. Both hypothermic and hyperthermic areas adjacent to the same lesion were visible in the other two cases.

All oligodendroglial tumors ($n = 10$) and mixed radiation necrosis/astrocytosis ($n = 1$) were hypothermic (Fig. 2A). Among non-neoplastic lesions ($n = 10$) eight of them were hyperthermic relative to their surroundings. Among astrocytic tumors ($n = 11$), eight glioblastomas were hypothermic, one mixed glioblastoma and two astrocytomas were slightly hyperthermic (Fig. 2D). Slight hyperthermia was observed also for single cases with falx meningioma and cavernous angioma. For metastatic tumors, the group average tumor-induced temperature gradient was 49% larger than that of oligodendroma group ($P = 0.001$), and 40% larger than that of glioblastoma group ($P = 0.014$).

Dramatic spatial reorganization of thermal gradients was observed after tumor resection ($n = 28$). Remote from the area of resection, multiple cortical sites and vessels previously nonvisible on preresection IR image (Fig. 3A) were seen on postresection IR images (Fig. 3B). Increased temperature after tumor resection indicated higher functional capillary density at the end of the operation, which is probably because of the reduction of intratumor pressure. Marginal tissue close to areas of resection (Fig. 3B) was cooler in comparison to the intact cortex in all patients. Reduction in the IR signal in these areas could potentially be used as a signal of reduced blood flow to the brain adjacent to the tumor. This may be of importance in maintaining the viability of the brain tissue when removing tumors in proximity to functionally eloquent cortex.

Thus, specific brain lesions showed distinctive temperature signatures that were manifestations of their blood flow, and a surrogate for their metabolic functional state. The correlation between IR images of the tumors and vascular density and distribution patterns confirmed by histology support the conclusion that the major factor contributing to IR signal intensity is the degree of functional microvascularization within tumor and normal brain.

The vascularity of a tumor presumably reflects a tumor's ability to induce the formation of new blood vessels (angiogenesis). As vessel density correlates with temperature, temperature gradients over the tumor might correlate to clinically significant tumor properties, such as tumor growth rate and the occurrence of metastasis. A thermal gradient associated with high perfusion of individual microvessels within the tumor may indirectly mark new, fast-growing vessels. Therefore,

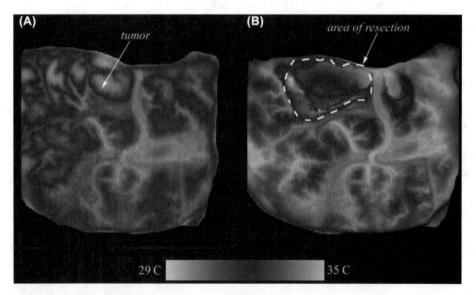

Figure 3 Reorganization of cortical thermal gradients after tumor resection. Cortical IR images obtained before tumor resection (**A**) and after tumor resection (**B**) are presented. Notice remotely from the area of resection that multiple cortical sites and vessels previously invisible in the pre-resection IR image (**A**) are visible in the post-resection IR image (**B**). (*See color insert.*)

the related temperature value can be an important prognostic indicator of metastasis and postoperative survival in several human cancers.

Intraoperative Near-IR Imaging During Tumor Resection

Another intrinsic optical signature of tumors—absorption changes because of the hemoglobin oxygen saturation—was explored as an intrinsic contrast for optical intraoperative imaging in the near-infrared (near-IR) wavelength. The ability of tumors to survive under hypoxic conditions is one of their hallmarks and helps differentiate them from normal tissues. Moreover, the degree of tumor oxygenation is now recognized as a strong prognostic indicator, as hypoxia dictates responsiveness to chemotherapy and radiation therapy.

To prove tumor sites can be recognized intraoperatively based on degree of oxygenation, a near-IR imaging spectroscopy attachment (OKSI, California, U.S.A.) to a surgical microscope (Carl Zeiss, Inc., U.S.A., Model OPMI CS-NC) was designed to visualize the human cerebral cortex in reflective mode. An advanced thermoelectrically cooled near-IR CCD camera (Pixel Vision, U.S.A.) (512×512 pixels, three frames/sec, 16 bit accuracy, dark current less than 1 electron/sec/pixel) was attached to a liquid crystal tunable filter (CR Inc., U.S.A.). The standard halogen lamp of the microscope was used. Custom optics were designed for these experiments. Three imaging sessions (24 images each) of different wavelengths (between 460 and 720 nm wavelength) and with different exposure time of the camera's shutter (50, 120, and 240 msec) were collected with spectral resolution of 10 nm and stored for off-line analysis. All images were coregistered, and after computing a continuum removed spectral cube, unsupervised classification (ENVI 3.0, Research Systems Inc., Boulder, Colorado, U.S.A.) was used to extract images for 640, 550, and 570 nm. A false color image is presented on Fig. 3C after calculation of spectral ratio 640 to 570 nm and application of mixture matched filters.

Distinctly different degrees of oxygenation and deoxygenation in normal and tumor cortical sites were shown in the near-IR image. Oxygen saturation was highest mainly within arteries of the normal cortex. Deoxygenation was highest predominantly in cerebral veins. Local hypoxia was observed at the tumor site and, was even more pronounced, at the posterior margin of the tumor. The decrease in hemoglobin oxygen saturation in the tumor might be related to the decrease in cerebral oxygen delivery or increased consumption of oxygen within the tumor. One can speculate that hypoxia demonstrated by the near-IR image is caused by the low blood flow depicted on the thermal IR image of the same tumor (Fig. 4B). That is not the case for the posterior cortical margin of the tumor, where maximal deoxygenation found on a near-IR image (Fig. 4C) colocalized with moderate blood flow found on a thermal IR image (Fig. 4B). Here, one might speculate that increased consumption of oxygen is responsible for the hypoxia rather than poor blood flow.

Thus, changes in tissue oxygenation represent a balance among oxygen delivery, consumption, and clearance and can be monitored intraoperatively with multispectral optical imaging. Because of its safety, speed, and low cost, IR and near-IR imaging can be performed continuously and may be particularly useful in measuring responses to new antiangiogenesis agents. The ability to visualize hypoxia intraoperatively may be important for estimating the degree of tumor differentiation, vascularity, and growth rate and, therefore, has the potential to influence treatment strategies.

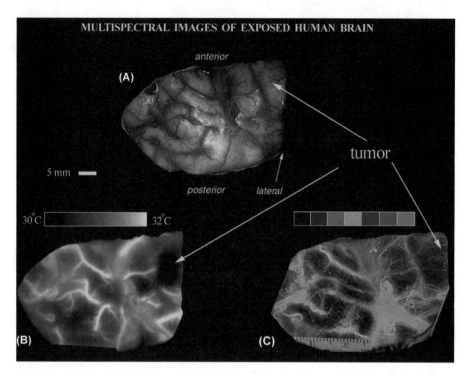

Figure 4 Multispectral imaging of human brain with tumor. Snapshot images were obtained intraoperatively during brain tumor surgery (patient with right frontal macroadenoma, 5 mm deep from the cortical surface). (**A**) High-resolution digital image of the exposed cortex. The arterial and venous vessels can be identified based on their color. There is no evidence of tumor on the surface. (**B**) Infrared image of exposed cortex. The coolest area on the image is at the tumor area. Largest IR signal coming from perfused arteries. (**C**) False color processed near-IR image of exposed cortex. Multiple vessels including those not seen on **B** show increased oxygen content (*arteries*) and decreased oxygen content (*venous*). The lowest signal in parenchyma is not colocalized with the tumor identified on **B**. (*See color insert.*)

In Situ Optical Imaging of Cancer

The optical properties of cancer cells, such as nuclear enlargement, pleomorphism, and increased chromatin content, can be utilized for imaging as another type of internal natural optical contrast. These inherent properties of cancer cells can be used to optically identify precancerous and early cancerous changes in various tissues. The technique, called light scattering spectroscopy (LSS), is capable of characterizing structural properties of tissue on the cellular and subcellular scale (9). LSS-based methods to measure epithelial morphology in living tissues do not require tissue removal. Such techniques can be used for noninvasive or minimally invasive detection of precancerous and early cancerous changes and other diseases in a variety of organs such as esophagus, colon, uterine cervix, oral cavity, lungs, and urinary bladder (10).

In dysplastic epithelium, the cells proliferate and their nuclei enlarge and appear darker (hyperchromatic) when stained (11). LSS can detect these changes as bulk optical characteristics of tissue. The details of the method have been published earlier (9) and will only be briefly summarized here. Consider a beam of light incident on an epithelial layer of tissue. A portion of this light is backscattered from the epithelial nuclei, while the remainder is transmitted to deeper tissue layers, where it undergoes multiple scattering and becomes randomized before returning to the surface.

Epithelial nuclei can be treated as spheroidal Mie scatterers with refractive index, n_n, which is higher than that of the surrounding cytoplasm, n_c (12). Normal nuclei have a characteristic size of $l = 4$ to $7 \, \mu m$. In contrast, the size of dysplastic nuclei varies widely and can be as large as $20 \, \mu m$, occupying almost the entire cell volume. In the visible range, where the wavelength $\lambda \ll l$, the Van de Hulst approximation (12) can be used to describe the elastic scattering cross-section of the nuclei

$$\sigma_s(\lambda, l) = \frac{1}{2} \pi l^2 \left\{ 1 - \frac{\sin(2\delta/\lambda)}{\delta/\lambda} + \left[\frac{\sin(\delta/\lambda)}{\delta/\lambda} \right]^2 \right\}, \tag{1}$$

with $\delta = \pi \, l \, (n_n - n_c)$. Equation (1) reveals a component of the scattering cross-section, which varies periodically with inverse wavelength (13). This, in turn, gives rise to a periodic component in the tissue reflectance. As the frequency of this variation (in inverse wavelength space) is proportional to particle size, the nuclear size distribution can be obtained from the Fourier transform of the periodic component.

To test this, the spectra of elastic light scattering from densely packed unstained monolayers of isolated normal intestinal epithelial cells (14) and intestinal epithelial T84 malignant cell line (15), affixed to glass slides in buffer solution and placed on top of a $BaSO_4$ diffusing plate, used to simulate the diffuse reflectance from underlying tissue. The diameters of the normal cell nuclei ranged from 5 to $7 \, \mu m$, whereas those of the tumor cells from 7 to $16 \, \mu m$. The spectra were then inverted to yield nuclear size distributions (solid curves, Fig. 5). A nucleus-to-cytoplasm relative refractive index of $n = 1.06$ and cytoplasm refractive index of $n_c = 1.36$ were used. The dashed curves in Figure 5 show the corresponding size distributions measured morphometrically using light microscopy. The extracted and measured distributions for both normal and T84 cell samples are in good agreement, indicating the validity of the above physical model and the accuracy of our method of extracting information (9).

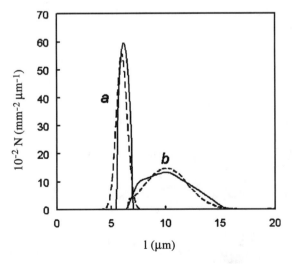

Figure 5 Nuclear size distributions from spectral data. (**A**) Normal intestinal cells; (**B**) T84 cells. In each case, the solid line is the distribution extracted from the data, and the dashed line is the distribution measured using light microscopy.

It has been observed that similar periodic fine structure in diffuse reflectance from Barrett's esophagus (BE) of human subjects undergoing gastroenterological endoscopy procedures. A schematic diagram of the proof-of-principle system used to perform LSS is shown in Figure 6. Immediately before biopsy, the reflectance spectrum from that site was collected using an optical fiber probe. The probe was inserted into the accessory channel of the endoscope and brought into gentle contact with the mucosal surface of the esophagus. It delivered a weak pulse of white light to the tissue and collected the diffusely reflected light. The probe tip sampled tissue over a circular spot approximately $1\,mm^2$ in area. The pulse duration was 50 msec, and the wavelength range was 350 to 650 nm. The optical probe caused a slight indentation at the tissue surface that remained for 30 to 60 seconds. Using this indentation as a target, the site was then carefully biopsied, and the sample was submitted for histological examination. This insured that the site studied spectroscopically matched the site evaluated histologically.

The reflected light was spectrally analyzed, and the spectra were stored in a computer. The spectra consist of a large background from submucosal tissue, on which is superimposed a small (2% to 3%) component that is oscillatory in wavelength because of scattering by cell nuclei in the mucosal layer. The amplitude of this component is related to the surface density of epithelial nuclei (number of nuclei per unit area). Because the area of tissue probed is fixed at $1\,mm^2$, this parameter is a measure of nuclear crowding. The shape of the spectrum over the wavelength range is related to nuclear size.

An example of nuclear size distribution extracted from the small oscillatory components for nondysplastic and dysplastic BE sites are shown in Figure 7. As can be seen, the difference between nondysplastic and dysplastic sites is pronounced. The distribution of nuclei from the dysplastic site is much broader than that from the nondysplastic site, and the peak diameter is shifted from ~7 μm to approximately ~10 μm. In addition, both the relative number of large cell nuclei (lesser than 10 μm) and the total number of nuclei are significantly increased. Further, it is noted that the method provides a quantitative measure of the density of nuclei close to the mucosal surface.

However, single scattering events cannot be measured directly in biological tissue. Because of multiple scattering, information about tissue scatters is randomized

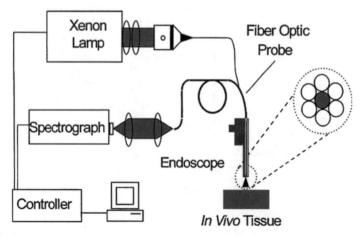

Figure 6   Schematic diagram of the proof-of-principle LSS system.

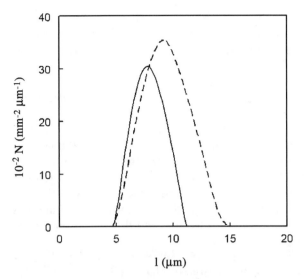

Figure 7 Typical BE nuclear size distributions extracted using LSS technique. Solid line: a non-dysplastic site; dashed line: dysplastic site (9).

as light propagates into the tissue, typically over one effective scattering length (0.5 to 1 mm, depending on the wavelength). Nevertheless, the light in the thin layer at the tissue surface is not completely randomized. In this thin region, the details of the elastic scattering process can be preserved. Therefore, the total signal reflected from a tissue can be divided into two parts: single backscattering from the uppermost tissue structures such as cell nuclei, and the background of diffusely scattered light. To analyze the single scattering component of the reflected light, the diffusive background must be removed. This can be achieved either by modeling (9,16) or by polarization background subtraction (17).

The pilot clinical study was conducted at the Brigham and Women's Hospital and the West Roxbury Veterans Administration Medical Center (10,18). Data were collected from 16 patients with known BE undergoing standard surveillance protocols. After informed consent, consecutive patients undergoing surveillance endoscopy for a diagnosis of BE or suspected carcinoma of the esophagus were evaluated by systematic biopsy. In surveillance patients, biopsy specimens were taken in four quadrants, every 2 cm of endoscopically visible Barrett's mucosa. In patients with suspected adenocarcinoma, biopsy specimens for this study were taken from the Barrett's mucosa adjacent to the tumor. Measurements were performed using the developmental LSS system (Fig. 6). Additional details can be found in Ref. 18.

Spectra were collected by means of an optical fiber probe, inserted in the biopsy channel of the endoscope and brought into gentle contact with the tissue. Each site was biopsied immediately after the spectrum was taken. Because of the known large interobserver variation (19) the histology slides were examined independently by four expert GI pathologists. On the basis of average diagnosis (20,21) of the four pathologists, four sites were characterized by the degree of light scattering.

To establish diagnostic criteria, eight samples were selected as a "modeling set," and the extracted nuclear size distributions were compared to the corresponding histology findings. among these, it was decided to classify a site as dysplasia if more than 30% of the nuclei were enlarged, with "enlarged" defined as exceeding a 10-μm threshold diameter, and classified as nondysplasia otherwise. Averaging the diagnoses of the four pathologists (20), the sensitivity and specificity of detecting dysplasia were both 90%, an excellent result, given the limitations of interobserver agreement among pathologists.

To further study the diagnostic potential of LSS, the entire dataset was then evaluated adding a second criterion, the population density of surface nuclei (number per unit area), as a measure of crowding. The resulting binary plot (Fig. 8) revealed a progressively increasing population of enlarged and crowded nuclei with increasing histological grade of dysplasia. Using logistic regression (21), the samples were then classified by histological grade as a function of the two diagnostic criteria. The percentage agreements between LSS and the average and consensus diagnoses (at least three pathologists in agreement) were 80% and 90%, respectively. This is much higher than that between the individual pathologists and the average diagnoses of their three colleagues, which ranged from 62% to 66%, and this was also reflected in the kappa statistic values (22).

These results demonstrate the promise of LSS as a real-time, minimally invasive clinical tool for accurately and reliably classifying otherwise invisible dysplasia in BE.

Thus, a new (23) biomedical imaging modality based on polarized light scattering spectroscopy, which is capable of providing morphological information about the epithelial cells in situ has been developed. In contrast to conventional images of cells or tissues, the LSS-based imaging provides quantitative images of the histological properties, such as cell nuclear enlargement, pleomorphism, and increased chromatin content. Methods for providing such quantitative, functional information without tissue removal are not currently available. It is important to emphasize that the pixel size and wavelength of light do not limit the resolution of the technique, in contrast to conventional optical imaging. For example, in our tissue images (Fig. 9) the nuclear size is determined with an accuracy exceeding 100 nm, whereas the pixel size is 25 μm and the light wavelength ~500 nm. Such accuracy is obtainable, because the information is derived from spectral variations of the backscattered light. The cell nucleus behaves as an optical interferometer. The resonant condition varies with

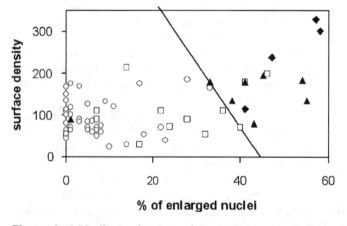

Figure 8 LSS diagnostic plots of Barrett's esophagus data. The decision threshold for dysplasia is indicated. Circles, squares, triangles, and diamonds mark different histological grades of dysplasia.

(A)

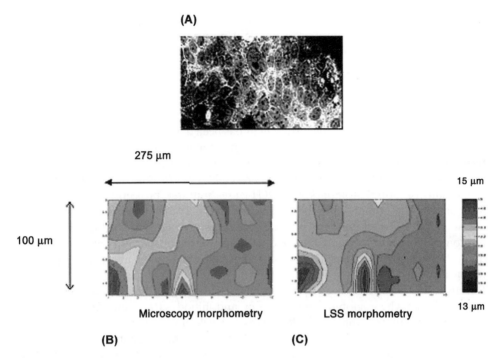

275 µm

100 µm

15 µm

Microscopy morphometry   LSS morphometry   13 µm

(B)   **(C)**

Figure 9 LSS imaging of a T84 colon tumor cell monolayer sample. Microphotograph of a portion of the sample. (**B**) LSS image of the spatial distribution of cell nuclear sizes. (**C**) Spatial distribution of nuclear sizes measured by standard morphometry. The color bar indicates nuclear size shown in (**B**) and (**C**). (*See color insert.*)

the wavelength of light. LSS makes it possible to observe these variations, and measuring them enables the nuclear size and refractive index to be determined. The results reported here indicate the promise of LSS-based imaging for clinical use as well as a biomedical research tool to study the dynamics of nuclear changes accompanying the progression of cancer and other diseases.

OPTICAL IMAGING BASED ON EXTERNAL CONTRASTS TO IDENTIFY CANCER

In view of the recent developments of novel external contrast agents and biocompatible fluorescent probes for probing molecular function, optical imaging methods may be used for noninvasive molecular imaging in vivo with high specificity and localization accuracy. Herein, key components of optical imaging in planar and tomographic modes as an investigational tool for carcinogenesis and focus on recent progress with optical tomography of tissues are briefly outlined.

Emission and reflectance imaging are suitable tools for clinical imaging, and offer simplicity of operation and high sensitivity for optical contrast of cancers close to the surface. On the other hand, both these imaging techniques have fundamental limitations since the penetration depths achieved (typically less than 1–2 cm) restrict their applicability. By obtaining a single projection in "photographic mode" the depth, size, and target concentration cannot be independently retrieved. Therefore, the application of theoretical models to correct nonlinear light propagation and to obtain quantification becomes problematic if no prior information exists.

Diffuse Optical Tomography

To overcome the limitations of emission and reflectance imaging, a set of technologies was developed that allows tomographic imaging using light. The general framework of reconstruction techniques using diffuse light has been developed during the last decade where rigorous mathematical modeling of light propagation in tissue, combined with technological advancements in photon sources and detection techniques has made possible the application of tomographic principles (24,25). The technique, generally termed diffuse optical tomography (DOT) uses multiple projections and measures light around the boundary of the illuminated body. It then effectively combines all measurements into an inversion scheme that takes into account the highly scattered photon propagation to model the effect of tissue on the propagating wave and allow quantitative reconstructions. DOT has been used for imaging of absorption and scattering as well as fluorochrome lifetime and concentration measurements (26,27). Recently, DOT has also been applied clinically to imaging breast cancer, targeting oxy- and deoxyhemoglobin concentration and blood saturation (28), which are representative of the abnormal blood-vessel development in breast tumors. DOT has been further used simultaneously with MRI to image contrast agent uptake (29). In a similar study, image-guided optical spectroscopy was implemented to obtain hemoglobin volume and saturation of breast tumors with higher quantification accuracy than stand-alone optical imaging (30).

DOT offers a set of intrinsic tissue contrast mechanisms not typically available to other medical imaging modalities. By directly targeting oxy- and deoxyhemoglobin, DOT may reveal significant information on function responses or pathological conditions. This is largely because of the association of these features with angiogenesis and hypoxia, two correlates of carcinogenesis. Nevertheless, imaging of intrinsic contrast (or vascular nontargeted contrast agents) is probably best suited for basic research studies and for cancer characterization (30,31) rather than early detection, since there is no evidence that hemoglobin signatures will be able to surpass in performance conventional cancer detection techniques such as X-rays, computed tomography (CT), or contrast-enhanced MRI. Furthermore, the technology suffers from relatively low resolution. Although currently available systems and reconstruction methods have not been exploited to the full potential of DOT, it has been postulated from simulations that in breast imaging applications, for example, the resolution will not be better than 5 mm (32). In larger organs, the resolution would worsen, while imaging tissues with smaller dimensions or small animals will probably attain better resolution. However, It should be noted that it would not be within DOT's capacity to provide anatomical images but rather it is used to sample the tissue for unique optical signatures, whereas a higher resolution may be provided by an anatomical imaging modality operating concurrently. It is possible that a hybrid combining anatomical, functional, and hemoglobin signatures during the same examination would be ideal (29,30). Penetration depth is another potential limitation for optical imaging. While penetration depths of several centimeters through the breast have been demonstrated, other organs, such as the liver or the lung, for example, are unlikely candidates for noninvasive optical tomography using transillumination projections because of the high absorption of the former and the large dimensions of the latter.

Fluorescence-Mediated Molecular Tomography

A particular class of optical tomography of tissues was developed specifically for molecular interrogations of tissue in vivo and is termed "fluorescence-mediated molecular tomography" (FMT) (33). In its optimal implementation, FMT combines measurements at both emission and excitation wavelengths to quantify and three-dimensionally reconstruct fluorochromes of high molecular specificity that are extrinsically administered and home to specific cancer-associated molecular events. The technique is used in conjunction with a fluorescent targeting probe specific to a gene expression product (34). Thus, specificity relies on the molecule and imaging requirements are less stringent than in DOT because even low-resolution detection of the fluorochrome would suffice to identify a specific marker to carcinogenesis. An example from animal imaging is shown in Figure 10. Other applications may imply noninvasive gene expression profiling and imaging treatment effects based on the molecular basis of the drug action (34).

FMT is a crucial technology for noninvasively studying the biological behavior of new classes of fluorescent molecular probes or fluorescent proteins in living systems. This is because it allows for quantitative 3D localization of fluorochromes and can enable molecular imaging at many different levels of gene expression. Of particular importance are "activatable" near-IR probes, i.e., appropriately engineered fluorochromes that are nonfluorescing in their base state but activate (fluoresce) only in the presence of a specific molecular target as described in the next section. A linear relation of reconstructed fluorochrome concentration and targeted molecule exist in biologically relevant concentrations (Fig. 11). Furthermore, it has been shown that penetration depths of more than 15 cm can be achieved for small tumor-like structures in the near-IR for breast and lung imaging (35), whereas penetration is closer to 6 to 8 cm for more vascular organs such as the brain or muscle (Fig. 12). These results were obtained assuming commercially available technologies and at the complete absence of background fluorochrome (ideal case). Furthermore, submillimeter resolutions have been demonstrated for

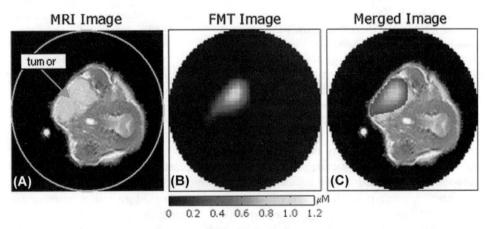

Figure 10 In vivo tomography of cathepsin B expression in cancers. While a single slice is shown, these results are part of a full three-dimensional reconstruction of the animal's upper body. (**A**) MRI image passing through an HT1080 tumor implanted in the mammary fat pad of a nude mouse; (**B**) corresponding FMT image; (**C**) superposition of (**A**) and (**B**). (*See color insert.*)

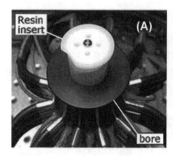 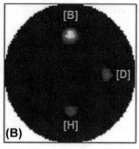 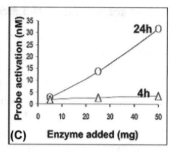

Figure 11 Correlation of reconstructed fluorescence concentration and underlying molecular activity. (**A**) Photograph of a turbid resin tube with the optical properties of mice inserted into an FMT imaging bore. The four capillaries (*open holes*) shown were filled with 1 μM of a cathepsin-B sensitive NIR activatable probe. (**B**) FMT reconstruction obtained from the middle slice of the resin tube at 24 hours after 25 μg of cathepsins (B, D, and H) were added in different capillaries as marked on the image. The fourth capillary did not contain any enzyme. (**C**) Fluorescent probe activation as a function of cathepsin B concentration obtained with FMT at 4 and 24 hours after enzyme addition demonstrates a linear correspondence between reconstructed concentration and amount of enzyme added.

small animal imaging using optimized systems (36). However, the same general performance characteristics are expected between FMT and DOT in terms of resolution. Potentially FMT could surpass DOT in the detection of sensitivity and specificity because of the contrast enhancement and fluorescence amplification achieved by targeted fluorochromes.

Near-IR Fluorochromes and Reporter Probes

Important to the application of advanced optical imaging methods to molecular investigations of tissue in a noninvasive manner is the recent development of targeted (near-IR fluorochrome attached to affinity ligand) and activatable (based on fluorescence resonance energy transfer, FRET) imaging probes (37). These probes have largely been used to detect early cancers or inflammatory diseases in mouse models. In the future, however, these probes could be developed into clinical imaging agents.

Detecting Early Cancers

A variety of agents have been used for enhanced detection of early cancers including somatostatin receptor–targeted probes (38,39), folate receptor–targeted agents (40), tumor cell–targeted agents (41–43), or agents being activated by tumor-associated proteases (37,44,45). Many of these agents accumulate (and thus enhance) tumors to a certain degree however, FRET-based agents can result in particularly high tumor-to-background ratios because of their nondetectability in the native state. For example, recent work has shown that highly dysplastic tumoral precursors are readily detectable by targeting cathepsin B (46), a protease capable of activating a model reporter (Table 2). In this particular study, the sensitivity and the specificity of optical intestinal polyp detection increased to over 95%. Similar approaches may be particularly useful for the early endoscopic detection and characterization of polypoid lesions and/or laparoscopic detection of residual/recurrent tumors such as ovarian cancer.

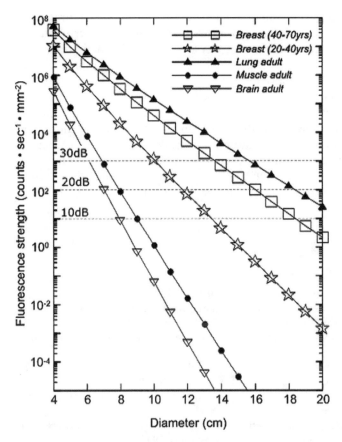

Figure 12 Average fluorescent photon counts predicted at the periphery of different human organs as a function of organ diameters, assuming a 100 μL volume containing 100 nM of Cy5.5 dye at the center of the corresponding organ. These results are simulations employing diffusion theory calibrated on experimental data from phantom measurements. The results depict the counts due to the fluorescent lesion only, i.e., in the absence of other fluorochromes. Three SNR levels for shot-noise limited detection are also plotted.

Molecular Therapy Assessment

One particularly interesting application of enzyme-activated imaging agents has been to use them as tools for objective target assessment of the new therapeutic agents. In one study, the efficacy of an MMP-2 inhibitor (dosing, timing, etc.) was revealed with an MMP-2 targeted imaging probe (47). Small molecule-induced target inhibition could be externally imaged as early as eight hours after therapeutic drug admin istration. It is clear that the other classes of imaging agents will be developed to image the growing array of different drug targets.

SUMMARY

Emission and reflectance imaging is becoming a useful clinical technique when probing superficial tissue during intraoperative imaging or probing deep tissue structures using an endoscopic approach. These optical techniques are unique and noninvasive, and can quantify functional vascularization and oxygen saturation of tumors. Furthermore, there is an intensified effort to produce fluorescent probes, especially for the near-IR region, that target physiological and genetic responses. These probes, combined with appropriate imaging planar or tomographic technologies could allow unprecedented insights into the biology of living tumors and the cellular circuitry underlying these observations. Optical methods further use non-ionizing radiation and are generally compatible with most other radiological imaging techniques for realizing combined modalities for simultaneous examinations that could yield a superior feature set. Furthermore, optical methods are economical and can acquire data continuously; hence, they may be used for real-time monitoring. It is believed that by assessing structural, functional, and molecular cancer characteristics noninvasively, optical imaging could play a major role in several clinical applications and cancer research.

REFERENCES

1. Otsuka KTT. Hippocratic thermography. Physiol Meas 1997; 18:227–232.
2. Foster K. Thermographic detection of breast cancer. IEEE EMB Mag 1998; 17:10–13.
3. Gorbach AM, Heiss J, Kufta C, Sato S, Fedio P, Kammerer WA, Solomon J, Oldfield EH. Intraoperative infrared functional imaging of human brain. Ann Neurol 2003; 54(3):297–309.
4. Gorbach AM. Infrared imaging of brain function. Adv Exp Med Biol 1993; 333:95–123.
5. Sessler D. Perioperative heat balance. Anesthesiology 2000; 92:578–596.
6. Mellergard P, Nordstrom CH. Intracerebral temperature in neurosurgical patients. Neurosurgery 1991; 28:709–713.
7. Stone JG, Goodman, RR, Baker KZ, Baker CJ, Solomon RA. Direct intraoperative measurement of human brain temperature. Neurosurgery 1997; 41:20–24.
8. Watson J, Gorbach A, Pluta R, Rak R, Heiss J, Oldfield E. Real-time detection of vascular occlusion and reperfusion of the brain during surgery by using infrared imaging. J Neurosurg 2002; 96:918–923.
9. Perelman L, Backman V, Wallace M. Observation of periodic fine structure in reflectance from biological tissue: a new technique for measuring nuclear size distribution. Phys Rev Lett 1998; 80:627–630.
10. Backman V, Wallace MB, et al. Detection of preinvasive cancer cells. Nature 2000; 406:35–36.
11. Cotran R, Robbins S, Robbins K. Pathological Basis of Disease. Philadelphia: WB Saunders Company, 1994.
12. Beuthan J, Minet O, Helfmann J, Herrig M, Muller G. The spatial variation of the refractive index in biological cells. Phys Med Biol 1996; 41:369–382.
13. Van de Hulst H. Light Scattering by Small Particles. New York: Dover Publications, 1957.
14. Blumberg RS, Terhorst C, Bleicher P, McDermott FV, Allan CH, Landau SB, Trier JS, Balk SP. Expression of a nonpolymorphic MHC class I-like molecule, CD1D, by human intestinal epithelial cells. J Immunol 1991; 147:2518–2524.
15. Dharmsathaphorn K, Madara JL. Established intestinal cell lines as model systems for electrolyte transport studies. Meth Enzymol 1990; 192:354–389.
16. Zonios G, Perelman L, Backman V. Diffuse reflectance spectroscopy of human adenomatous colon polyps in vivo. Appl Optics 1999; 38:6628.
17. Backman V, Gurjar R, et al. Polarized light scattering spectroscopy for quantitative measurement of epithelial cellular structures in situ. IEEE J Select Topics Quantum Electron 1999; 5:1019–1027.

18. Wallace M, Perelman L, Backman V. Endoscopic detection of dysplasia in patients with Barrett's esophagus using light scattering spectroscopy: a prospective study. Gastroentorology 2000; 119:677–682.

19. Reid BJ, Haggitt RC, et al. Observer variation in the diagnosis of dysplasia in Barrett's esophagus. Hum Pathol 1988; 19:166–178.

20. Riddell RH, Goldman H, et al. Dysplasia in inflammatory bowel disease: standardized classification with provisional clinical applications. Hum Pathol 1983; 14:931–968.

21. Haggitt RC. Barrett's esophagus, dysplasia, and adenocarcinoma. Hum Pathol 1994; 25:982–993.

22. Landis JR, Koch GG. The measurement of observer agreement for categorical data. Biometrics 1977; 33:159–174.

23. Gurjar RS, Backman V, Perelman LT, Georgakoudi I, Badizadegan K, Itzkan I, Dasari RR, Feld MS. Imaging human epithelial properties with polarized light-scattering spectroscopy. Nat Med 2001; 7:1245–1248.

24. Schotland J-C. Continuous wave diffusion imaging. J Opt Soc Am 1997; A-14:275–279.

25. Yodh A, Chance B. Spectroscopy and imaging with diffusing light. Physics Today 1995; 48:34–40.

26. Hawrysz DJ, Sevick-Muraca EM. Developments toward diagnostic breast cancer imaging using near-infrared optical measurements and fluorescent contrast agents. Neoplasia 2000; 2:388–417.

27. Ntziachristos V, Chance B. Probing physiology and molecular function using optical imaging: applications to breast cancer. Breast Cancer Res 2001; 3:41–46.

28. Pogue BW, Poplack SP, McBride TO, Wells WA, Osterman KS, Osterberg UL, Paulsen KD. Quantitative hemoglobin tomography with diffuse near-infrared spectroscopy: pilot results in the breast. Radiology 2001; 218:261–266.

29. Ntziachristos V, Yodh AG, Schnall M, Chance B. Concurrent MRI and diffuse optical tomography of breast after indocyanine green enhancement. Proc Natl Acad Sci USA 2000; 97:2767–2772.

30. Ntziachristos V, Yodh AG, Schnall MD, Chance B. MRI-guided diffuse optical spectroscopy of malignant and benign breast lesions. Neoplasia 2002; 4:347–354.

31. Tromberg BJ, Shah N, Lanning R, Cerussi A, Espinoza J, Pham T, Svaasand L, Butler J. Non-invasive in vivo characterization of breast tumors using photon migration spectroscopy. Neoplasia 2000; 2:26–40.

32. Boas D, Oleary M, Chance B, Yodh AG. Detection and characterization of optical inhomogeneities with diffuse photon density waves: A signal-to-noise analysis. Appl Optics 1997; 36:75–92.

33. Ntziachristos V, Tung CH, Bremer C, Weissleder R. Fluorescence molecular tomography resolves protease activity in vivo. Nat Med 2002; 8:757–760.

34. Weissleder R. A clearer vision for in vivo imaging. Nat Biotechnol 2001; 19:316–317.

35. Ntziachristos V, Ripoll J, Weissleder R. Would near-infrared fluorescence signals propagate through large human organs for clinical studies. Optics Lett 2002; 27:333–335.

36. Graves E, Ripoll J, Weissleder R, Ntziachristos V. A sub-millimeter resolution fluorescence molecular imaging system for small animal imaging. Med Physics 2003. In press.

37. Weissleder R, Tung CH, Mahmood U, Bogdanov A Jr. In vivo imaging of tumors with protease-activated near-infrared fluorescent probes. Nat Biotechnol 1999; 17:375–378.

38. Licha K, Hessenius C, Becker A, Henklein P, Bauer M, Wisniewski S, Wiedenmann B, Semmler W. Synthesis, characterization, and biological properties of cyanine-labeled somatostatin analogues as receptor-targeted fluorescent probes. Bioconjug Chem 2001; 12:44–50.

39. Becker A, Hessenius C, Licha K, Ebert B, Sukowski U, Semmler W, Wiedenmann B, Grotzinger C. Receptor-targeted optical imaging of tumors with near-infrared fluorescent ligands. Nat Biotechnol 2001; 19:327–331.

40. Tung CH, Lin Y, Moon WK, Weissleder R. A receptor-targeted near-infrared fluorescence probe for in vivo tumor imaging. Chembiochem 2002; 3:784–786.

41. Ballou B, Fisher GW, Waggoner AS, Farkas DL, Reiland JM, Jaffe R, Mujumdar RB, Mujumdar SR, Hakala TR. Tumor labeling in vivo using cyanine-conjugated monoclonal antibodies. Cancer Immunol Immunother 1995; 41:257–263.

42. Neri D, Carnemolla B, Nissim A, Leprini A, Querze G, Balza E, Pini A, Tarli L, Halin C, Neri P, Zardi L, Winter G. Targeting by affinity-matured recombinant antibody fragments of an angiogenesis associated fibronectin isoform. Nat Biotechnol 1997; 15:1271–1275.

43. Muguruma N, Ito S, Hayashi S, Taoka S, Kakehashi H, Ii K, Shibamura S, Takesako K. Antibodies labeled with fluorescence-agent excitable by infrared rays. J Gastroenterol 1998; 33:467–471.

44. Bogdanov AA Jr, Lin CP, Simonova M, Matuszewski L, Weissleder R. Cellular activation of the self-quenched fluorescent reporter probe in tumor microenvironment. Neoplasia 2002; 4:228–236.

45. Tung CH, Mahmood U, Bredow S, Weissleder R. In vivo imaging of proteolytic enzyme activity using a novel molecular reporter. Cancer Res 2000; 60:4953–4958.

46. Marten K, Bremer C, Khazaie K, Sameni M, Sloane B, Tung CH, Weissleder R. Detection of dysplastic intestinal adenomas using enzyme-sensing molecular beacons in mice. Gastroenterology 2002; 122:406–414.

47. Bremer C, Tung CH, Weissleder R. In vivo molecular target assessment of matrix metalloproteinase inhibition. Nat Med 2001; 7:743–748.

Index